HEALTH AND DISEASE

CURRICULUM FOR THE 21ST CENTURY MEDICAL STUDENTS

PUBLIC HEALTH IN THE 21ST CENTURY

Additional books in this series can be found on Nova's website
under the Series tab.

Additional e-books in this series can be found on Nova's website
under the e-book tab.

HEALTH AND DISEASE

CURRICULUM FOR THE 21ST CENTURY MEDICAL STUDENTS

PAUL GANGULY
EDITOR

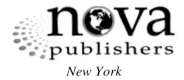

nova
publishers

New York

Library of Congress Cataloging-in-Publication Data

ISBN: 978-1-63463-052-8

Library of Congress Control Number: 2014950601

Published by Nova Science Publishers, Inc. † New York

This book is dedicated to the Dean, Professor Khaled Al-Kattan for his vision, incredible work and excellence in education at College of Medicine, Alfaisal University.

CONTENTS

PREFACE

According to experts in education the definition of curriculum is, "a study course, or an integrated course of academic studies". This definition outlines courses, coursework, and any other content dealing with courses at a primary scholastic level or university. In a medical setting, the goal of a curriculum is to use various modalities to define parameters of medical education. With this goal in mind, the outlines of the curriculum should encourage students to pursue a wide range of careers. These include, but or not limited to, becoming outstanding practitioners, medical educators or investigators. We as educators, expect our graduates to be leaders in patient care. Thus it is the ultimate goal of medical curriculum to educate and empower medical students to succeed in their respective medical careers.

In the past, a study course in medicine was developed to ensure individuals were able to accommodate subjects related to basic science followed by clinical science. However, such concept arguably forms the foundation of medicine; preclinical courses were introduced before students had encountered patients and strategically learned medicine, surgery, gynecology and obstetrics. The experts in medical education questioned the efficacy of such system. It was apparent that students were not able to integrate a medical problem as they were also refrained from acquiring longtime, lifelong learning. Thus educationists around the globe made several changes in medical curriculum in the late 20th century. The introduction of newer systems such as problem-based learning, integrated curriculum, hybrid curriculum and team-based learning were challenging but very successful in many modern medical schools.

Medical schools of the 21st century are looking for innovative approaches. These schools have a general mandate outlining teaching medical subjects in the presence of decreased contact hours to fulfill the curricular need of more integration. The question thus remains as to how best can we teach medical students? What is the best medical curriculum? How much integration is acceptable to students? How can we monitor the system? To answer these questions American University of Barbados (AUB), a new medical school organized a symposium on January 20th, 2014 on a theme of 21st century medical curriculum. Dr. Gary Brar, CEO, AUB invited me to speak on how best we can teach anatomy in a modern curriculum. The idea of synthesizing a book on medical curriculum thus came into existence.

The present book entitled "Health and Disease: curriculum for the 21st century medical students" addresses the above questions so as to ensure that a medical school can select a curriculum based on its mission, vision and objectives. The book highlights the evolution of medical curriculum and describes a state-of the-art approach that indicates the essential points behind designing a curricular map. Care has been taken to bring a concept that no particular curriculum may fit to the need of a medical school and thus it is necessary to fine tune of a system that is ever rolling and dynamic in the context of medical education. At the end of the study, the students should appreciate the facts of health and disease through a well-described curricular outcome. I sincerely hope that this book will bring many answers that are presently needed. Thus I am indebted to all the contributors in this book.

The book is dedicated to Dr. Khaled Al-Kattan, Dean and Professor of Surgery, College of Medicine, Alfaisal University. Dr. Khaled is also the founding Dean who made Alfaisal University very proud by bringing the College in the map of excellence. In fact, the College of Medicine has surpassed many of the expectations within the span of six years mainly due to Dr. Khaled's hard work and right vision from the very beginning. His message to the students is simple- "when you join the College you will understand from the first day, that we are a student-centered university and we are prepared to provide you with all the knowledge and skills you will need to graduate as an outstanding doctor, who would serve the community with best practice in patient care, together with excellence in research ability and academia". College of medicine believes that Dr. Khaled is an outstanding Dean in true sense of the word. His personal contribution to fine tuning of the curriculum has also a pivotal influence and remains center to ongoing activities and success at the College.

It has been a particular privilege to have continued support from outstanding faculty, staff and students at the College of Medicine, Alfaisal University for the past several years. Many of our colleagues have had a long standing interest in the medical education and contributed several chapters in this book. I am grateful to my wife Rina and children, Riya and Rishi for encouragement and motivation for completing and editing this book in time.

Thank you,

Paul Ganguly, MBBS, M.D., FACA
Professor and Chairman of Anatomy
College of Medicine
Alfaisal University
Kingdom of Saudi Arabia
Tel: +966503092964
E-mail: pganguly@alfaisal.edu
July 1, 2014

In: Health and Disease   ISBN: 978-1-63463-052-8
Editor: Paul Ganguly   © 2015 Nova Science Publishers, Inc.

Chapter 1

HISTORY OF THE MEDICAL CURRICULUM

S. Schofield*

Centre for Medical Education, University of Dundee, Scotland, UK

ABSTRACT

In this chapter I follow the fascinating course of medical education through the ages, starting with our first written record, the Yellow Emperor's Classic of Internal Medicine. The journey proceeds through the centuries to the current time, drawing parallels between curricula then and now. I draw on the contributions of Galen, Hunayn ibn Ishaq, Trotula de Ruggiero, Culpepper, the Hunter brothers, Flexner and Osler to name but a few, and there will be many I have not mentioned due to only having one chapter. However I have picked out what I feel to be key figures and key dates, not least the influence of inventions such as paper, the printing press and the World Wide Web, which have directed not only the content but also the process by which we deliver curricula. I finish with the challenge I know will be taken up by subsequent authors: how do we provide our students with the tools of their future trade when we don't know what their trade will look like ten years hence?

I'm often asked 'why medical education, why not just education?' Indeed our new lecturers in the College of Medicine, Dentistry and Nursing at the University of Dundee, UK are offered the choice between the Post Graduate Certificate in Higher Education run by the University's School of Education or our own Post Graduate Certificate in Medical Education. So why would a University go to all the extra expense of running two courses? Why do over 3,000 delegates attend the annual conference of the Association of Medical Education Europe (AMEE) each year? Why is developing a curriculum for medical and other health professionals considered so different from developing curricula in other disciplines that it warrants its own specialty? Indeed why was my own Centre for Medical Education created in Dundee by Professor Ronald Harden in 1974 [1]?

---

* Dr S Schofield s.j.schofield@dundee.ac.uk

The Mackenzie Building where CME is now based is named after Sir James Mackenzie, a General Practitioner who transformed cardiology in the early 20th century. In his memoires of working with Dr Mackenzie, Wilson [2] quotes Mackenzie's own reminiscences of working with Dr Briggs: '*Unhappily Dr Briggs was quite unable to impart or hand on his secret. He didn't know how he knew. His experience was entirely personal to himself*'. Health professionals across the globe are now recognising the importance of a workforce equipped with educational skills tuned to the needs of the 21st century health service. Although the very word 'Doctor' comes from the Latin *Docere* (to teach), the skills of teaching are not inherent, as recognised by the GMC: '*Teaching skills are not necessarily innate, but can be learned. Those who accept special responsibilities for teaching should take steps to ensure that they develop and maintain the skills*' [3], yet this could be said of any discipline. In the preface to 'Problem-based learning: An approach to Medical Education', Robyn Tamblyn encapsulates what is special about medical education: '*the need to actively apply knowledge to the assessment and care of patients and the ability to continue to identify areas where further learning would enhance or improve the practice of these skills*' [4]. The price of such training is not insignificant. In 2012 a national newspaper reported that it cost the tax payer £250,000 to put one student in the UK through medical school [5], and of course the cost to patient health, if badly done, goes beyond money.

So how did we get to where we are today in medical education, and where are we going next? The majority of this book deals with the curriculum now, but in this chapter I want to take you on a journey starting hundreds of years ago and, certainly for me, hundreds of miles away. It's a fascinating journey, with some surprises, and many themes you'll recognise in current curricula. Of course it is very much informed by written records since sadly I don't have a time machine. That's not to say medical education didn't happen before – we can assume it did in an oral tradition – but we have no record. And so our journey must start with the first writings we still have evidence of.

ANCIENT CHINA

Huang Ti Nei Ching Su Wen (The Yellow Emperor's Classic of Internal Medicine) [6] is reputed to be the oldest medical text in existence, credited to Huang-ti (the Yellow Emperor who reigned c. 2697 – 2597 BCE) and his chief minister Chi'I Po (also translated as Qu Bo). It formed the basis of Chinese medicine and is based on a series of dialogues between the two men. Handed down from generation to generation in the oral tradition, it is thought to have been first written down in the Chou dynasty (1000 BCE). Dr Ilza Veith's translation of part of the work published in 1966 is thought to be of a version completed about 762 CE. The following is an example of the discourse from a later edition of Veith's book [7].

"about human growth and life cycle, The Yellow Emperor asked, How people grow old and when people grow old why they cannot give birth to children?

The divinely inspired Health Minister Qu Bo answered, 'in normal growth when a girl is 7 years of age, the production of Kidney Qui (that is, producing female hormones) becomes abundant, she beings having physical changes. Her teeth and her hair grow longer. When she reaches her 14th year, she begins to menstruate and is able to become pregnant and the circulation and the flow of Qi to Ren and Chong meridians are strong.

When the girl reaches 21, she is fully grown and is able to bear a child. When the woman reaches age 28, her muscles and bones are strong, her hair has reached its full strength and her body is flourishing and fertile.

When the woman reaches the age of 35, the Ren and Chong meridians Qi begin to deteriorate, her face begins to wrinkle and her hair begins to fall. When she reaches the age of 42, her hair begins to turn white, and her entire face is wrinkled. When she reaches the age of 49 she can no longer become pregnant and the circulation of the Ren and Chong meridians Qi is further decreasing; her menstruation is exhausted, her body deteriorate and she is no longer able to bear children"

From a medical education point of view, I find this particularly interesting for its engaging nature and the reasoning given behind each stage. Reading the book we can get a very clear feeling for the curriculum followed by the apprenticed medical student. Chinese medicine is very much intertwined with Chinese philosophy, the flow of Qi, the Yin and Yang. Good health was thought to be when the body was in balance of the five elements – fire, earth, metal, water and wood.

Another influential figure in Chinese medicine was the philosopher Confucius (551 – 479 BCE). Learning was a key part of Confucianism, done not for material reward but rather for *Jen*, the love of men. Confucius believed that the teacher was a transmitter of knowledge, not an innovator; devoted to antiquity rather than questioning it. In his excellent book looking at the history, present and future of medical education, Sir Kenneth Calman [8] suggests this is why after such promising beginnings the development of Chinese medicine slowed down, the curriculum stagnating. Yet some Confucian quotes still inform our teaching today. Take for example 'I hear and I forget. I see and I remember. I do and I understand' [9]. How many of us endeavour to make our lectures more interactive; ensure our curriculum combines instruction with observation of patients and practice in the clinical skills centre?

Formal medical education started in the Imperial Court of the T'ang dynasty (618 – 906 CE). The curriculum was divided into three subcategories: disorders of adults (da fang ke); acupuncture (zhen ke) and inner lesions (jin yang) [10]. In 657 CE Emperor Gaozong of Tang commissioned *materia medica* which listed 833 different medicinal substances, and learning in medicine was delivered in imperial medical colleges, with publications of forensic manuals and state examinations for doctors [11]. The following Song dynasty (960- 1279 CE) saw schools being set up firstly in the capital then beyond. The Imperial College, set up in 1076 CE, enrolled 300 students to learn medicine, surgery and acupuncture [8]. The Chinese medical curriculum of the Imperial Court included disorders of adults (da fang ke); disorders related to wind (feng ke); disorders of children (xiao fang ke); obstetrics (chan ke); disorders of the eyes (yank ke); mouth, teeth, pharynx, throat (kou chi yan hou ke); sore, swollen, broken, wounded (chuang zhong zhe yang ke); acupuncture and moxibution (zhen jui ke); and inner lesions and incantations (jin yang shu jin ke) [10]. Students were examined orally on *materia medica*, typhoid fever, action of drugs, modes of infection and causes of diseases. Clinically they were examined on justification of their choice of patient management and the results of the treatment. Those being awarded the top grades were given official appointments, writing medical books and / or teaching. Those attaining a pass were licensed to practise; those failing were ordered to change profession. Teaching was seen as an important job to be done by the top achievers, and teachers were held to account for the success of their students, with fines being imposed on the teacher for non-attendance of his students.

Selection of students was on their medical knowledge, high moral character and esteem by their friends, the first two echoed by e.g. today's UKCAT in the UK [12] and references. Entry examinations were held in the capital.

BABYLONIA

Medicine in Bablyonia was exclusively the property of the priests who trained in treating diseases. Medical knowledge was to be kept secret within the priesthood '*may he who knows instruct him who knows and may he who knows not, not read this.... He who does not keep the secret will not remain healthy. His days will be shortened*' [13]. There were three types of physician: the baru ö a seer who specialised in divination, the ashipu ö who specialised in exorcism, and the asu ö who were knowledgeable in charms, drugs and surgical procedures. The physician priests were very powerful because of their social status, their knowledge of medicine and their interpreting of omens. In order to reduce the risk of malpractice and exploitation the Code of Hammarabi was written (c. 2000 BCE).

ANCIENT EGYPT

Physicians in Ancient Egypt were renowned for their skills and knowledge, with specialist Egyptian physicians travelling to other lands to attend royalty. A large range of materials on ancient medical education survives in papyri, statues and inscriptions. For example the Ebers Papyrus (1550 BCE) is among the oldest and most important Egyptian medical papyri and contains extensive detail of both physiology and pathology [14]. The Edwin Smith Surgical Papyrus (3000 BCE) is attributed to a high priest of Heliopolis, Imhotep [15]. William Osler, himself considered to be the father of modern medicine, recognised Imhotep as the father of medicine [16]. Imhotep was considered to be a magician as well as a physician, and was so famous for his skill in healing disease that he eventually became the Egyptian God of Medicine.

There were four classes of Egyptian priest: the highest ranked wabw (pure priest) was entitled to examine patients; the swnw (lay physician) practised surgery and medicine; the sa. u (magician) used charms; the wt (nurses) assisted the physicians including bandaging. Physicians weren't exclusively priests, but the priests were considered the guardians of medicine. All physicians were highly revered and handsomely rewarded. Students, selected for their industriousness and abilities, lived in houses attached to the medical schools, under the watchful eye of their tutors. The schools were known as 'Houses of Life' and provided physicians with practical experience. The sick, brought to the temple for relief, were a ready source of patients for instruction alongside care. Ethical duties such as kindness and not abandoning or ignoring patients were expected of physicians. All physicians were able to write, but memory was also heavily relied on, with proverbs and question / answer statements to be rote-learned. Temples had their own collections of books and manuscripts, including those relating to medicine, stored in the 'per-ankh'. Students and visitors could visit these to read and copy texts. The curriculum included surgery, procedures and use of drugs, and scribe training. There were also apprenticeships where medicine was passed from father to son [13].

Much of the ancient Egyptians' life revolved round understanding of the flow of the Nile, and it seems they transferred this to their belief in how the body worked. The heart was considered to be the main organ of the body, a mirror to the soul. The Egyptians introduced the concepts of diagnosis, prognosis and medical examination, with great detail on these being contained in the Edwin Smith Papyrus. Hesy-Ra (270 BCE) was known as the chief of dentists and physicians [17], and Peseshet the 'Lady Overseer of the Lady Physicians' [18], the latter training midwives at Sais.

ANCIENT GREECE

Ancient Greece brought us the writings of Hippocrates (460 to 370 BCE) which tell us much about the teaching of medicine, including the difficulties. For example: *'finally, medical teaching is subject to the difficulty which besets all doctrine, that is indeed to say what should be done in a particular case when one is confronted by it, but that one cannot give general advice about what should be done without seeing the particular case'*. In his 'The Law' [19] Hippocrates talks of medicine as being the most noble of the arts but far behind due to lack of punishment for those guilty of malpractice. He likens teaching to cultivation, whereby the teacher sows the seed which is cultivated by diligent study. He values experience and self-reliance in physicians.

Once more there is the air of secrecy: *'those things which are sacred are to be imparted only to sacred persons; and it is not lawful to impart them to the profane until they have been imitated in the mysteries of the science.'*

Unlike the ancient Egyptians, practising medicine did not require an examination nor a fixed period of study. Reputation was built on 'good business', and the secret craft of healing often passed from family to family. Without easy access to books knowledge was passed on orally, making the teacher a key person. Any free man could be selected to be a student, with the traits of a natural disposition to both the subject and prolonged industriousness being listed in Hippocrates' canon. The teacher, even if not a family member, was urged to treat the student as a son, teaching them the art of medicine without fee or indenture. Teaching was almost exclusively oral, with huge amounts of rote learning, and teaching communication skills seen as an important part of medical education. Reputations of potential physicians could also be made by being a pupil of a good teacher. Good schools were able to attract the best teachers and pupils, and so probably the birth of school league tables. Medical education included the impact on health of diet, physical condition, housing, lifestyle and age [19].

The writings reveal an understanding of best evidence medicine, with observations being meticulously recorded to generate recommendations for management, emphasis on case studies, and a belief that scientific method assists understanding of disease. Gask [20] says of him *'Hippocrates gave to the world a sound approach to medicine. He and his followers popularised, if they did not invent, the approach known as the 'inductive method' that is to say, the practice of inferring a general law or principle from the observation of particular instances.*' From his works (though all attributed to him, scholars believe they are by him and his followers) we can build up a clear idea of the curriculum his students would have followed. Prognosis was also recognised as key to a physician's reputation, as was knowing his own limitations as can be seen in his oath. Indeed amongst lay people Hippocrates is perhaps most famous for The Oath [19]. The oath has historically been taken by physicians and other healthcare professionals, and is important not only for its content but also for the concept of a physician taking such an oath. It speaks of medicine as an art whose secrecy is to be upheld. It also talks of doing good regardless of class of patient, not doing harm, and knowing one's own limitations. These three are certainly all very familiar to us in the modern curriculum.

ANCIENT ROME

The Romans initially saw health as very much the responsibility of the family and a private affair and were distrustful of physicians though large Roman households had their own medical staff. The army however saw things differently, perhaps because the men were by necessity miles away from their family. Every Roman legion had medical staff (the doctor *medici* and their assistants *capsarii)*, and the legion's hospital (*valetuduniari)* was part of the fort. The army was an excellent place to learn medicine, not only via care of wounds, but also via learning from the inhabitants of the regions they moved into. Knowledge of public health such as clean water and dealing with sewage increased, and the history books show us many examples of sophisticated ways of dealing with these matters as well as heating. Preventative medicine was part of the curriculum alongside nutrition, pharmacology and surgery. Here we see evidence of professionalism, with codes of practice outlining how the physician should appear (well-dressed, sweet smelling), and their demeanour (serious but not harsh) [21].

The Greek physician Archagathus of Sparta arrived in Rome in 219 BCE when he started to introduce Greek medical practice into Rome [22]. He specialised in battle wounds and skin complaints, and taught that disease should be treated speedily, safely and agreeably (though with Pliny labelling him three centuries later *carnifex* (the executioner) one wonders agreeable to whom). Diagnoses were reduced in number, each with a prescribed management resulting in a curriculum which could be taught in six months. This put his teachings at odds with the prominent Greek physician, surgeon and scholar Galen of Pergamon (129 – c. 216 CE), a polymath who had learnt his trade in a gladiator school. Galen's own studies had taken 11 years, perhaps prompting him to write '*it is not the doctor who is most skilful in his profession but the one who knows best how to flatter who enjoys the regard of the multitude*' [23].

Through Galen's prolific writings we learn of his claim to have developed a systematic approach to medicine. He continually refined his work based on observation, and felt physicians should be skilled in logic, physics (the study of nature) and ethics. His writing 'That the Best Physician is also a Philosopher' demonstrated the importance of an understanding of philosophy to Galen. Does this again strike chords with the tensions of today's curricula, trying to balance a need for efficiency with a broader education? Galen enjoyed teaching, allowing not only medical students but also others interested in the human body to attend his dissections. One can certainly imagine a charismatic teacher, the sage on the stage. However he also recognised the importance of doing and of repeating this learning:

Young students must see specimens not once or twice but often. For it is only by applying oneself with intelligence to these things and by examining them frequently that one get a thorough knowledge of them. [23]

He also recognised the value of books for sharing knowledge, and in his later years invested a lot of his not inconsiderable wealth employing scribes to copy books from other libraries.

Celsus (25 BCE – c. 50 CE recognised the uncertainty in the art of medicine:

… the art of medicine is conjectural, and such is the characteristic of a conjecture, that though it answers more frequently, yet it sometimes deceives. A sign therefore is not to be rejected if it is deceptive in scarcely one out of a thousand cases, since it holds good in countless patients [24], Book II

He was also unhappy with what he perceived as the simplistic classifications by the Greeks into chronic and acute, and one remedy for one disease:

There is another point which should be borne in mind, that the same remedies do not suit all patients. [24] Book III

And expressed concern about patient to doctor ratios:

… it is not possible for many patients to be cared for by one practitioner, and provided that he is skilled in the art, he is a suitable one who does not much absent himself from the patient. [24], Book III

As to the teaching of the Art of Medicine, he considered dissection of the dead a necessity to teach the positions and relations of the internal organs, and wasn't adverse to the use of condemned criminals for vivisection.

As for the remainder, which can only be learnt from the living, actual practice will demonstrate it in the course of treating the wounded in a somewhat slower yet much milder way. [24], preamble

By the 2nd century BCE Greek doctors were well established in Rome, but weren't always favourably looked upon by their Roman counterparts. Pliny the Elder (23 – 79 CE) was a strong critic, complaining of their unethical behaviour and high fees. Physicians were recommended to avoid serious injuries such as to the brain or heart with little hope of a positive outcome to protect their reputations – the beginnings of risk avoidance? Dioscurides of Anazarbus' influential *Materia Medica* was an enduring reference on drugs. Yet for all that there was no official medical training or qualifications, and no orthodox approach to medicine. Learning was by apprenticeship, and individual practitioners gained their reputations through accurate diagnoses and prognoses of patients. The work of Roman physicians and medical scholars would, however, remain dominant for another millennium [25].

MEDIEVAL ISLAM

With the collapse of the Roman Empire the knowledge-base of medicine moved to the Islamic world and the *lingua franca* of medicine moved from Greek to Arabic [26]. Islamic medicine was initially based on Hellenic medical practice, and likewise medieval Europe drew upon Islamic works and practice. The Islamic scholars produced commentaries and encyclopaedias, including Avicenna's *Canon of Medicine*, itself translated into Latin and disseminated across Europe. Learning papermaking from China, the Islamic paper-producers used linen in place of mulberry bark, producing paper more durable than papyrus and more cheaply than parchment [27]. The first paper factory built in Baghdad 794 CE furthered book production. Islamic scholars combined the theory and practice of medicine, integrating it with philosophy, religion, natural science, astrology, alchemy and mathematics.

The most prolific of translators of Greek medical and scientific texts was Hunayn ibn Ishaq (809 – 873 CE). He also wrote a number of works including one for medical students, Questions on Medicine for Beginners (Kitāb al-Masā'il fī al-ṭibb lil-muta'allimīn), which attracted a number of commentaries, the most important being by Ibn Abi Sadiq. The copy housed in the Bodleian Library in Oxford was copied 1235 CE and used for teaching by the famous physician Muwaffaq al-Din Ya'qub al-Samiri (d 1281 CE), and contains a certification that one of his pupils had studied and mastered its contents [28]. Abu Bakr Muh al-Razi (c. 845-930 CE) reworked the teachings of Hippocrates to make them easier to commit to memory. Recognising the importance of the patient – doctor relationship he created a checklist for practitioners to follow, giving a systematic process to diagnosis and management, and ensuring the patient understands the prognosis.

Snan ibn Thabit ibn Qurra (880 – 943 CE) saw the necessity for rigorous examination and licensing of physicians. Jumai' (1153 – 1198 CE) in his Treatise to Ṣalāḥ ad-Dīn on the revival of the art of medicine [29] outlined three areas of concern: the selection of teachers who should have excellent knowledge and skills to educate the students and train them in the care of the sick under their supervision; the selection of students who should be intelligent, of good character, hard-working and desire excellence; and examination of physicians which should be on all aspects of the art of medicine. El Hakim (1135 – 1204 CE)'s *Book of Knowledge* talks of the student / teacher relationship, encouraging teachers to treat their pupils as they would their children. Something that particularly strikes a chord with me is: '*much wisdom I have learned from my masters, more from my friends, but most from my pupils. Even a small twig kindles a great fire so a little pupil stimulates the rabbi and there goes out from his questions marvellous wisdom*' [30], recognising both peer-learning and the incredible journey of learning our students take us through if we are open to it.

By the 11th century there were three types of medical school: firstly those associated with hospitals with lecture theatres, libraries and pharmacists; secondly the private medical schools such as that run by al-Razi whose fame attracted many students; and thirdly the apprenticeship model where a student would be apprenticed to a physician. Avicenna's Canon

[31] was enormously successful and influential. Avicenna saw learning as key to being a doctor, the practice of medicine being the ability to give opinion based on that learning. As the knowledge base did not change much during this period the book remained a best-seller for some time, yet this reticence to challenge the words of the ancients meant Islamic medicine stagnated.

EUROPE

The first recognised University in Europe was Salerno in Southern Italy. Salerno itself had been conquered by Robert Guiscard in 1076, putting it under Norman rule [32]. Twenty years later Solerno Medical School *Scuola Medica Salernitana* was formed. As such it was the most important source of medical knowledge in Western Europe [33]. The nearby abbey of Montecassino, founded in 529 CE, had already become home to one of the most significant libraries of the Western world [34]. Medical knowledge was part of the monks' plan of studies *(ordo studiorum)*, and their work included translating the important Arabic medical works such as those by Avicenna into Latin. The library also housed the 9th century *Codex 69*, a collection of practical remedies and recipes for different trocisci (forerunners to tablets). The medical school developed from the monastery's dispensary which had been founded in the 9th century, and was enormously important to both medical knowledge and medical education between the 10th and 13th centuries. People came from all over the world to Solerno, both to be cured and to study medicine.

The school kept to the Greek-Latin medical tradition, with its curriculum synthesizing Arab and Jewish medical traditions. Indeed it is said the school was founded by four masters: the Jewish Helinus, the Greek Pontus, the Arab Adela, and the Latin Salernus. The school welcomed males and females, irrespective of religion and nationality, both as students and teachers. The most famous female doctor was Trotula de Ruggiero who also authored several books on gynaecology and cosmetics around 1100 CE. Applicants had to be 21 and have completed five years study of logic, and the medical course was itself a five year curriculum plus one year supervised practice. Rather akin then to the MBChB degree followed by a registrar post. On passing the exam students swore an oath including elements relating to upholding both the school and the profession, and were entitled to call themselves Magister or Doctor. Although the library was unrivalled, students still had to commit much to memory.

Medicine and surgery were seen as two separate areas of expertise, with the former more book-based, the latter based on practice. For this reason physicians were seen as educated, and knowledgeable in the wisdom of the ancients. Surgeons on the other hand were regarded as academically inferior and kept away from the seats of power. De Chauliac (1300 – 1368 CE), a French physician and surgeon credited with introducing traction for treating fractures, wrote a lengthy treatise on surgery *Chirurgia Magna* [35], earning him the title 'restorer of surgery'. Two surgeons of note from Salerno were Roger, author of *Practica* in about 1170 and Roland who edited the book in around 1240. Roland notes the book is not just for practising surgeons but also for those learning. Roland's purpose in editing Roger's book is to clarify its content for the learner, as is evident from his note: '*whatever I have been able to glean from his* (Roger) *writing, I have put into order, so that his ideas may more clearly be grasped*'. Teaching was not only by lecture but also by observing operations. Practical experience was recognised as key, with learning from experience essential – what today we might call reflection in action and reflection on action.

Other important universities in Europe at this time were Bologna and Padua in Italy and Montpellier and Paris in France. Students selected their University by the reputation of the teachers and the University's library. Some Universities restricted teaching to their own graduates, something recognised as potentially stifling by Guillem VIII in 1180 who decreed this should not be the case at Montpellier. The rapid expansion of the European Universities gave rise to a market for text books and a need for mass production. Student texts were split into sections so that scribes could work on portions, with quality control rules drawn up by the Universities, a system known as the *Pecia* system [36]. For the first time students could access relatively cheap books for their own private study.

THE RENAISSANCE

The Renaissance (from the French for rebirth) was a movement starting in 14th century Italy which would sweep across Europe focusing on creativity and invention. The ancient work of Galen was found to not always match everyday observations, and a curriculum shift was seen from Aristotelian natural philosophy to chemistry and biological sciences. Copernicus, himself medically trained, questioned the motions of the sun and earth. Medicine was about to become transnational with Colombus' discovery of the New World in 1492. Leonardo da Vinci (1452 – 1519) who originally trained as a painter was apprenticed to Andrea del Verocchio who insisted all his students learn anatomy. Da Vinci's skill as a medical illustrator was recognised and he was given permission to dissect human corpses in hospitals in Florence, Milan and Rome. Working with Doctor Marcantonio della Torre, he made over 240 detailed drawings, including that of a foetus in the womb (c. 1510). Although da Vinci planned to publish his diagrams with della Torre's help, the latter died before the project got underway and da Vinci's pictures had to wait another 200 years [37].

Just as the Islamic development of cheap and durable paper had influenced medical education in the 8th century, so did another technological advance in the mid 15th century with the advent of the printing press. Interestingly just as paper was invented in China, so was printing technology, with its invention credited to the Han Chinese printer Bi Sheng around 1040 (38). In Europe a German goldsmith Johannes Gutenberg developed his press in 1452, allowing mass production of books by the Pecia system to be replaced by the far faster printing press. One Renaissance printing press could produce 3,600 pages per workday [39]. Pictures could be reproduced with no reduction of accuracy and no reliance on the drawing skills of a scribe. Without this massive technological advance would Andre Vesalius' *Fabrica* in 1543 have become such a widely respected atlas of human anatomy? The drawings are credited to John Stephen of Calcar, a pupil of Titian, under the direction of Vesalius who regularly dissected human bodies in front of audiences of 500 people. Published in one volume *Fabrica* consists of seven books: the bones; muscles; veins and arteries; nerves; organs of nutrition and generation; heart and lungs; and the brain and organs of sense [40]. Many inaccuracies introduced by Galen and propagated through the centuries by a profession immersed in the classical tradition were exploded by Vesalius who wrote: *'I myself cannot wonder often enough at my own stupidity and too great trust in the writings of Galen and other anatomists.'*

A shorter version of the atlas, *Epitome* was developed for students and had a profound impact on the education of students in the field of anatomy. This had a stronger focus on the illustrations, with the grandiose Latin text from *Fabrica* being abridged for the *Epitome* [41]. The layout of the Fabrica and Epitome informed Gray's anatomy, well known to countless medical students since its original publication in 1918.

Another graduate from Padua, the Englishman William Harvey questioned the Galenic view that blood was continuously created by the liver [42]. His experimental methods showed instead that blood circulated ceaselessly, changing both the medical curriculum and the way the secrets of nature could be uncovered by experiment. Harvey also clearly valued education, donating a large library and museum of anatomical works to Merton College in Oxford.

THE REFORMATION

The reformation started with Luther's publication of the 95 theses in 1517. He felt keeping the bible in Latin kept it in the hands of the priests whereas translating it into the language of the people would make it more accessible. His translation of the New Testament was first published in 1522 and the complete bible in 1534. The recently invented printing press allowed him to print and disperse these. Why was this important to medical education? Well up to this point the language of medicine had been unified – from Greek to Arabic to Latin. Just as Luther felt the words of the bible would be more accessible to the layperson if it was in their own language so an Englishman Nicholas Culpeper (1615 – 1654) felt medicine was similarly inaccessible in Latin. Although not qualified by degree he began practising medicine in Cambridge. Here he published Physical Directory in 1649, his unauthorised translation of the College of Physicians' *Phamacopoaeia*. He was an outspoken critic of his contemporaries' work, writing: "*This not being pleasing, and less profitable to me, I consulted with my two brothers, DR. REASON and DR. EXPERIENCE, and took a voyage to visit my mother NATURE, by whose advice, together with the help of Dr. DILIGENCE, I at last obtained my desire; and, being warned by MR. HONESTY, a stranger in our days, to publish it to the world, I have done it.*" [43]. He also deplored learning by rote '*...in the School of tradition, and to teach them just as a parrot is taught to speak*', and felt the physicians were guilty of keeping secret the art of medicine. His use of the vernacular for medical guides aimed at the poor who could not afford expensive physician fees could be seen as a form of patient-centred care. Indeed, his subsequent publications included a manual on childbirth and another entitled 'The English Physician' which he deliberately sold cheaply and went far beyond the shores of England.

At this time in Europe some attempt was being made to regulate medical practitioners, with guilds and colleges. The London College of Physicians had been set up by Henry VIII in 1518 but was prescriptive and restrictive, only recognising degrees from Oxford and Cambridge and only allowing physicians to practise in London. It set exams, had a library, and provided a place for physicians to meet and discuss, but its elitism kept its numbers down to no more than 30 physicians during the 17th century.

The Royal College of Surgeons of Edinburgh was established in 1505 as: *'The incorporation of barber surgeons with examinations in anatomy and the nature and complexion of man's body'*. Surgeons had long been associated with barbers, the first reference to the London Barbers Company being 1308 when Richard the Barber had been instructed by the Lord Mayor and Aldermen to oversee and maintain the integrity of the Company. The first recording of a surgeon in the group was 1312, barbers frequently performing minor surgical skills including dentistry and bleeding (an almost universal procedure for medical conditions at that time). In 1497 they granted the first Diploma in Surgery in England, approved by both the Company and the Guild of Surgeons. In 1540 an Act of Parliament amalgamated the Surgeons Guild and the Company of Barbers, the newly formed Barber-Surgeons Company being allotted annually the bodies of four executed criminals for dissections.

The trades of barber and surgeon were separated, neither being allowed to perform the tasks of the other. The Company remained united till 1745 when the Surgeons created their own Company which in 1800 became the Royal College of Surgeons in England. To this day barber shops in the UK have a red and white pole outside representing the blood and bandages of their earlier association with surgery [44].

Padua was probably the most reputed medical school of the 16th and 17th centuries. Students came from across Europe, and spread their knowledge across Europe upon graduation. The Padua curriculum emphasised clinical education, and the first botanical garden for medicine was founded there in 1545 (though it should be noted monasteries had had their own herb gardens for medical purposes before that, passing the knowledge apprenticeship-style from monk to novice). The medical school was organised as colleges of doctors, with students paying for instruction and examination including a written dissertation. In 1543 Giovanni Battista da Monte introduced bedside teaching at St Francis' Hospital, instructing students to first observe, then talk to the patient about the symptoms, then examine. This innovation in University-delivered medical education from scholastic to practical was taken to Leiden by Dutch graduates, then beyond to other medical schools in Europe.

France was another centre for medical education in the 17th century. The work of the ancients, in particular Galen, was especially revered by Paris, and students questioning these works were frowned upon. The first degree in medicine had no clinical element, with graduates and young doctors learning their clinical skills on their first patients. This led Diderot to observe: *'As a result the young doctor makes his first essays on us, and only becomes skilful by dint of murder'*. Graduates wishing to practise in Paris were required to take a second degree. For this they needed to deliver lectures to demonstrate their knowledge, pass a number of oral examinations, and complete an apprenticeship.

The medical faculty at Vienna was founded in 1389. In 1520, at student request, an introduction to medicine was printed: *Liber do modo student seu legend in medicine*, an early example of a study guide. It consisted of seven parts including guidance on how to study, and covered all five years of the curriculum.

Students were examined by two doctors in the presence of all the doctors at the faculty after the required years of study. On graduation the young doctor was required to lecture in the faculty for at least one year.

THE AGE OF ENLIGHTENMENT

The 18th century brought with it revolution – America in 1776 and France in 1789. Often referred to as the Age of Enlightenment it brought about its own revolution in attitudes to and understanding of public health. Despite the reformation and Culpepper's attempts, the language of medical education continued to be Latin for both lectures and examination, though this slowly started to change mid 1700s onwards. The centre for medical education in Britain was Scotland, with 2600 students receiving degrees in medicine between 1750 and 1800. The degree was open to all classes, with lower class and poor students encouraged. The degree was three years long and, unlike England at that time, integrated medicine and surgery. Edinburgh Medical School was established in 1726 by Drs Sinclair, Rutherford, Plummer and Innes who had all studied at Leiden. Chemistry became an important subject within medicine. A fascinating document *'A guide for Gentlemen Studying Medicine at the University of Edinburgh 1792'* gives a description of the medical institutes in Edinburgh at that time. Of a Dr Gregory who lectured on the practice of medicine it says: *'As he has not yet made out a perfect plan of lectures, very little can be said respecting this course'*, echoing perhaps the complaints of today's students if a particular lecturer's notes are not available on the institutional vle (virtual learning environment). The document also gives suggested curricula dependent on their future career plans. Lecturers received no salary and relied on attracting students to their lectures for which there was a fee – a very direct quality control of lectures.

A notable Scottish teacher of the time, William Cullen, was professor, firstly at Glasgow Medical School then Edinburgh. He sought to instill in his students active learning rather than passive, preparing them for what we would now term lifelong learning. His hour-long lectures were followed by an hour of discussion about the previous lecture. Whereas we might think discussion should be on the current lecture, this would ensure students revisiting the previous lecture in a considered way, perhaps discussing amongst themselves. He was engaging in his teaching, using anecdotes to illustrate, and connecting topics much as we encourage in today's integrated curricula. A great mentor to his students, he was involved with the students' Royal Medical Society in Edinburgh which had been set up in 1734 and attracted its Royal Charter in 1778.

Another renowned Scottish 18th century medical educator was William Hunter, resident pupil of fellow Scot William Smellie, obstetrician and author of Treatise on Midwifery, in London. He assembled a large collection of anatomical and pathological specimens to support his teaching of surgery and anatomy, and set up his own school of medicine in Great Windmill Street, London. Here he was a prodigious lecturer, preferring to share his ideas orally than by publication. His introductory lecture was a history of anatomy, following very much the path we have so far in this chapter: China, Greece, Rome, Arabia to the 18th century; his second an introduction to the role and values of anatomy. A sentiment I hear echoed by the anatomists of today, he saw such study vital for the profession: *'Who then are the men in the profession, that would persuade students that a little anatomy is enough for a physician, and a little more too much for a surgeon? God help them'*.

His brother John was also a medical man committed to teaching. His first motive, he wrote in 1793, was to serve St George's Hospital, his second to spread his knowledge which he felt was *'the highest office in which a surgeon can be employed'*. He was very much of the opinion that medicine and surgery could not and should not be learnt separately, and his lectures on surgery included physiology and the concepts of health. A great thinker, he valued experimental method for establishing surgical principles, something he passed onto his pupils, including Philip Physick, dubbed the father of American surgery.

THE BODY SNATCHERS

Private schools such as Hunters flourished, but there was little regulation. Anatomy became central to the curriculum but cadavers were scarce. Good money could be made securing bodies for dissection, as evidenced by the infamous Burke and Hare in Edinburgh. The legitimate source of cadavers for teaching anatomy in Britain's medical schools was executed criminals, but the number of executions was declining just as the needs of medical schools was increasing. Institutions such as Edinburgh Medical School increasingly relied on body-snatchers who would steal recently deceased bodies from graves. The first body Burke and Hare sold to the School did not make it to the grave, the pensioner having died of natural causes owing Hare £4 rent. Hare recouped his losses by filling the coffin with bark and selling the body for £7.10s.0d to Dr Robert Knox. Able to advertise his lectures on anatomy as 'a full demonstration on Anatomical Subjects' Knox's lectures regularly drew audiences of over 400, each paying him for the privilege. Motivated by the money, Burke and Hare moved onto murder, often intoxicating the victim first, then transporting the body to Surgeons' Hall in a tea-chest. Burke was found guilty on 16 counts of murder and hanged in 1829, his body being publicly dissected in the University's Old College anatomy theatre by Professor Monro. Hare was given immunity from prosecution for turning King's evidence and released, fleeing from the mob. Knox was not prosecuted despite public protestations as Burke swore that Knox had no knowledge of the origin of the cadavers, but he left Edinburgh to take up a post as anatomy demonstrator in London. The public's view of the three players in the tragedy is clear in this 19th century Edinburgh skipping rhyme:

> Up the close and doun the stair,
> But and ben wi' Burke and Hare.
> Burke's the butcher, Hare's the thief,
> Knox the boy that buys the beef.

Of particular relevance to medical education is the subsequent passing of the Anatomy Act 1832 which stated that the person with legal custody of a dead body could send it to a medical school before burial for the study of anatomy and practice of surgery. If there were no known relatives this power was devolved to Public Health Authorities, Parish Councils and Boards of Guardians. The Lancet in an editorial dated 1828 stated *"It required no extraordinary sagacity, to foresee that the worst consequences must inevitably result from the system of traffic between resurrectionists and anatomists, which the executive government has so long suffered to exist. Government is already in a great degree, responsible for the crime which it has fostered by its negligence, and even encouraged by a system of forbearance."* [45]. The Act also ended the practice of sending the body of executed prisoners to the anatomy hall.

JOURNALS

This is perhaps a good time to mention medical journals which soon became another foundation of medical education. The Lancet itself was launched in 1823, founded by the English surgeon Thomas Wakley. From the very start it published lectures (not always with the authors' permission) and commentaries on lectures (not always in a flattering light). The *New England Journal of Medicine and Surgery and the Collateral Branches of Medical Science* was founded by the Boston surgeon John Collins Warren and physician James Jackson in 1812. Unlike the weekly Lancet, this was originally a quarterly journal. Another medical journal, *The Boston Medical Intelligencer* was launched in 1823 but ran into financial troubles in 1827. The editors of the *New England Journal of Medicine and Surgery and the Collateral Branches of Medical Science* purchased *the Boston Medical Intelligencer,* merging the two publications to form *the Boston Medical and Surgical Journal* which was published weekly. In 1921 the Massachusetts Medical Society purchased the journal, renaming it in 1928 the *New England Journal of Medicine,* arguably the oldest medical journal albeit with a name change.

After the French revolution a government report (1794) resulted in three new schools of health to be set up in Paris, Montpellier and Strasbourg, with more following. Medical education saw integration of medicine and surgery, licensing of different levels of doctors, and employment of full-time teachers. Students received state scholarships, and the idea that doing nothing was better than something doubtful became the new maxim. France developed the clinical method of observation, palpation, percussion, auscultation, linking these to the pathology of the autopsy room. By the 1850s Germany started to dominate medical education with its focus on scientific medicine. The polymath of previous centuries gave way to the specialist, and universities transformed into specialist scientific institutes built on two freedoms: Lernfreiheit (the freedom to learn) and Lehrfreiheit (the freedom to teach). Academics were expected to research and teach, increasing the number of teachers needed. In his book *The Medical Sciences in the German Universities* (1876), Billroth urges medical students to choose smaller universities for their earlier studies, where the teachers can become well-acquainted with each student. Interesting when one considers the large lecture hall of the 1st year undergraduate (UG) compared to the educational supervision of the trainee today.

The 19th century industrialisation of much of Europe had led to overcrowding and epidemics such as cholera. The physician John Snow's plotting of cholera cases in Soho led to his conclusion that the public water pump was the source, arguably the birth of epidemiology. By the end of the 19th century there were around 120 journals. There was concern that such journals might confuse the public (parallels to the internet?) yet from a continuing professional development perspective they were an invaluable tool, providing up-to-date knowledge, a platform for debate, information on conferences, and as a vehicle for campaign both within the profession and for social reform.

AMERICAN MEDICAL EDUCATION

The first medical students to be granted degrees in America graduated in 1768. Medical colleges opened in Harvard (1783), Dartmouth (1798) and Yale (1817), with students apprenticed to masters. By 1827 concern was being expressed about the quality of the teaching, and a convention to discuss medical education was held in Northampton, Massachusetts in 1827. Little reform resulted, and in 1846 an association was formed which a year later became the American Medical Association (AMA), its journal being launched in 1883.

By this time Paris was the European centre for medical education, so it was natural that AMA should recommend the French emphasis on clinical teaching for their own curriculum. Perhaps due to the civil war little actual reformation happened and schools shot up everywhere granting unregulated diplomas. Chicago Medical College, founded in 1859, saw the need to maintain high standards. Harvard medical school reformed in 1871 with a three-year graded curriculum and salaried faculty, and two years later a banker named Johns Hopkins established a board of trustees to construct a hospital to rival the best in Europe. The university medical school was established in 1876 and, with the appointment of John Shaw Billings as Dean, the appointed faculty made Hopkins' hospital central to their medical degree along with laboratories. One of the four founding professors of the Johns Hopkins Hospital was the "Father of Modern Medicine" Canadian physician Sir William Osler (1849 – 1919). Following his medical degree at McGill University he took post-graduate training in Europe, returning to McGill as professor and is credited with creating the first formalised journal club. He was one of the founding members of the Association of American Physicians, created in 1885 which was dedicated to 'the advancement of scientific and practical medicine'. At Johns Hopkins University School of Medicine he gained the reputation of being an excellent clinician and teacher, and was a strong advocate of bedside clinical training. He created the first residency program for specialty training, whereby a hospital's medical staff would have many interns, fewer assistant residents, all overseen by a chief resident for a specialty. Residency programmes were open-ended, usually lasting seven to eight years, and residents would live in hospital accommodation, working long hours. He also brought in clinical clerkships where third and fourth year students took patient histories on the wards.

Still though, there was a need for educational reform and the Council on Medical Education was set up in 1906. A massive change in how medical education was viewed came with the Flexner report [46]. Abraham Flexner was an educator based at the Carnegie Foundation. His previous report on The American College led the Carnegie Foundation president Henry S Pritchett to ask Flexner to review medical education. The report was a comprehensive assessment of medical education in North America, for which he surveyed all 155 medical and osteopathic educational institutions across the United Stated and Canada that granted MDs (Medical Doctor) or DOs (Doctor of Osteopathy). He concluded there were too many institutions, many driven by profit rather than quality of students and graduates, and that the quality of the education was often substandard. He recommended reducing the number of institutions from 155 to 31, minimum admission standards, a four year curriculum of two years' basic sciences followed by two years' clinical, and that all schools should be assimilated into universities. His vision was for scientifically-sound students to complete their clinical education in academically-oriented hospitals where clinicians would pursue research in addition to their clinical duties. He saw research as core to improved clinical care and teaching, and, as for quality of teaching, championed quality of research 'Think much; publish little'.

In the following 25 years, 89 medical institutions closed, of which many were osteopathic institutions. The number of physicians fell from 172 to 125 per 100,000 of population as schools sought to produce fewer better doctors. Perhaps a less anticipated impact of this report was the focus on research rather than teaching and a 'publish or perish' culture as research productivity became the measure of 'worth' of academics. With advances in understanding, medical research has moved away from whole organism to molecular, and from ward to laboratory [47].

America wasn't by any means alone in its concerns about medical education and licensing. The UK's General Medical Council (GMC) completed its own report in 1881, starting with entry examinations and the subjects to be included, length of study (professional study should be at least four years), subjects to be studied, and testing of those subjects. Reports followed in 1890, 1909, 1922 (which extended the curriculum to five years), 1936 and 1947. It did not recommend uniformity of teaching, rather that individuality of Universities was a good thing. It was however clear on one thing: 21 should be the earliest a doctor should be licensed to practise.

Sir George Newman, Chief Medical Officer for England 1919 – 1935, had a keen interest in medical education, seeing universities as a place where students not only formed close associations with their teachers but also worked with each other. He also recognised the importance of good teachers, those who were not only knowledgeable about their subject but also skilled in teaching, and that a good learning environment was needed. Newman felt examinations were not always a good thing, encouraging cramming and what we would now term shallow learning.

Having taken a chair at Oxford in 1905, Osler set up the Postgraduate Medical Association in 1911 which merged with the Fellowship of Medicine in 1919. The importance of continuing medical education was recognised, with courses and publications produced.

In the UK the Beveridge Report (1942) had recommended creating 'a comprehensive health and rehabilitation services for prevention and cure of disease'. The Labour Government, elected in 1945, had committed to implementing this across the UK by 1948 with services free to patients at the point of use, the service being funded by national insurance payments. The Goodenough report (1944) was commissioned by the Ministry of Health and the Department of Health for Scotland to report on the facilities for medical teaching and research in preparation for this service. The report recognised the need for *'highly developed and vigorous systems of general and professional education for members of the medical and allied professions, and it must evoke the enthusiastic and intelligent cooperation of the general public'* (p9). It made strong recommendations for student selection, including their education before entry, that students should be interviewed, and that unsuitable students should be weeded out at the earliest opportunity, preferably in their first year. Graduates were required to complete a pre-registration year as a junior house officer at one or more approved hospitals. It also recognised the needs of the teacher, recommending guidance on teaching methods. The 'intelligent cooperation of the general public' extended to an expectation that the public would help medical education and research. It also recommended that women be given the same opportunities as men with respect to postgraduate (PG) education, though it should be noted at this time many medical schools had a maximum quota of female UGs e.g. in the USA until the 1970s no medical school had more than 6% female admissions [48].

The GMC responded to the Goodenough Report in 1947 with its own recommendations. In response to Goodenough's worry that the curriculum was overcrowded the GMC recommended that licensing bodies and schools ensured there was nothing being taught unnecessarily or prematurely. Goodenough had recommended that the curriculum not exceed 4.5 years: the GMC responded this was not reasonable though did recognise the strain this might put on students of limited means. With the arrival of the NHS medical education at both UG and PG levels could now be planned. Regional PG centres were developed and training could be coordinated with the availability of specialties locally, regionally and nationally. The following year the Medical Education Committee of the British Medical Association brought out their report on the training of doctors. It recognised the importance of lifelong learning, student selection, an overcrowded curriculum, and the reliance on rote learning of facts rather than understanding and ability to apply principles. It also recognised the duty of the student and practitioner for a life-work balance *'Time must be available for healthy exercise and recreation and for independent reading and leisurely reflection'*. Following on from Goodenough's urging to weed out students unsuited to medical training it suggested interviews be done by committee and that that committee reviewed student progress at the end of both first and second year. With regard to good teachers, the report noted that teaching ability was not high on the majority of appointment panels' criteria, and that most with educational roles would benefit from some teacher training. This was picked up by Lauwerys (1950) who recommended junior teachers be observed by more experienced ones, and that there be staff meetings on educational matters.

The Royal College of Physicians in 1955 reported that: contemporary students started their studies with less cultivated minds; qualifying as a doctor did not entitle that doctor to practise unsupervised; and that the GMC should create a broad statement of educational objectives for medical schools to follow. They also recommend the GMC inspect both the schools and the examinations to meet their statutory obligations.

Meanwhile in the USA Joseph Wearn had been appointed Dean to a failing school, the Western Reserve University. His vision was for a student-focused curriculum where students and medical teachers were involved in educational planning. This change in philosophy soon spread across the western world and Australia, the latter through the Commonwealth Fund. It was no longer enough for teachers to just deliver; now they were expected to meet regularly for seminars on medical education. The first to take this approach to a formal evaluation and development of the teaching role was the University of Buffalo. There was a recognition that being a content expert was not enough – educational principles were to teaching as basic sciences were to clinical medicine. These principles should be integral to the curriculum and there should be a Masters in Medical Education. The importance of an understanding of student learning was being recognised, and perhaps no surprise that a need for research in medical education soon followed. One of the most influential players in this move was Dr J Hillis Miller, President of the Medical College of Virginia in Richmond, who stated: *'what needs most to be acquired in medical school is not a vast body of knowledge, much of which will be outmoded by graduation, but a set of attitudes and values that will persist throughout a professional career'*. This is something very much recognised in today's higher education attributes – the skills for lifelong learning. In 1953 the first World Conference in Medical Education was held around four themes: entry requirements, curriculum content, curriculum delivery, and social medicine. Across the 90 papers presented disagreement can be seen as to the need for teacher training, but general agreement on the need for student selection strategies in a field oversubscribed by applicants.

John Ellis, Sub-Dean of the London Medical School made a tour of the leading medical education centres in the USA and reported back his findings in the 1956 Goulstonian Lecture to the Royal College of Physicians which he entitled Changes in Medical Education. Of particular interest regarding curriculum-design is the lack of integration between preclinical and clinical, and the need for full-time appointments in medical education. Western had taken integration to its extreme by introducing clinical teaching from the start of the curriculum though Ellis thought this a step too far. He did however identify a need for research into learning and teaching. Ellis' report also influenced the GMC 1957 report which recommended interdepartmental teaching throughout and the need to foster critical study of principles and independent thought rather than cramming facts.

The 60s saw further changes in curricula as schools took on board the recommendations for integrated curricula. In the UK a survey of Higher Education teachers (across all subjects) found the majority would have liked a period of instruction in teaching. The Robbins Report (1963) recommended: *'all newly appointed junior teachers should have organised opportunity to acquaint themselves with the techniques both of lecturing and of conducting small group discussions'*. The Royal Commission on Medical Education: the Todd Report (1965-68) again picked up on the need for rigorous research into medical education and PG education comprising an intern year, general professional training, further professional training, and continuing education and training.

The 60s and 70s was a time of enormous growth in medical schools, with new schools being set up across the globe, including my own, the University of Dundee which in 1967 separated from its parent, the University of St Andrews. The Association for the Study of Medical Education (ASME) launched its journal the *British Journal of Medical Education* (now *Medical Education*) in December 1966 with articles on ASME, the history of British medical education, student selection, UG paediatric teaching, the use of closed-circuit television in teaching UG surgery, teaching psychodynamic aspects of psychiatric, the future role of computers in the doctor's job, student travel, the MD by thesis, and the University of Malaya Medical Centre. Indeed looking at the titles of papers in the discipline's leading journal gives a fascinating insight into the themes of each decade [49].

In 1981 the *Medical Education: Fourth Report from the Social Services Committee*) highlighted the thorny issue of how many doctors should be trained and what the career structure should look like. As stated at the very beginning of this chapter training a doctor is not cheap – training too many would waste resources and lead to unemployed doctors, training too few may seriously compromise the health service. Another point raised that we've seen throughout this chapter is the age of entry to UG training – the report recommends medical schools consider more mature students. In 1980 the Association of Medical Schools in Europe (AMSE) was created, its first annual conference being in Groniger.

THE SPREAD OF THE GLOBAL CURRICULUM

Concern was raised about the growth in the number of medical schools around the world, some established under questionable conditions, and a need to safeguard the quality of healthcare systems at a time of increasing mobility of medical practitioners. The World Federation for Medical Education (WFME) was set up in 1972 to enhance the quality of medical education world-wide, covering all stages of medical education from basic (UG) to PG (including vocational training, specialist training and research doctoral education) and continuing medical education and continuing professional development (CPD) of medical doctors. In 2004 WFME teamed up with the World Health Organisation (WHO) to create the WHO-WFME Joint Task Force on Accreditation of Medical Education Institutions and Programmes. Its purpose was to develop a set of quality assurance guidelines to assist national authorities and agencies responsible for the quality of medical education. The task force of 26 members from 23 countries covering all six WHO-WFME regions developed the guidelines to be viewed as recommendations, recognising the importance of national sovereignty over education and policy-making. However, there was also the offer to assist countries and regions without accreditation systems to set these up. The report [50] emphasises that it did not accredit medical schools, but accreditation according to the WHO-WFME guidelines would be noted in the WHO Health Academic Institution Database.

THE BOLOGNA PROCESS

Following a series of meetings between European ministers the European Higher Education Area was created and the Bologna declaration (named after the University where the declaration was proposed) was signed in 1999 by 29 countries. The purpose was a major higher education reform in response to a need for globalisation and mobility. Its aims were to allow students to move amongst countries within the European Higher Education Area and to create greater alignment between USA and European higher education. In subsequent years more countries joined and the process now has 47 signed up. Bologna actions included: adoption of a system of easily recognised and comparable degrees; establishment of a universal system of credits; promotion of mobility; attractiveness of the European Higher Education Area; cooperation in quality assurance; focus on lifelong learning; and inclusivity. A two-cycle model was created whereby students were prepared for the labour market after a first cycle of studies which would last a minimum of three years. It has been extensively argued that the two-cycle model does not fit well with medical training, and that the medical degree is already well-recognised across Europe, negating the need for adapting medical curricula to the Bologna declaration [51].

A statement on the Bologna process and medical education (52) is a good summary of the issues and challenges of applying such a process to medical education. Written in consultation with the AMSE and WHO Europe (WHO-Euro), the report summarises three primary characteristics of European medical schools at the start of the 21st century. Firstly, they recognised the recent reforming of curricula to take into account social responsibility, content / outcome / competencies at graduation, pedagogical methods (in particular student-centred e.g. problem based) to inculcate lifelong learning habits, assessment methods, integration of basic sciences and clinical disciplines, early contact with patients, improving communication and clinical skills, and integrating research options. Secondly, they raised the issue of the low level of knowledge about the Bologna process and implications amongst the 236 medical schools canvassed. Thirdly, they highlighted the lack of homogeneity across the

European region with regard to disease patterns, health care delivery systems, and the differences in health workforces. The report did not feel this diversity had been adequately taken into account. For me this chimes with the American model of the 19th century where Flexner [46] recommended local schools for local training, though is at odds with the earlier European history where scholars travelled large distances to attend the best schools, taking the knowledge and methods back with them. The European Credit Transfer System (ECTS), the report goes on to conclude, should not cause problems provided schools new to the credit system are supported. The credit system reflects the effort involved measured in hours for an activity within the curriculum, though clearly needs to be alongside outcomes / objectives if used for credit transfer. Mobility though was recognised as challenging, particularly with the move to integrated curricula. Also the authors did not feel focussing mobility within Europe was enough, recommending a wider remit to encompass regions such as America, Africa, Asia and the Middle East. This accreditation should be done in conjunction with the professional bodies, and the criteria and standards need to be specific, such as the WFME Global Standards for Quality Improvement in Basic Medical Education. By 2007 seven countries had opted to adopt the two-cycle system within all their medical schools, 19 had opted not to, four had devolved the decision to their medical schools, and 11 had made no formal decision [53].

In 2013 the MEDINE2 (Medical Education in Europe) final report came out [54]. The authors concluded that despite efforts via legislation and funding streams, mobility of medical students and doctors in Europe remained quite low, due not only to language barriers but also incomplete application of the Bologna principles in medical education. They also looked at modern curriculum trends and the Bologna Process, including enhancing sharing best practice and joint thinking on future directions of medical education, with an emphasis on communication with all medical schools. They recognised the importance of exploring and documenting potential barriers to coordinated curriculum change, and the importance of developing quality lifelong learning in education, research and innovation.

GOING ELECTRONIC

Throughout this chapter we've seen how technological advances have changed the course of the medical curriculum or certainly its delivery. It may surprise you to learn the first email was developed in 1971 by Ray Tomlinson who also came up with the @ symbol. The same year Project Gutenberg was started. Named after the inventor of the European printing press its vision was to make a global repository of books and documents made into electronic format for wide distribution freely. 1977 saw the arrival of the first PC modem, allowing home users to go online. The first virtual community of developers was The WELL, an open and 'remarkably literate and uninhibited intellectual gathering'. And then in 1991 a huge innovation – Tim Berner's Lee created the first webpage and the World Wide Web was born. This same year the first webcam was developed (deployed at a Cambridge University computer lab to monitor a particular coffee maker so that lab users could avoid wasted trips to an empty coffee pot). Although I find it hard to imagine life without, Google didn't make an appearance till 1998, revolutionising the way in which people find information online. 2001 saw the launch of Wikipedia, loved and despised in equal measures by academics the world over. Anyone who can access the site can edit most of its articles, causing concerns about its writing, vandalism and the accuracy of information (though a 2005 investigation by Nature found it to be close to the level of accuracy in the Encyclopaedia Britannica). On February 9, 2014, *The New York Times* reported that Wikipedia is ranked fifth globally among all websites stating, '*With 18 billion page views and nearly 500 million unique visitors a month, according to the ratings firm comScore, Wikipedia trails just Yahoo, Facebook, Microsoft and Google, the largest with 1.2 billion unique visitors.*'

2003 saw Skype launched, giving a user-friendly interface to VoIP (Voice over IP calling). The Web, once the home of the geeks, was becoming more and more accessible to the not so computer-obsessed, and 2004 saw Web 2.0 really take off, allowing users to create web content without needing to know html. Facebook launched in 2004, though at the time it was only open to college students. Flickr was launched in 2004, YouTube in 2005, Twitter in 2006. The biggest innovation of 2007 was arguably the iPhone, which was almost wholly responsible for renewed interest in *mobile web* applications and design though this was also the year of Dropbox and Kindle. The following year the term MOOC (Massive Open Online Course) was coined by Dave Cormier, University of Prince Edward Island and Bryan Alexander, National Institute for Technology in Liberal Education. The first 'MOOC' was CCK08 *Connectivism and Connective Knowledge* led by George Siemens, Athabasca University and Stephen Downes, National Research Council. It has 25 tuition-paying students attending the University of Manitoba and over 2,200 online students who paid nothing. Course content was available through RSS feeds and online students could participate through blog posts, threaded discussions in Moodle and Second Life. In May 2011 Amazon (launched in 1994) announced that its e-book sales in the US exceed all of its printed book sales for the first time.

So what does that mean to us as medical educators and to our curricula, both with regards to delivery (e.g. blended, distance, flipped classroom) and content (e.g. professionalism online, electronic records systems, telemedicine)?

AND NOW

And what of other curriculum changes? The move from traditional to integrated, the spiral curriculum, didactic to student-centred, problem-based and team-based learning, the move from content to process, inclusion of the 'softer' social topics such as communication skills and empathy, changing modes of delivery, interprofessional education, the needs of the students we teach and the wider community we serve. How does the move to patient-centred care affect our curriculum? And perhaps the most challenging question of all: how do we provide our students with the tools of their trade when we don't know what their trade will look like ten years hence? These are all challenges for the curriculum developers of today to produce the health professionals of tomorrow.

REFERENCES

[1]   CME. Centre for Medical Education Dundee: University of Dundee; 2014. Available from: http://medicine.dundee.ac.uk/medical-education-centre/centre-medical-education.

[2]   Wilson RM. The beloved physician: Sir James Mackenzie, London: John Murray; 1926

[3]   General Medical Council. *The Doctor as a Teacher.* London: GMC, 1999.

[4]   Tamblyn RM. Problem-based Learning. An Approach to Medical Education. In: Barrows H, Tamblyn R, editors. Problem-based Learning An Approach to Medical Education. New York: Springer; 1980.

[5]   Smith R. The NHS will train fewer doctors to avoid future brain drain, report warns. *The Daily Telegraph.* 2012 6 Dec 2012.

[6]   Saunders J. Huang Ti Nei Ching Su Wen. *California Medicine.* 1967:125-6.

[7]   Veith I. *The yellow emperor's classic of internal medicine.* Berkley, CA: University of California Press; 2002.

[8]   Calman KC. *Medical education past, present and future: handing on learning.* London: Churchill Livingston Elsevier; 2007.

[9]   Smoot B. *Conversations with great teachers.* Bloomington, IN: Indiana University Press; 2010.

[10]   Hsu E. *The transmission of Chinese medicine.* Cambridge, UK: Cambridge University Press; 1999.

[11]   Adshead S. *T'ang China: The Rise of the East in World History.* New York, NY: Palgrave Macmillan; 2004.

[12]   UKCAT. UK Clinical Aptitude Test: UKCAT; 2014 [cited 2014 June]. Available from: http://www.ukcat.ac.uk/.

[13]   Rozina YV. Medical practice in the ancient world 1998 [cited 2014 June]. Available from: http://humweb.ucsc.edu/gweltaz/courses/techno/papers/doctors.html.

[14]   Ebbell B. *The Papyrus Ebers: the greatest Egyptian medical document.* Copenhagen: Levin and Munksgaard; 1937.

[15]   Breasted J. *The Edwin Smith surgical papyrus: Hieroglyphic transliteration, translation and commentary.* Whitefish, MT: Kessinger Publishing; 2006.

[16]   Osler W. *The Evolution of Modern Medicine.* Whitefish, MT: Kessinger Publishing; 2004.

[17]   Selin H, Shapiro H. Medicine Across Cultures: History and Practice of Medicine in Non-Western Cultures. New York, NY: Springer; 2003.

[18]   Harer WB, el-Dawakhly Z. Peseshet- the first female physician? Obstetrics and Gynecology. 1989;74(6):960-1.

[19]   Adams F. Hippocrates: Of the epidemics (translation) 2005 [cited 2014 June]. Available from: http://www.greektexts.com/library/Hippocrates/Of_The_Epidemics/eng/index. html.

[20]   Gask DGE. *Essays in the history of medicine.* London, UK: Butterworth; 1950.

[21]   Jackson R. Doctors and diseases in the Roman Empire. London, UK: Britsh Museum Publications; 1988.

[22]   Beasley AW. The origins of othopaedics. *Journal of the Royal Society of Medicine.* 1982;75:648-55.

[23] Puschmann T. *History of Medical Education* (History of Medicine). London, UK: HK Lewis; 1891.

[24] Celsus AC. *De Medicina Book* V 1962.

[25] Cartwright M. Roman medicine 2013 [updated 26 October 2013; cited 2014 June]. Available from: http://www.ancient.eu.com/Roman_Medicine/.

[26] Pormann PE, Savage-Smith E, Hehmeyer I. *Medieval Islamic medicine*. Edinburgh: Edinburgh University Press; 2007.

[27] Anon. Islamic medical manuscripts 2013 [cited 2014 June]. Available from: http://www.nlm.nih.gov/hmd/arabic/med_islam.html.

[28] al Qāsim A, al Raḥmān A, I.A. Ṣ. Commentary on 'The Questions on Medicine for Beginners' by Ḥunayn ibn Isḥāq 2013 [cited 2014 June]. Available from: https://www.nlm.nih.gov/hmd/arabic/C2.html.

[29] Jumai' HAiI, H. Fh. Treatise to Ṣalāḥ ad-Dīn on the revival of the art of medicine (Vol. 46, No. 3). Herndon, VA: Steiner; 1983.

[30] Maimonides M. *The book of knowledge: From the Mishneh Torah of Maimonides*. Jersey City, NJ: KTAV Publishing House, Inc.. 1981.

[31] Gruner OC. A treatise on the Canon of Medicine: Of Avicenna, Incorporating a Translation of the First Book, by O. Cameron Gruner. Brooklyn, NY: AMS Press; 1930.

[32] Turismoninsalerno. Town of Salerno nd. Available from: http://www.turism oinsalerno.it/salerno_e.htm.

[33] de Divitiis E, Cappabianca P, de Divitiis O. The "Schola Medica Salernitana": The Forerunner of the Modern University Medical Schools. *Neurosurgery*. 2004;55(4):722-45.

[34] Himetop. *The library of Montecassion 2011* [cited 2014 June]. Available from: http://himetop.wikidot.com/the-library-of-montecassino.

[35] Ogden MS. The Galenic Works Cited in Guy de Chauliac's Chirurgia Magna. Journal of the history of medicine and allied sciences. 1973;28(1):24-33.

[36] Norman J. Introducton of the Pecia System 2014 [cited 2014 June]. Available from: http://www.bl.uk/catalogues/illuminatedmanuscripts/GlossP.asp.

[37] Gross CG. Brain, vision, memory: *Tales in the history of neuroscience*. Cambridge, MA: MIT Press; 1999.

[38] Pan J. On the origin of printing in the light of new archaeological discoveries. *Chinese Science Bulletin*. 1997;42(12):976-81.

[39] Wolf H-J. Geschichte der Druckpressen (1st ed.). Arnsberg, Germany: Interprint; 1974.

[40] Karger. At the heart of the Fabrica nd [cited 2014 June]. Available from: http://www.vesaliusfabrica.com/en/original-fabrica/inside-the-fabrica/contents.html.

[41] Kemp M. A drawing for the Fabrica; and some thoughts upon the Vesalius muscle-men. *Medical History*. 1970;14(3):277-88.

[42] Key JD, Keys TE, Callahan JA. Historical development of concept of blood circulation: an anniversary memorial essay to William Harvey. *The American Journal of Cardiology*. 1979;43(5):1026-32.

[43] Culpeper N. The English physitian, or an astrologo-physical discourse of the vulgar herbs of this nation being a compleat method of physick, or cure himself being sick for three pence charge, with such things only as grow in England. Ann-Arbor, MI: EEBO, Pro-Quest; 1652.

[44] Durrant P. The history of the company: The worshipful company of barbers; 2013 [cited 2014 June]. Available from: http://www.barberscompany.org/historical_group.html#The history of the company.

[45] Wakley T. Mr Warburton's Bill. *The Lancet.* 1829:818-21.

[46] Flexner A. Medical education in the United States and Canada: a report to the Carnegie Foundation for the Advancement of Teaching (No. 4). Carnegie Foundation for the *Advancement of Teaching.*, 1910.

[47] Cooke M, Irby DM, Sullivan W, Ludmerer KM. American Medical Education 100 Years after the Flexner Report. *The New England Journal of Medicine.* 2006;355(13):1339-44.

[48] Wirtzfeld D. The history of women in surgery. *Canadian Journal of Surgery.* 2009;52(4):317–20.

[49] Medical Education [Internet]. Wiley Online Library; 1966 [cited 2014 June]. Available from: http://onlinelibrary.wiley.com/doi/10.1111/med.1966.1.issue-1/issuetoc

[50] WHO/WFME. WHO/WFME guidelines for accrediation of basic medical education. Geneva/Copenhagen: WHO/WFME, 2005.

[51] GMC. Bologna Process Update. London: GMC, 2009.

[52] WFME AMEE. *Statement on the Bologna process and medical education.* 2005.

[53] Patricio M, den Engelsen C, Tseng D, ten Cate O. Implementation of the Bologna two-cycle system in medical education: Where do we stand in 2007? Results of an AMEE-MEDINE survey. *Medical Teacher.* 2008;30(6):597-605.

[54] Cumming A. *Medical education in Europe 2.* Edinburgh: University of Edinburgh, 2013.

In: Health and Disease   ISBN: 978-1-63463-052-8
Editor: Paul Ganguly   © 2015 Nova Science Publishers, Inc.

Chapter 2

STATE-OF-THE ART CURRICULUM FOR THE 21ST CENTURY MEDICAL STUDENTS

*Ahmed Yaqinuddin**, Wael Al-Kattan and Khaled Al-Kattan*

College of Medicine, Alfaisal University,
Riyadh, Kingdom of Saudi Arabia

ABSTRACT

Over the years, the changing health care needs of the society have greatly influenced the expectations from the graduating physician. The main objective of the health care system has shifted from individualized hospital-based care to promoting generalized health of the community.

There is now more emphasis on continuous professional development of health professionals and evidence based medical practice. This has a major impact on design and structure of medical training in the medical schools around the world. Various curricular models have been introduced with an emphasis on active learning and introducing strategies which will encourage inquiry based learning. These are more flexible curricular models where in multiple educational strategies have been utilized and students have a central role in their learning process.

These programs are developed keeping in mind the final product "a competent physician". Herein, we have discussed the evolution of different curricular models in medical education, briefly highlighting their strengths and weaknesses.

Finally, we have discussed a curriculum model which could be adopted as a model for 21st century undergraduate medical education.

---

* Correspondence: Dr Ahmed Yaqinuddin, MBBS ,Ph.D. Assistant Professor of Anatomy and Cell biology, College of Medicine, Alfaisal University, Riyadh, 11533, KSA. E-mail: ayaqinuddin@alfaisal.edu. Phone: +966-2157669.

INTRODUCTION

The burden we place on the medical student is far too heavy and it takes some doing to keep from breaking his intellectual back.

Thomas Huxley, 1876

The key question each medical student has to ask himself when graduating from medical school is has the medical curriculum he/she took at the medical school prepared him/her aptly to meet the challenges of 21st Century medical practice ?

There is no doubt that the content and delivery of medical curricula are under immense pressure due to several external factors [1]. The changes in life styles and patterns of diseases have significantly modified society's expectation from a physician. Moreover, educational systems, healthy delivery systems and regulations of regulatory bodies are continuously changing and will continue to do so [1].

Our young generation of doctors will face several newer challenges like 1) adults will be expected to live relatively disease free well into their 80's 2) Young children will be expected to have disease free childhood 3) Cancers will be expected to be cured 4) they will encounter patient who would be very knowledgeable of their conditions through internet learning 5) Sequencing of Human genome (Human Genome project) will change current mode of medical practice significantly [1].

As these and many other factors will impact the life of new generation of doctors, it is imperative to prepare them adequately to meet these challenges. The 21st Century health care systems have a revolutionized approach where it is aiming at 1) community care rather than individualized care 2) health preservation & disease prevention rather than curing disease 3) comprehensive and continuous care rather than incidental care 4) single physician based care to a team based care. Experiential based practice is changing into evidence based medical practice. Health systems around the world are now emphasizing on reaccreditation, revalidation and continuous professional development of health professionals [2-4].

Aforementioned changes in the society and health systems have significantly impacted the methods of teaching and learning in medical institutes around the world. The newer medical curricula have shifted their emphasis to learning concepts, applying active learning process, and developing problem solving skills.

In these curricula, learning is in context and efforts have been made to integrate interdisciplinary knowledge [1]. More flexible programs of curriculum delivery have been adopted with emphasis on professional and clinical skills and attitudes which are complementary to core medical knowledge. Student centered approaches have taken the place of teacher oriented methods in modern medical curricula.

The following part of this chapter will describe the strengths and weaknesses of different medical curricular models and the reasons why newer models were adopted in a chronological order. In the final section of this chapter, we will describe a medical curricular model which could meet the educational requirements of 21st century physician.

APPRENTICESHIP BASED CURRICULUM MODEL

In early 1800's, this was the first curricular model which was adopted by approximately 40 medical schools across United States. It consists of two four months long semesters, where most of teaching was done by didactic lecture based system [5]. Five days a week, students received five to six lectures, one hour long, on courses including anatomy, physiology, chemistry, medicine, surgery, obstetrics and gynecology, pathology and pediatrics. There was hardly any emphasis on basic sciences, as main focus of instruction was to deliver content which has clinical importance [6]. Rote memory and note taking skills were of prime importance, as lectures given in first semester were repeated in second semester [6]. In-addition, there was no availability of textbooks till 1850s [6]. Most of this curriculum was taught by 7-8 unlicensed physicians with training in internal medicine.

The critical component of this model was 3-4 years apprenticeship, with a physician of student's choice [7]. Every day, the student will "shadow" his mentor in his routine clinical practice and learn clinical history and physical examination skills. The level of training was solely dependent on the expertise and training of the mentor [6].

Strengths

    I.   Early introduction of clinical sciences
    II.   Contextual learning (learning basic science in clinical context)
    III.   One to one teaching and learning method

Weaknesses

    I.   No emphasis on basic science
    II.   Knowledge content of the curriculum was very weak (The whole curriculum is taught in one semester)
    III.   Emphasis on rote memory rather than critical thinking and problem solving
    IV.   Non availability of textbooks, with only reliance on note taking skills of students
    V.   Non availability of active learning strategies.
    VI.   Training depends on the expertise of an unlicensed practitioner

Reasons for Change and Recommendations

In 1910, Flexner's report, Medical Education in the United States and Canada: A report of Carnegie Foundation for Advancement of Teaching, described the following problems in this model [8]:

    1.   *Lack of standardized and rigorous curriculum*: The report recommended that there should be four years of premedical courses as entry requirement to medical school.

The medical school curriculum should be divided into two years of basic sciences and two years of clinical sciences [8].

2. **Integration:** integration of laboratory science teaching with clinical sciences. The clinical teaching should be performed in University teaching hospitals [8].

3. **Habits of inquiry and improvement:** Physicians need to be trained like scientist as "Problem solvers and critical thinkers". Medical curriculum should be taught by scientifically trained faculty [8].

4. **Identity formation:** Medical education should be a part of the University culture. There should be a close interaction between medical students and trained faculty mentors [8].

THE DISCIPLINE-BASED MODEL

In the late 19th century and early 20th century the ignorance and incompetence of an average American physician has become a norm which led to the following observation by Charles Elliot, then President of Harvard University

"The ignorance and general incompetence of the average graduate of American Medical Schools, at the time he receives the degree which turns him loose upon the community, is something horrible to contemplate" [9].

These statements and observations from leading educationists, led to Flexner's movement and adoption of discipline based curriculum model by universities around United States of America [6].

The discipline based model was developed based on best practices in Europe, especially in France and Germany [6]. The first change was that the medical schools were housed within the university. The faculties in these schools were segregated in discipline based-departments [6]. Second, the length of the formal training was increased from two four-month-long, repetitive semesters to two six-month-long, distinct semesters [6]. The length of formal training eventually changed from one year to two years and finally to four years. This four year medical training had two exclusive basic science and two clinical years [6]. Third, as the basic science was given parity with clinical sciences, it was hoped that the physicians graduating through this curricular structure would have more reliance on laboratory derived clinical sciences [6]. Finally, it was hoped that basic scientist would serve as role models for budding physicians and this would help these physicians to inculcate key skills like "hypothetical-deductive reasoning" in their practice.

Strengths

I.   The length of formal training was appropriate

II.   The knowledge content of the curriculum become stronger with emphasis on basic science

III.   Hypothetical-deductive reasoning was emphasized rather than rote-memory

Weaknesses

I. Segregated basic science and clinical years, barred students from early exposure to the patients

II. Knowledge content expanded enormously without any consideration of what a physician would need in his/her clinical practice.

III. No attention was given to the temporal sequence of basic or clinical subjects.

IV. Basic science was taught in isolation from clinical science with no horizontal or longitudinal integration.

V. Departments started to control the amount of knowledge a medical student would be expected to know from each discipline.

These and other issues led to development of less segregated and more integrated "Organ-systems based model"

ORGAN SYSTEMS BASED MODEL, (1951)

In the middle of 1900's a wide-spread dissatisfaction with the discipline-based curriculum model surfaced with calls from leading educationist to reduce the "details" of basic science content [10]. Sinclair professed that teaching details of science subjects through different departments in a repetitive, non-sequential and disjointed manner is of little value to medical students [11]. Sinclair was of the view that basic, preclinical and clinical sequence of instruction in the medical school led to a sense of dissatisfaction among medical students who aspired to be healers from the outset [11].

These issues culminated in a paradigm shift where a curricular model was proposed wherein the discipline specific information is reduced. Moreover, the curriculum content should be delivered in more integrated and coherent manner. The organ systems based model had the following salient features.

1. An integrated system was introduced where departmental control of the educational system was replaced by a multidisciplinary curriculum committee [10]. This committee supervised several topic committees and departmental role in curriculum management and delivery was reduced to mere supportive.

2. The first organ-system based curriculum was introduced at the medical school in Western Reserve University in 1951 [12, 13]. The key feature of this curriculum was to integrate basic sciences (Anatomy, Physiology and Biochemistry) around a focus of single organ system. Even with this change students viewed the curricular content as disjointed. This led to further modification of organ systems based model where basic science (structure & function), pathophysiology of disease (mechanism of disease) and clinical sciences were integrated together with focus on single organ system. It also included a few clinical encounters so that students would understand the relevance of knowledge they are acquiring.

3. During the clerkship years students were exposed to more specialists rather than generalists [6]. The clinicians believed that the integrated knowledge which students

have acquired through organ systems based approach could easily be utilized in diagnosing diseases. However, it quickly became apparent that the students' knowledge gained through this approach was neither sufficient nor efficient for clinical utility.

Strengths

    I.   Integration of basic science with clinical sciences within a modular frame work of organ systems.

    II.   Control of curriculum development and management placed under supervision of multidisciplinary curriculum committee.

    III.   Well defined learning objectives enhanced the learning process as expectations from the students became clearer.

    IV.   The model encouraged students to develop self-directed and problem solving skills.

Weakness

    I.   Integration or synergistic delivery of content of different disciplines in an organ system based approach does not necessarily translate into integration of content by the learners.

    II.   Inability of medical students to use integrated knowledge to solve clinical problems in clinical years.

Around 1970's cognitive science studies made it evident that knowledge imparted without the context of application would be difficult for learners to retain or apply [14]. Growing quantities of medical literature, with little application utility, pushed medical educationist to develop a curricular model taking a lead from cognitive science theories [15].

PROBLEM BASED CURRICULUM MODEL (1971)

The main flaw in the organ-system based approach was that all learning was centered around an organ system rather than a disease. The main task of a physician is to diagnose and treat diseases. Given this premise and taking lead from cognitive science studies, Dr. Howard Burrows, from MacMaster University, recommended a medical curriculum which is structured around clinical problems and delivered through small group discussions [16]. The first Problem based learning (PBL) curriculum was developed at Macmaster University, medical school [16]. It had the following salient features:

1. In this approach clinical problems like joint pains, hypertension and stroke etc. became the core of medical curriculum around which all basic and clinical sciences were learned.

2. The mode of delivery of instruction also changed from large class room format to small group tutorials.
3. Active learning and student centered learning was emphasized with introduction of non-expert tutors to facilitate small group tutorials. The students were given a clinical case as a problem and they had to use their prior knowledge to hypothesize and identify their learning needs. They were then encouraged to actively use literature resources to acquire contextual knowledge to address them. It was hoped that active learning and learning in context will help learners to retain better.
4. Discovery learning was one of the key elements of PBL method. It was thought that by this form of learning, problem solving and hypothetical deductive reasoning skills would be inculcated in the learners, which is essential for clinical diagnosis.

Strengths

I.   Contextual clinically relevant knowledge would improve retention and its utility among learners.
II.   Small group tutorials would improve attitude and interest of the learners towards learning
III. Active learning aids in retention
IV.   Discovery learning helps in developing problem solving and hypothetical deductive reasoning.

Weaknesses

I.   The main theory behind the PBL was that knowledge is better retained when learned in context. Colliver and other leading educationist have challenged this theory and termed it as "weak" [17]. He argued that learning around a PBL case does not give a substantial advantage to a student to learn clinical practice, as type written cases cannot substitute for clinical encounters in a clinical setting. Thus, although the context of traditional curriculum versus PBL curriculum are different, neither of them is the same as a clinical setting [17]. He asserted that because of this reason: the PBL school graduates would have no substantial advantage in clinical contextual learning over traditional school graduates [17].
II.   As problem solving is a generalizable process, so cases used to learn this skill would have equal value. Given this premise the cases used in the PBL curriculum needed to be carefully defined in-order to serve the mission of the institution (e.g., relevant to primary care or tertiary care) [6].
III. In a PBL curriculum students in different groups do not cover all the learning objectives as identified by the faculty. This may results in gaps in the knowledge base of a learner.
IV.   PBL curriculum uses non-expert tutors as facilitators of PBL process. This may lead to misconceptions in understanding mechanisms, which remain uncorrected [6].

V.   Typical PBL curriculum focuses on a "single clinical problem" chosen to represent classes of diseases. For example, a single problem could be "Chest pain" which represents several disease classes like myocardial Infarction, esophagitis, pulmonary embolism etc. So, it is not sufficient to learn about chest pain by using a single problem related to myocardial infarction. It is further complicated by the fact that it has been shown by studies that students' ability to arrive at correct diagnosis largely depends upon typical presentation of disease in the case [6].

VI.   Use of small group teaching as the main strategy in PBL curriculum is extensively resource intensive. In the setting of a class of 200 medical students, a medical institute would require 30 trained PBL tutors and as many small class rooms [6].

OUTCOME BASED CURRICULUM MODEL (1990S)

Ever growing medical knowledge, changing demands from the society towards a physician, the medical education is in revolutionary mode [18]. In the industrialized countries like United States, Canada and United Kingdom there is a movement towards defining competencies/outcomes which physician needs to possess as a medical graduate [19-21]. So the main idea behind this approach is that all learning activities, content, assessments of a medical curriculum will be defined based on pre-defined outcomes and competencies [22]. It has been envisaged that the road to become a competent physician starts from a medical school; there should be a continuum of medical education from a medical student to the final product as a "competent physician" [23]. This can only be achieved if there are clearly defined outcomes at each level (i.e. medical students, residents, fellows and consultants). The main features of this approach are given below:

1.   The educational outcomes of a medical curriculum are identified and made explicit to all stake holders including, curriculum developers, faculty, students etc. [22].

2.   The content of the curriculum, methods of teaching and learning, time allocation to different courses, assessments would be guided by the learning outcomes of the course [22]. For example, a course of medicine may have learning outcomes related to content of knowledge required for practice of medicine but in-addition may have learning outcomes related communication skills, prevention and health promotion.

Strengths

I.   This approach makes a relationship between the curriculum and capability of a future physician [22].

II.   This approach is readily acceptable on political, social, educational and ethical grounds readily acceptable by faculty, administration and regulators. [22].

III.   This model of curriculum sets up a powerful frame work for accountability. The graduating physician is judged against predefined competencies/outcomes [22].

IV.   Well defined learning outcomes provide the learners freedom to develop their own learning methods and plans to achieve desired outcomes [22].

V.   This approach is relatively flexible and does not enforce any particular educational philosophy or strategy [22].

VI.   This approach helps to make the assessments more standardized [22]. So students have to achieve certain standards to graduate as set up by learning outcomes.

VII.   This approach also provides a frame work (outcomes) through which the curriculum can be assessed [22].

VIII. It provides a frame-work for continuous medical education from a medical student to a competent physician [22].

Weaknesses

I.   It is a teacher-directed approach rather than student centered approach [25].

II.   It conflicts with certain educational strategies like PBL, wherein students are required to develop their own learning needs [25].

III.   "Competencies" or outcomes are complex multifaceted phenomenon [26]. Thus, competencies cannot be divided into measurable tasks or sub-competencies. For example, if a student successfully learns steps of taking history and examination of patient with chest problem does not necessarily makes him/her competent chest physician.

IV.   This approach narrows down the content of the curriculum in two ways and can lead to gaps in knowledge and skills among learners. First, by narrowing the content of the curriculum to the expected tasks to be completed [26]. Second, it limits the curriculum to what can be directly measured [26].

V.   This educational approach is often criticized for teaching the students for an examination [26]. As students are only taught those aspects of the medical curriculum which are defined in the outcomes and only those will be tested.

VI.   As this approach provided the frame work for evaluation of curriculum, it has at the same time pushed educators to become more and more form filling bureaucrats. It has diverted them from devoting their energies in developing and implementing educational strategies to a paper chase [26].

ALFAISAL CURRICULUM MODEL AS AN EXAMPLE OF 21ST CENTURY MEDICAL CURRICULUM

The medical curriculum of Alfaisal University was developed in 2008 taking up a "hybrid" approach. The key to this approach was that no single educational strategy or instructional method was used as a core to develop this curriculum. This hybrid curriculum was viewed as a program of study developed where whole should have a bigger impact than sum of parts of the curriculum (figure-1).

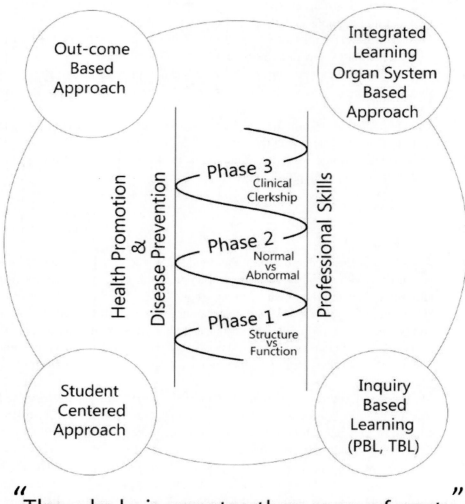

Figure 1. The Curricular Model of the Alfaisal Medical School.

The following are the salient features of this curriculum.

1. Spiral curriculum: A spiral approach to curriculum development was taken, where the curriculum had three interconnected phases. An outcome based approach was taken where outcomes of each phase builds on to develop the final product "a competent intern". The phase -1 of the curriculum dealt with normal structure and function of human body. In the phase-2 of the curriculum the normal versus abnormal relationship is sorted out, in-addition clinical skills for clinical practice were introduced. The third phase of the curriculum is the clinical clerkship phase, where students learnt the practice of medicine. These phases of curriculum are not

distinct but rather interlocked so that knowledge gained in one is used to learn the knowledge and skills in the successive phases. For example, the structure and function of the heart learned in phase-1 is revisited and reassessed when learning about mechanism of heart diseases in phase-2. Moreover, the disease mechanisms are revisited and reassessed when students learn the management of heart diseases in phase-3 of the curriculum.

2. The modules of study have been divided according to organ systems based approach. In-addition longitudinal modules of community oriented courses and professional skills were included in the curriculum.

3. The educational methods included myriad of strategies including problem based learning, team based learning, large group discussions and community based approaches to learning.

4. A community based approach to curriculum has been adopted where in, the curriculum was developed keeping in mind most prevalent diseases in the community. The students were encouraged to participate in disease prevention and health promotion programs from the beginning.

5. The student centered approach was emphasized where students take responsibility for their own learning. They were provided by well-structured guides which helped them to develop their own plan of study including "what to study" and "how to study". Development of active learning and self-study skills was core to this curriculum.

6. The curriculum was managed by an eight member curriculum committee which included five year chairs, PBL coordinator, TBL coordinator and a Professional skills coordinator. Each year chair runs a year committee, which included module directors from that particular year of curriculum. Further, module committees included discipline representatives and were chaired by module chair.

7. The curriculum is continuously reviewed internally by an independent curriculum review committee and externally reviewed by "Partners Harvard International" (a renowned group of medical educationists).

Strengths

I. The spiral design of the curriculum where basic science knowledge gained in earlier phase is revisited and used to build concepts of next phase of the curriculum. We have found that use of this approach has helped our students to "build up" knowledge as they progress through different phases of curriculum. This is evidenced by a nationwide progress test where our students had consistently shown substantial improvement as they progress through the successive years of the medical curriculum (figure -2).

II. Organ systems based approach was used to ensure that integration of different disciplines.

III. PBL and TBL based educational strategies were introduced throughout the curriculum to ensure adult principles of learning were inculcated within the curriculum including 1) active learning 2) contextual learning and 3) small group learning.

IV.   Students centered approach was used where students were given control of their learning. This included providing them with 1) self-study time 2) well-structured study guides 3) well equipped learning resource centers and empowering them by giving them membership in various educational committees. The school also had a well-structured medical students association which continuously provides feedback regarding students learning needs to the Dean of the medical school through its representatives.

Figure 2 shows the mean percentage scores of medical students throughout the five years of medical curriculum on a nation-wide progress test participated by 12 medical schools. The scores of College of Medicine, Alfaisal University students are represented by bar "J"

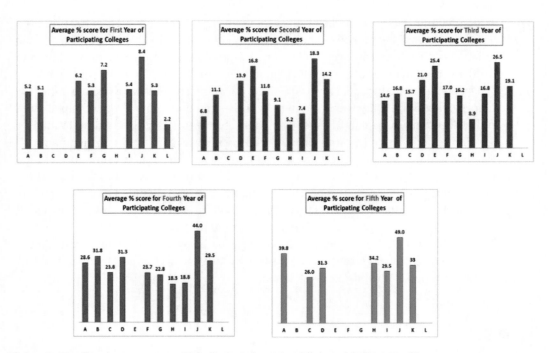

Figure 2. The Percentage scores of Medical students in a Nationwide Progress Test.

Improvements Being Implemented

I.   Although the spiral curriculum design is robust, we have found that there should be an interface as students' transition through one phase to the other.
II.   We are in the process of writing the final outcomes of the program and mapping these with each phase, year and module of the curriculum.
III.   An adaptive curriculum model needs to be implemented, wherein the students are given chances to retrain until required standard is met.

CONCLUSION

We have presented herein several curricular models including an example of 21st century curriculum. We believe that with ever growing demands of medical practice in the 21st century, the medical curricula of this age should 1) provide high degree of flexibility towards achieving standardized outcomes, 2) provide processes for integrated and active learning 3) encourage students to develop analytical and self-learning skills, and 4) provide students with a conducive environment. Collectively, these attributes should help the students not only employ self-study skills but to work for improving health care needs of the society.

REFERENCES

[1]   Jones R, Higgs R, de Angelis C, Prideaux D. Changing face of medical curricula. *Lancet.* 2001;357(9257):699-703.

[2]   du Boulay C. Revalidation for doctors in the United Kingdom: the end or the beginning? *BMJ* (Clinical research ed. 2000;320(7248):1490.

[3]   Newble D, Paget N, McLaren B. Revalidation in Australia and New Zealand: approach of Royal Australasian College of Physicians. *BMJ* (Clinical research ed. 1999;319(7218):1185-8.

[4]   Dauphinee WD. Revalidation of doctors in Canada. *BMJ* (Clinical research ed. 1999;319(7218):1188-90.

[5]   WG R. *Ameican Physicians in the Nineteenth Century: from Sects to Science.* Baltimore: The John hopkins University Press; 1972.

[6]   Papa FJ, Harasym PH. Medical curriculum reform in North America, 1765 to the present: a cognitive science perspective. *Acad Med.* 1999;74(2):154-64.

[7]   Shryock RH. European backgrounds of American medical education (1600-1900). *Jama.* 1965;194(7):709-14.

[8]   Irby DM, Cooke M, O'Brien BC. Calls for reform of medical education by the Carnegie Foundation for the Advancement of Teaching: 1910 and 2010. *Acad Med.* 2010;85(2):220-7.

[9]   Eliot C. *Annual Report of President of Vard college 1870-71.* Cambridge: Havard University; 1972.

[10] Dornhorst AC, Hunter A. Fallacies in medical education. *Lancet.* 1967;2(7517):666-7.

[11] Sinclair. *Basic Medical education.* London: Oxford University Press; 1972.

[12] Patterson JW. Western Reserve. 3. Interdepartmental and departmental teaching of medicine and biologic science in four years. *Journal of medical education.* 1956;31(8):521-9.

[13] Caughey JL, Jr. Western Reserve. 4. Clinical teaching during four years. *Journal of medical education.* 1956;31(8):530-4.

[14] Schmidt HG. Problem-based learning: rationale and description. *Medical education.* 1983;17(1):11-6.

[15] Ausubel D. The use of advanced organizers in learning and retention of meaningful verbal material. *J Educ Psychol.* 1960;51:267-72.

[16]   Barrows H. *How to design a Problem -based Curriculum for the Preclinical Years.* New York: Springer Publishing Company 1985.

[17]   Colliver JA. Effectiveness of problem-based learning curricula: research and theory. *Acad Med.* 2000;75(3):259-66.

[18]   Norman G. Editorial - outcomes, objectives, and the seductive appeal of simple solutions. *Adv Health Sci Educ Theory Pract.* 2006;11(3):217-20.

[19]   Scientific foundations of future physicians: Report of the AAMC-HHMI committee. Washington, DC: Association of American Medical Colleges; 2009.

[20]   Tomorrow's doctor: Outcomes and standards for undergraduate medical education. London: *General Medical Council*; 2009.

[21]   CanMEDS 2000: Extract from the CanMEDS 2000 Project Societal Needs Working Group Report. *Medical teacher.* 2000;22(6):549-54.

[22]   Harden JRCMHDMFRM. AMEE Guide No. 14: Outcome-based education: Part 5- From competency to meta-competency: a model for the specification of learning outcomes. *Medical teacher.* 1999;21(6):546-52.

[23]   Albanese MA, Mejicano G, Anderson WM, Gruppen L. Building a competency-based curriculum: the agony and the ecstasy. *Adv Health Sci Educ Theory Pract.* 2010;15(3):439-54.

[24]   Spady W. Oragnization for results: the basis of authentic restructuring and reform. *Educational leadership.* 1988:4-8.

[25]   Rees CE. The problem with outcomes-based curricula in medical education: insights from educational theory. *Medical education.* 2004;38(6):593-8.

[26]   Malone K, Supri S. A critical time for medical education: the perils of competence-based reform of the curriculum. *Adv. Health Sci Educ Theory Pract.* 2012;17(2):241-6.

In: Health and Disease   ISBN: 978-1-63463-052-8
Editor: Paul Ganguly   © 2015 Nova Science Publishers, Inc.

Chapter 3

MEDICAL CURRICULUM: DOES ONE SIZE FIT ALL?

H. Thomas Aretz, *

Vice President - Global Programs, Partners HealthCare International, Boston, MA, US
Associate Professor of Pathology, Harvard Medical School, Boston, MA, US

ABSTRACT

Healthcare needs and healthcare delivery are changing dramatically across the world, and medical education planning needs to provide specific solutions for the various needs, cultures and environments. "One Size Fits All" is not an acceptable and meaningful solution. Curriculum planners will need to use a systematic organizational and pedagogical approach to assure that future programs are desirable and needed, feasible, and sustainable. This chapter outlines a three step planning approach to create programs that address practical needs by teaching and developing relevant competencies, and instill values through the development of operating principles that guide the curriculum planning process and the organization. As the healthcare workforce is being redesigned and restructured throughout the world, medical education needs to collaborate with the other healthcare professions and help the process by aligning itself to the needs of societies and their stakeholders.

INTRODUCTION

A Brief Historical Perspective

In order to begin to answer the question in the title of this chapter, "Does One Size Fit All?", it may be useful to provide some historical perspective on the evolution of medical education to date, focusing on its variability. Medicine, like many other professions, was originally a family business, and later, as strangers became students, was taught as an apprenticeship. Students would follow a master physician and learn from him (physicians were invariably men) [1], which by its very nature induced quite a significant amount of variability into the learning process. When medicine became part of the medieval universities in Europe, its design followed the structure of the medieval university: its theory and

---

* Corresponding author: H. Thomas Aretz, MD. E-mail address: taretz@partners.org, Aretz.Tom@mgh.harvard.edu.

philosophy being taught based on established texts [2], thereby providing some uniformity in the teachings. The apprenticeship model, however, persisted well into 19th century North America and is still the model for clinical training virtually everywhere, especially in postgraduate education. [3]. A notable exception was the more holistic and institution based medical education in the Middle East, where academic medical centers were established as early as the 10th century [4]. The scientific revolution and the subsequent creation of the discipline-based model [3], which made the basic sciences paramount to the understanding of medicine, required more rigor in the studies of medicine. With the publication of the Flexner report [5], the discipline-based model became the norm, which has essentially not changed until now [6]. Most medical education changes (e.g. organ system based models; problem based learning; disease presentation based models; the outcomes/competency based models [3]) have been variations on this theme, some exhibiting more substantial changes than others. Fundamental changes and unique approaches, however, are still rare.

Figure 1 outlines the essential commonalities and differences of medical education across the world. The major distinctions are:

- Entry into medical school directly out of high school (in some countries after a special preparatory year), called the undergraduate model, which is dominant in the world;
- Entry into medical school after a college degree, called the postgraduate or North American model, which includes certain required courses in college;
- The requirement of a general internship or foundation courses (e.g. UK) rather than direct entry into specialty residencies;
- Length of study.

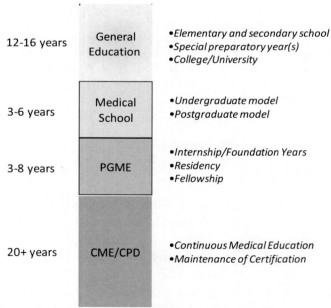

PGME = Postgraduate Medical Education; CME = Continuous Medical Education; CPD = Continuous Professional Development.

Figure 1. Common and distinctive features of medical education in the world.

Once in medical school, however, the subjects taught are remarkably similar, dictated by the historical departmental structures of universities and hospitals, and often specified by detailed regulations, which take their origins in the Western discipline-based models. The absence of meaningful patient interactions, at least for the first, and often for the initial three to four years [6], is another common feature.

In essence, the pre-clinical - clinical divide and the continued emphasis on the basic sciences are still the norm virtually everywhere in the world, and thereby provide a rather unified theme to medical education, often bolstered by international accreditation efforts. It should be noted that, while advocating a scientific approach to the teaching of medicine, Flexner always intended medicine to be a profession grounded primarily in practice [7].

MEDICAL EDUCATION IN CONTEXT

The Need to Align Education to the Provision of Care – Why One Size Does Not Fit All

The need for fundamental changes to medical education have been written about extensively, in essence stating that it is time to align medical education to the changing needs of healthcare around the globe and the societies they serve [8, 9].

Figure 2 tries to give a high-level overview of the various aspects of healthcare, outlining the various determinants of health, the different elements of healthcare systems, the various levels of healthcare, the points of interactions experienced by patients and their families, and the ultimate measures of success for any healthcare system.

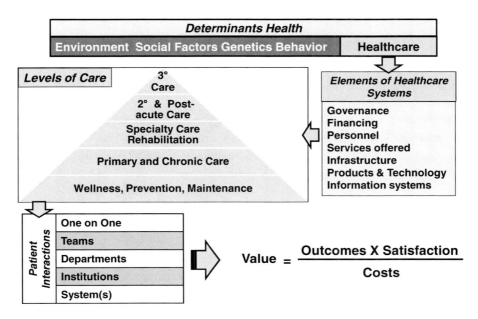

Figure 2. Figure 2 illustrates the various determinants of health, the elements of healthcare systems, levels of care in them, patient interactions with healthcare and the essential metrics of success.

Figure 2 tries to illustrate that healthcare is complex, and subject to multiple influences, stakeholders and outside forces affecting how physicians and patients interact. It should therefore not be a surprise that there are many differences in healthcare around the world and within regions and nations.

Healthcare is only one *determinant* of health on a personal and population basis, and there are many other important factors that influence health [10]:

- The *environment*, natural or man-made;
- *Social factors* such as education, economic status, race, ethnicity, and marital status;
- *Genetics,* in terms of susceptibility to disease, the environment and lifestyle choices;
- *Behaviors and lifestyle* choices, such as drug use, risk taking (e.g. reckless driving), smoking, alcohol use, sexual behaviors, and diet.

While physicians may not be able to influence many of these factors, they should understand their effects and try and provide inputs into the modification of these various risk factors. They at least need to understand where and how patients and their families can find help and support. Recent data indicate such provider efforts reduce the costs and improve the quality of care [11].

There is a finite number of *elements* that can be influenced and controlled in the provision of healthcare, and they vary profoundly from nation to nation, region to region and place to place.

- *Governance* is crucial in the functioning of healthcare systems and no two healthcare systems in the world are structured alike. Governance structures, processes and policies influence how decisions are made, the level of autonomy of the various stakeholders in the system and its overall effectiveness and efficiency. Medical students have traditionally not been taught much about governance principles and systems.
- *Financing* strategies and insurance and financing schemes are crucial in determining access to quality care. Medical schools rarely teach relevant healthcare economics and the prudent use of resources.
- The creation of a relevant *healthcare workforce* has become increasingly important in developed and emerging economies around the world [8, 12], and novel approaches that challenge traditional healthcare professional roles have emerged, especially in resource constrained environments [13]. Established hierarchies and traditional professional boundaries, however, have provided significant barriers to implementation [14]. Medical education needs to address these issues head-on and become a leader and active participant in the creation of a flexible and suitable healthcare workforce, including the roles of physicians.
- The *services* that are offered in healthcare systems are driven by a variety of factors including commercial interests, needs of the population, and availability of personnel, technology and infrastructure. Both undersupply and oversupply of certain services are issues that will require system level approaches, but customized education programs can help train physicians who understand the specific needs of the societies they serve [9].

- *Infrastructure* involves more than just buildings, it also includes the means of access to healthcare providers and facilities. This varies widely from place to place and physicians should understand the implications and minimum requirements, and how specific physical barriers and infrastructures affect the care of their patients.

- *Products and technology* are often developed based on research efforts by physicians and in many instances, supported by public funds. Commercial entities, however, are necessary to bring products and technology to the market, and physicians should understand the basic elements and economics of this process, the determination of needs, the assessment of new technologies and products, and how their own behaviors influence the usage of technologies. The need for and use of specific technologies, especially in resource-constrained environments, varies widely.

- *Information technology* plays an ever increasing role in the delivery of healthcare, not only in its administration and record keeping, but also in decision support, quality management, performance improvement, and patient involvement and engagement. Similarly, educational technologies are reshaping medical education, and are yet to be used in their most effective and efficient manner. Education and healthcare are two industries that have yet to realize significant increases in productivity [15]. The availability and applicability of information and communications technology varies widely around the world, and within countries. Education programs should address the effective and efficient use of these technologies to address specific needs of the populations served.

The listing above and the brief descriptions are merely an outline of the many differences and distinct elements that distinguish healthcare delivery around the globe. Education programs clearly cannot be "generic" and assume that they will address these special needs.

There are multiple *levels* at which care is delivered across healthcare systems, with academic medical centers, the predominant site of medical education, principally operating at the tertiary care level. The traditional role of academic medical centers has been to provide highly specialized and complex care, train the healthcare workforce, and conduct research. Yet the vast majority of medical care is provided outside academic medical centers [16], especially as ambulatory and chronic care becomes increasingly important. In addition, most healthcare providers at the various levels are operating independently, making education across the spectrum difficult. Education programs need to address the specifics of the various regional and local healthcare systems in order to create physicians who can function in them and, more importantly, help shape them to be more effective.

Patients and their families find themselves having to interact with this vast array of providers, trying to navigate a maze of options, barriers and obstacles. The traditional education of physicians has focused almost exclusively on the one-to-one interaction between patients and their physicians. Only recently has the medical establishment begun to realize that teamwork, communications, practice based improvement and systems/population based thinking are required competencies for physicians in today's complex medical landscape [17].

Recent studies in the context of the implementation of the Affordable Care Act in the US have shown that the provision of coordinated, longitudinal, personal and holistic care to patients and their families requires significant transformations of medical practices, for which physicians are ill prepared [18].

If we are to align personal care with efficient and effective population health, physicians will need to be educated differently and specifically in the context of their healthcare systems and their future roles.

Finally, healthcare, like many other service industries, is being increasingly scrutinized and reimbursed based on *"value"*, defined as the outcomes achieved for the amount of resources expended [19], patient satisfaction being an important component. Physicians have traditionally not thought of themselves as providing customer service or being part of a service industry; they have traditionally viewed themselves as individual professionals serving their specific patient population.

As quality concerns are rising and as the cost of healthcare is becoming prohibitive, physicians will need to understand how to provide services efficiently at high quality, which will require operational changes, process improvement strategies and reorganization of medical practice at all levels and across levels, including appropriate collection of data over time [20]. In addition, as payment models begin to reimburse based on performance and cost, physicians' and providers' incomes will depend on their ability to provide value. The present medical education is ill equipped to address these issues and will need to develop specific programs to address the local relevant issues of access, quality and cost.

The above discussion highlights some of the issues concerning the content and structure of the existing medical education programs virtually everywhere in the world. The purpose of this chapter is not to address how to teach these specific content areas, or suggest specific new structures or pedagogies to address these shortcomings and future challenges. The purpose is rather to outline a curriculum development approach that allows for the design and implementation of the appropriate medical education programs that address the needs of the relevant healthcare system(s) and take into account emerging technologies and pedagogical advancements in support of the objectives. The following section outlines some existing models, innovations and experiments that try to better align education with the practice of medicine.

Present Innovations Addressing Better Alignment with the Healthcare System

Some of the present areas of experimentation in medical education are related to its length, addressing specific needs in the healthcare system, alignment of academic and clinical institutions, and educating professionals as teams. All of these efforts, however, still have to conform to existing accreditation and regulatory requirements, often leading to add-ons, rearrangement of subjects and adjustments of pedagogy to existing norms, i.e. "tweaks" rather than radical restructuring.

1   *Length:* The length of medical education is very much under pressure due to the need for physicians and the cost of education, whether borne by the public or the individual student. In times of need, such as war, medical education was shortened in the past, and fast track programs were instituted. There is now a renewed call to shorten medical education [21, 22], and multiple programs have been started in recent years or are offering fast track options in various parts of the United States. It is not clear how these schools or programs will perform in the long run, but warnings

are already being sounded [23]. Length may very well have to become a function of the curriculum planned, demonstrable student achievement, and local needs and circumstances, rather than being rigidly preordained.

2 *Healthcare needs:* While community based medical education as part of a standard medical curriculum has led to a better appreciation by students of the roles and responsibilities of community healthcare providers, primary care physicians and the unique needs of community based care [24], schools and programs designed specifically to address care in the community and rural settings were felt to better address those unique requirements. One analysis showed that these types of programs attract a greater number of practitioners to the rural setting [25], while others did not show such positive results [26]. The creation of medical schools, where clinical teaching is entirely accomplished in dispersed community healthcare facilities, practices and institutions was originally met with significant regulatory push-back, requiring the use of technology and well coordinated quality management efforts to assure comprehensive, comparable and satisfactory learning experiences for the students [27]. Given that medical care is increasingly moving into the community and increasingly involves patients and their families and caregivers, this type of education will only increase in the future, tailored to local communities.

3 *New alignments of healthcare and academic institutions:* Rather than creating new medical schools and their associated teaching hospitals, as still required in many regulatory jurisdictions (e.g. India), existing, often non-academic medical institutions have aligned or contracted with existing universities or medical colleges to form new programs or schools governed by joined supervisory and planning boards. These types of programs are trying to address specific needs in healthcare by the creation of these very specific programs and educational environments. Below are some examples of such associations and collaborations between various types of institutions:

- Private for-profit health care provider and a public university. The Semmelweis University Medical Faculty Asklepios Hamburg [28] is collaboration between Asklepios, a large for-profit German healthcare provider chain, and Semmelweis University, a public university in Budapest, Hungary, offering a medical curriculum in German. Students complete their preclinical work in Budapest, and their clinical work in Hamburg in the Asklepios hospitals and clinics. The intent is to train clinicians who can function in large healthcare systems.
- Private non-profit healthcare provider and a public university. The University of Queensland - Ochsner Clinical School [29] similarly combines a degree granting institution with an existing healthcare provider organization. Students spend two preclinical years in Brisbane, Australia, and two clinical years at the Ochsner Clinic in New Orleans, USA. The intent is to specifically train future physicians in a group-practice environment, which is becoming increasingly common.
- Public universities and public health districts. The so-called Bachelor of Medicine - Joint Medical Program (JMP) [30] is a five-year medical degree program aimed at creating practitioners for rural health in Australia. It is jointly offered by the School of Rural Medicine at the University of New England and the University of Newcastle in partnership with the Hunter New England and Central Coast Local Health Districts.

- Private non-profit healthcare organization and private non-profit university. The Cleveland Clinic Lerner College of Medicine of Case Western Reserve University [31] is collaboration between the Cleveland Clinic, a private non-profit healthcare system and the Case Western Reserve University, private non-profit university, both in Cleveland, OH, US. The five-year program is designed to educate clinician investigators and scientists.

These are just a few examples of a growing trend of healthcare system based academic endeavors or "modular academic medical centers"[1], where the healthcare institutions rather than the universities are the drivers of the educational programs in order to achieve specific results and outcomes. Regulatory issues and cultural and operational alignment present barriers for programs of this type, but using existing resources to support novel programs aimed at providing specific or better trained healthcare professionals will continue to provide an impetus for future creative and cost-effective alliances.

4   *Interprofessional education* efforts are another recent attempt at providing educational experiences that align with clinical practice [32]. There are no universities of health sciences in existence yet that have been designed on a pure interprofessional model, but significant programs do exist [33] and interprofessional competencies have been defined by pertinent regulatory agencies [34]. Results are not conclusive yet, and barriers to implementation clearly exist [35], but given the increasing interdisciplinary nature of healthcare, programs specifically designed to train physicians for collaborative clinical practice will need to be developed

As the above examples show, there is an increasing number of efforts to create very different and specific medical education programs that address the specifics of the healthcare context. The following section outlines a model for academic program planning to assure the creation of relevant and cost-effective medical education programs.

A MODEL FOR MEDICAL EDUCATION PLANNING

A Value and Needs Based Planning Approach to Create Medical Education Programs Suitable to Their Environments

In 1938, when the architect Ludwig Mies van der Rohe became the director of the Armour Institute in Chicago, he told the students and his audience in his inaugural speech that "true education is concerned not only with practical goals but also with values... Our aims assure us of our material life, our values make possible our spiritual life" [36]. The following model outlines a three-phase approach to curriculum planning based on this principle, which has been used in the planning of new institutions and programs [37]. The three phases address the following questions crucial to the long-term success of any project:

---

[1] The author's term.

1   Is the program desirable/needed?
2   Is the program feasible?
3   Is the program sustainable?

While these may seem like rather general questions, the answers require very specific and well researched solutions and a thorough understanding of the issues listed above, as they pertain to very specific aspects of the healthcare and societal context of the planned program. Needs and desirability will not be the same from place to place, and the requirements for implementation and sustainability of the programs will vary widely based on circumstances. Hence – "One Size Does Not Fit All".

Phase 1: Is the Program Desirable/Needed? Addressing the Needs of the Healthcare System and Imbuing the Program with Values

The Rolling Stones famously asserted that "You can't always get what you want, and if you try sometime you find you get what you need". The main objective of this first phase is to fulfill this premise, in providing at least what is needed, but strive to also develop programs and institutions that are desirable and go beyond mere needs and requirements. Any medical education program development, therefore, has to start with a thorough understanding of the local needs and environment. This step has been widely acknowledged in standard textbooks of medical curriculum development, as being the essential starting point [38, 39]. Needs to be indentified include:

- Gaps or imbalances in local, regional or global healthcare delivery, including specific diseases, populations (e.g. rural, urban, underserved, elderly), regions or fields (e.g. clinical investigation, healthcare management, quality assurance)
- Gaps or imbalances in knowledge, skills, attitudes and behaviors in the profession that are needed to accomplish the desired outcomes (e.g. management skills, information technology, data analysis, interprofessional competencies).
- Gaps in the quantity and quality of available faculty and administrators.
- Gaps in a suitable student population, their prior education and selection processes.
- Gaps in available resources, infrastructure and systems (e.g. patients and populations suitable for teaching, hospitals)
- Gaps in educational programs, pedagogy and existing content.
- Gaps and imbalances in regulations and existing competency frameworks.

A thorough analysis of all these factors allows the curriculum planners to clearly define the desired metrics of success, including a list of measurable outcomes not only on an individual, but also on a curriculum and an institutional level aligned with each of the identified needs. Having done so, competencies that characterize a successful graduate can be defined. The other side of the equation requires the creation of a "spiritual inventory"[2] that defines values unique to the program or institution. These values should characterize the culture of the institution and shape the attitudes and behaviors of students, faculty and staff

---

[2] The author's term.

alike, while being the basis of the operating principles that guide how the organization functions and conducts its business [40], and thereby defining a unique corporate identity. About two years ago, the author and his colleagues developed a model, curricula and concept for a new interprofessional university of health sciences, in the process of which a set of operating principles based on values was developed.

To give a specific example, one of the values was "Diversity", and one of the resulting operating principles was that " [we will select and support the] student body to be as diverse as possible in all aspects (cultural, ethnic, religious and socioeconomic) going beyond the requirements in existence, as diversity enriches the learning environment and campus life"[3].

This particular operating principle mostly applied to admissions and selection processes and student life, but other principles were developed in support of diversity to govern faculty selection, content and educational experiences.

Figure 3 tries to summarize how this two-pronged approach helps develop a meaningful strategy form a practical as well as spiritual point of view. Phase 1 is often shortchanged in curricular development as planners rush to define content and timetables. Business studies have shown that a lack of attention to this particular phase of "product development" leads to inadequate solutions, increased costs and delays during the subsequent phases of development [41]. It is here, where the unique purpose and distinguishing characteristics of a program are forged and defined.

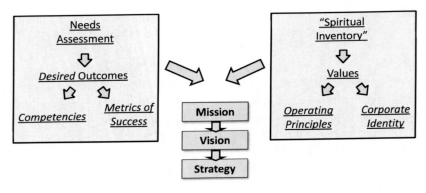

Figure 3. Both practical needs as well as values need to be addressed to create a meaningful strategy.

Phase 2: Is the Program Feasible?

Figure 4 summarizes this next phase. The strategy developed in Phase 1 now needs to be translated into a curriculum and the various structures and functions that will support its implementation and viability.

This development does not take place in a vacuum, but is developed in the background of the needs to be addressed, the values of the organizations to be created or preserved, and the services to be provided to the various stakeholders and society.

Available resources define what is ultimately feasible and where trade-offs need to be made.

---

[3] Due to the proprietary nature of the work, specifics cannot be disclosed.

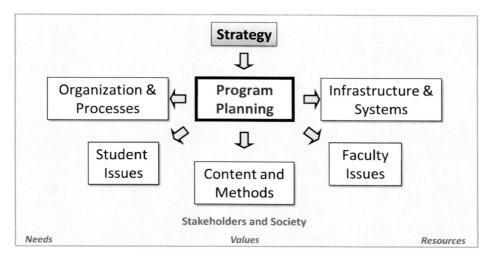

Figure 4. Program planning (Curriculum development) translates strategy into reality.

As figure 4 indicates, program planning plays the central role in translating strategy into reality. Designing a timetable and determining content is only one, albeit important aspect of academic program planning. Significant changes are not possible without changing the various elements indicated in figure 4, and they are guided by the operating principles developed for each area in phase 1. Below is a brief overview of the items not related to content development and educational methods, which will be discussed in greater detail in the following section.

1   As structure follows function, *organizational* structures, processes, policies and functions need to be aligned with the academic program planned. Clark and Wheelwright pointed out in their classic studies that the structure of an organization is mirrored in its products [42]. New programs, whose aims and structures depart significantly from established programs, need new organizational structures and processes to develop, implement and operate them [27]. For instance, it is not possible to create meaningful interdisciplinary and interprofessional programs if the established departmental structures and processes persist. Barriers include unwillingness to change, and often rigid regulations.

2   *Infrastructure and systems* similarly need to change or be designed to serve new programmatic elements, pedagogies and technologies. Case method rooms in business schools were designed to support case-based teaching, clinical skills labs and simulation labs are new infrastructures supporting clinical education and team training in medical environments, the latter having been used for years in military training and the aviation industry. Barriers here are mostly related to resources and an agreement that such efforts are needed and useful.

3   *Student issues* are often not considered when creating new schools or programs. For instance, if rural medicine is the focus of the program, recruitment and admissions criteria will need to change to accomplish the programmatic goals, as the general student population may not provide suitable candidates for such a program [43].

If "student-centeredness" is an espoused value of the organization, not involving students meaningfully in planning and operations would not be appropriate.

4   Similarly, *faculty* recruitment, promotion and development may all need to be designed quite differently for unique and novel programs, not only to address new content areas, but also in support of the institutional culture. Faculty structures and attitudes are crucial in the ability to create the right kind of environment and culture supportive of the programmatic goals [44]. Traditional departmental structures, faculty reward systems and general resistance to change all constitute significant barriers.

Educational Content, Methods and Technology: Much of academic program planning focuses on what to teach, when and how, and how to assess the outcomes and competency of the learners. Figure 5 summarizes schematically how goals and objectives relate to outcome, assessment and evaluation. For the purposes of this chapter, "assessment" refers to the testing of student competence, while "evaluation" is equivalent to program evaluation.

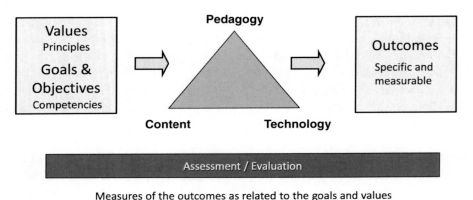

Figure 5. Content and pedagogy links goals to outcomes, and assessment and evaluation measure the results.

●   *Content:* The outcomes and competency movement across the world has resulted in the development of minimal competencies in virtually every country in the last 20 years [e.g. 45]. In addition, there have been efforts to create minimal global competencies, applicable anywhere in the world [46, 47]. These minimum competencies are useful in establishing minimum guidelines as to the desired outcomes of education and minimum content to be learned. Often standardized national licensing exams further dictate minimum content and skill development. These minimum requirements, however, need to be seen as such, a minimum baseline. While academic institutions are increasingly expected to produce graduates that have general minimum qualifications, they still need to develop programs specific to their mission as defined by specific needs and values. As described previously [37], Mercer University School of Medicine (MUSM) in Georgia, USA, for instance, has the very specific mission "to educate physicians and health professionals to meet the primary care and health care needs of rural and medically underserved areas of Georgia" [48]. MUSM chose to adopt the general ACGME competencies [17] as the basis for its curriculum development and content, but modified them to "reflect the knowledge, skills, behaviors, and attitudes expected of MUSM graduates." [49]. The acronym "BASKETS"[4] tries to capture major aspects of content and pedagogy development.

- **B** What new and specific *behaviors* need to be fostered to address individual and population needs, which may be quite different depending on the specific context? All learning is essentially about changing one's behavior – doing things differently or better as a result of an educational intervention. Educational programs are increasingly being evaluated based on change of behavior, performance and outcomes in the practical setting, not in an academic environment [50].

- **A** What are the *attitudes* that need to be inculcated to support these new behaviors and that fit the cultural context of a particular society and healthcare system? There has been much discussion about ethics and professionalism in the medical education literature, but ultimately, most attitudes are transmitted by example. Creating the appropriate educational environment and culture to align with societal norms and values is crucial.

- **S** What new *skills* need to be learned and applied to attain the goals and support the new behaviors? This category is often thought of as being restricted to traditional clinical skills, but modern medicine requires cognitive, organizational, technological and interpersonal skills not relevant in past practice settings. Educational programs must therefore be specifically designed to teach the relevant skills.

- **K** What is the new *knowledge* to be learned? Traditionally this meant learning mostly facts, but as information has increased enormously and becomes more ubiquitous and easily accessible, knowledge has taken on a new meaning, making the ability to find the information, analyze it, synthesize it and apply it much more important. How to do that requires new knowledge and cognitive skills [52].

- **E** What relevant learning *experiences* need to be provided? Experiential learning has always been the foundation of medical education. Unlike many other professions, much of learning takes place in the actual professional care environment. That environment, as discussed above, needs to reflect where and how clinical care takes place. Since the healthcare environment is different from place to place, and is in constant, often dramatic flux, medical education needs to align, just as it does when it comes to the advances of science.

- **T** What *technology* will support and enhance the learning experience? The discussion below will address some of the suggested changes in medical education.

- **S** How will learning be *sustained*? Sustainability is not meant to just preserve what was learned, given that knowledge constantly changes. Sustainability relates to the long-term process of learning, something that in and of itself

---

[4] This acronym was developed by the author and has been used in curriculum development and faculty development workshops. It has not been published.

requires certain knowledge, skills, attitudes, behaviors and most recently, technology [53].

- *Pedagogy:* Just as the medicine has changed dramatically, so has education. Advances in the understanding of the learning process [54] and technological advances have all provided great opportunities to tailor pedagogy to individual, institutional, societal and cultural needs, and resource constraints. A discussion of pedagogical methods and their use is beyond the scope of this chapter, but curriculum planners need to be cognizant of the fact that educational methods are a means to an end, and need to support the desired outcomes and the operating principles and values defined in phase 1 of the planning process. There is not one way to teach anything, and academic planners should critically evaluate their methods, rather than merely follow present fads or fashions.

  As an example, the author and his colleagues adopted the multistation technique originally developed to teach radiology in a clinical context to second-year medical students at Harvard Medical School [55].

  In the context of a multi-organ system course that included problem-based learning as a mainstay, this technique lent itself to help students integrate concepts requiring far fewer resources.

  It has been adapted to teach specific important skills to small groups in a limited amount of time with few faculty members [56].

  Similarly, active learning does not require small groups, but can be done quite successfully using case-based large group discussions [57]. These are just two examples to illustrate that schools need to be inventive in the use of pedagogy to address their specific needs and values.

  "One Size Fits All" certainly does not apply to individual students, especially when institutions espouse "student-centeredness" as being one of their important values and operating principles. Student populations the world over are quite different when they start their medical education. Methods need to take into account the developmental trajectory of students, not only in terms of knowledge and skills, but also in the way they learn and their readiness for more independent learning strategies [58]. Teachers, therefore, need to understand the various levels of expertise and create curricula that allow students to achieve the required levels [59]. Medical education is still rigidly proscribed in terms of its length, but the emergence of models based on demonstrable milestones challenges the notion that all students need to be educated for the same amount of time and in lockstep [60]. Resource constraints in the past necessitated one-room school houses, where children of all ages learnt together, requiring self-directed independent learning, tailoring of materials to the individual students and allowing advancement beyond one's years.

  It is interesting that the lessons learned and methods used in that historical context are now being used to design more seamless and continuous educational experiences with or without modern technology [61]. It will require increased flexibility by regulators and accrediting agencies, but if outcomes-based education is truly a goal, processes will need to be able to be tailored to local requirements.

- *Technology.* Not only do present-day students use technology every day and most often, more expertly than their teachers, the millennial learners or "selfie generation" also require different pedagogical approaches [62]. The ability to search and find information in a fraction of a second; to have access to the information of portable devices anywhere there is cell phone service; to be able to communicate with almost anyone anywhere at any time; to share information across the world; to collaborate online and asynchronously; to crowd source solutions; to monitor distant sites; to create virtual patients; to be able to train on simulators; and many more technological advances have created a set of possible educational tools that are yet to be fully utilized in medical education. There are increasing calls to "reimagine" medical education [63, 64]. These articles suggest techniques like "flipped classrooms", massive open online courses (MOOCs) and digital badges. The new technologies are presently evaluated, and the results are not conclusive [65], but many experts maintain that "disruptive changes" will come to education, regardless of the subject or profession [66]. A comprehensive discussion of educational technology and its use is beyond the scope of this chapter, but one of the advantages touted for educational technologies is their ability to create personalized learning experiences. They could therefore be major tools in solving the "One Size Does Not Fit All" issue.

In the end, comprehensive and relevant systems of *assessment* of student achievement, and program, curriculum and institutional *evaluation* will tell whether the academic planning was successful. If different outcomes are desired, then assessment needs to be different as well. Traditional metrics of success for medical education may also not be appropriate for unique and special programs [37].

Resources – What Can Really Be Done? Much of the early planning in phase 1 creates ideal solutions, which are often not realistic based on the available resources. Academic planning, at every stage, needs to take into account the existing resource constraints, which by necessity lead to different solutions. Business planning needs to accompany academic planning to assure the feasibility of the project. Resources that may vary widely, include:

- Human resources:
  - *Faculty:* The availability of quality suitable faculty varies widely, and recruitment may be difficult, requiring innovative incentives, structures and faculty development programs, especially for unusual programs and locations. The number and types of faculty being able to be recruited will influence the types of programs that can be delivered and the teaching methods.
  - *Staff:* Similarly, support staff may be difficult to obtain, especially if novel untried technologies are being used.
  - *Patients:* The types of patients and their diseases and demographics will determine what can be taught in a patient setting, and what may have to be supplemented by using virtual patients, standardized patients or affiliations with other institutions.
  - *Students:* Students may be difficult to attract to certain programs or locations, and the school should understand the market, which in many countries includes the students' parents. Certain professions may not be attractive to students and their parents due to local culture and economics, and schools will need to develop specific marketing and retention strategies for such programs.

- *Facilities:* The need for adequate infrastructure was briefly discussed above. Simulation and clinical skills laboratories, for instance require the appropriate infrastructures, as does small group teaching.
- *Technology:* There needs to be a clear understanding of the types of technology that will be useful and cost-effective for the planned programs. While technologies require initial investments, they can provide cost savings and efficiencies by decreasing the need for space (virtual library, virtual labs [67], etc.), personnel and materials if used appropriately. It is important that faculty and students alike understand how to use the technology and accept its use, in order to assure its successful implementation.
- *Funding:* Planners should have a solid understanding of the costs of the various options when discussing the academic programs, and check at multiple steps of the planning, whether the programs as envisioned are still feasible.
- *Affiliations:* Collaborations with other institutions, such as sharing of standardized patients, online learning programs [63], clinical facilities, teaching space, laboratories, faculty, teaching resources, administrative systems, library resources, etc. can all enrich the programs while helping to save money, time and efforts.

Knowing the available resources at the beginning of the planning process is crucial, as it provides a realistic basis for academic and business plans and can lead to creative solutions.

Phase 3: Is the Program Sustainable? – How to Stay Alive and Grow

Being sustainable means not preserving the status quo, but to create a robust governance and monitoring system that constantly evaluates and reevaluates the alignment of the program or institution with the changing needs and values of its stakeholders and the society it serves. Having a clear specific definition of what constitutes success from the beginning, is an absolute must to set the stage for this phase.

Principles of quality management apply to education as much as they do to other industries [68] and they have been applied successfully in multiple settings [69-72]. In this context, accreditation requirements should be seen as a bare minimum that allows the school to operate and achieve its goals. Accreditation and regulations may actually be a barrier to the creation of novel programs and institutions [27]. The regulators are therefore important stakeholders in the process of designing unique and suitable programs and schools, and need to be engaged form the beginning. Questions that schools should ask themselves, and for which they should collect the appropriate data, may include:

- Have our programs had the desired impact for society, students and faculty?
- Have the stakeholders changed or are there new stakeholders and rules?
- How have the needs and the environment changed requiring changes in programs/ processes or new programs/processes?
- Is the institution meeting its mission and business goals, while continuing to innovate?
- Is the institutional culture still supportive of its mission?

- Do the institutional governance structures, processes and policies still support its function?
- Does the curriculum continue to evolve, support the mission and adapt to the changing environment?
- Are faculty members thriving and growing intellectually and professionally, including in their educational and institutional roles and responsibilities?
- Are students successful and content in their careers, and are they making the impact in the healthcare system that aligns with the school's mission? Are they contributing to the intellectual life and culture of the organization?
- Are infrastructure and technology up-to-date to support changes and new needs?
- Are resources adequate to affect the changes and support operations and needed investments?
- What is the corporate identify and the reputation of the program/school?

Each item will be answered quite specifically for differing schools based on their specific purpose and mission. It is also clear that the above list goes much beyond the usual list of success metrics, which focus on ranking, graduation rates, test scores, publications, etc., all of which are important, but not sufficient to shape an ongoing and meaningful strategy [37].

CONCLUSION

Healthcare systems, healthcare delivery, patients, diseases, technology and the roles of healthcare professionals are all changing. While many issues may be global, solutions need to be specific to serve the local needs and culture, while meeting international standards.

Just as the need to have disease management guidelines does not eliminate the tailoring of care to individual patients and their circumstances, a global approach to the development of standards and guidelines [73], while necessary, does not mean that schools and programs will not need to have the flexibility and opportunity to create specific programs for their students and society.

Ultimately, medical education needs to be aligned with the overall development of the healthcare workforce. It is increasingly clear that approaches and strategies for healthcare delivery require very specific solutions, such that models that are successful in one part of a country may not work at all in another part of the same country [74].

Figure 6 tries to illustrate that the needs determine the workforce for the various levels of care provision and across the system, which in turn translate into programs of various lengths, taught at various levels.

Medical education moving forward will need to develop development models that create physicians that can serve their constituents, while fitting into the ever evolving healthcare workforce, and "One Size Fits All" will not be an acceptable solution.

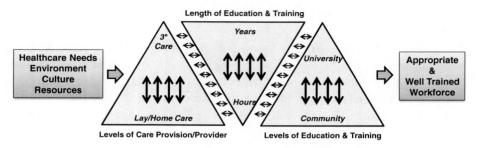

Figure 6. Model of education and training for a workforce that fits its environment[5].

REFERENCES

[1]   Kudlien, F. Medical education in classical antiquity. In: C. D. O'Malley (ed.) *The History of Medical Education.* UCLA Forum in Medical Sciences, Number 12. Berkeley: University of California Press; 1970; 3-37.

[2]   Talbot, C. Medical Education in the Middle Ages. In: O'Malley, C. D. (Ed.). *The History of Medical Education.* U.C.L.A. Forum in Medical Sciences No. 12. Berkeley: University of California Press; 1970; 73-87.

[3]   Papa, F. J., Harasym, P. H. Medical curriculum reform in North America, 1765 to the present: a cognitive science perspective. *Academic Medicine,* 1999, 74, 154-164.

[4]   Hamarneh, S. 1970. Medical Education and Practice in Medieval Islam. In: O'Malley, C. D. (Ed.). *The History of Medical Education.* U.C.L.A. Forum in Medical Sciences No. 12. Berkeley: University of California Press; 1970; 39-71.

[5]   Flexner, A. *Medical education in the United States and Canada: a report to the Carnegie Foundation for the Advancement of Teaching.* New York: Carnegie Foundation for the Advancement of Teaching; 1910; Bulletin No. 4.

[6]   Hostetter, M., Klein, S. In Focus: Modernizing medical education to advance new care models and foster continuous quality improvement. [online] *Quality Matters. Innovations in Health Care Quality Improvement,* April/May 2014, The Commonwealth Fund, [cited 2014 April 23] Available from: http://www. commonwealthfund.org/publications/newsletters/quality-matters/2014/april-may.

[7]   Flexner, A. *Medical Education: a Comparative Study.* New York, NY: MacMillan; 1925.

[8]   Frenk, J., Chen, L., Bhutta, Z. A., et al., Health professionals for a new century: transforming education to strengthen health systems in an interdependent world. *Lancet,* 2010, 376, 1923-1958.

[9]   Aretz, H. T. Some thoughts about creating healthcare professionals that match what societies need. *Medical Teacher,* 2011, 33, 608-613.

[10] WHO. Health Impact Assessment. *The Determinants of Health [online].* [cited 2014 May 27] Available at: http://www.who.int/hia/evidence/doh/en/

---

[5] The figure is adapted and modified from Mehta, M. C., Daly, I. E., Aretz, H. T., McCarthy, E. J., Mudge, G. H. Healthcare in the high growth emerging markets and developing economies: a rapidly transforming landscape. Periodical of the Hitachi Research Institute, Tokyo, Japan; 2014, 9(1), 24-35.

[11] Bachrach, D., Pfister, H., Wallis, K., Lipson, M., Manatt Health Solutions. Addressing patients' social needs: an emerging business case for provider investment [online]. *The Commonwealth Fund, May 29, 2014.* [cited 2014 May 29]. Available at: http://www. commonwealthfund.org/publications/fund-reports/2014/may/addressing-patients-social-needs?omnicid=EALERT480081andmid=taretz@phmi.partners.org.

[12] Rickets, T. C., Fraher, E. P. Reconfiguring healthcare workforce policy so that education, training, and actual delivery of care are closely connected. *Health Affairs* 2013, 32, 1874-1880.

[13] Rao, G. N., Khanna, R. C., Athota, S. M., Rajshekar, V., Rani, P. K. Integrated model of primary and secondary eye care for underserved rural areas: The L V Prasad Eye Institute experience. *Indian J. Ophthalmol.* 2012, 60, 396-400.

[14] Nancarrow, S. A., Borthwick, A. M. Dynamic professional boundaries in the healthcare workforce. *Sociology of Health and Illness* 2005 ISSN 0141-9889, pp. 897-919 [cited 2013 June 15]. Available at: http://onlinelibrary.wiley.com/doi/10.1111/j.1467-9566. 2005.00463.x/pdf.

[15] Triplett, J. E. *Output and productivity measures for medical care and education.* [Online] Brookings Institution; 15 September 2009; [cited 2014 May 20] Available at: http://www.brookings.edu/~/media/research/files/papers/2009/4/medical%20measures %20triplett/04_medical_measures_triplett.pdf.

[16] Green, L. A., Fryer, G. E. Jr, Yawn, B. P., Lanier, D., Dovey, S. M. The ecology of medical care revisited. *N. Engl. J. Med.* 2001, 344, 2021-2025.

[17] Accreditation Council for Graduate Medical Education. *ACGME Common Program Requirements [online].* [cited 2014 May 12] Avalable at: http://www.acgme.org/ acgmeweb/Portals/0/PFAssets/ProgramRequirements/CPRs2013.pdf.

[18] Nutting, P. A., Crabtree, B. F., Miller, W. L., Stange, K. C., Stewart, E., Jaén, C. Transforming physician practices to patient-centered medical homes: lessons from the national demonstration project. *Health Affairs* 2011, 30, 439-445.

[19] Porter, M. E. What is value in health care? *N. Engl. J. Med.* 2010, 363, 2477-2481.

[20] Institute of Medicine. *Performance measurement: accelerating improvement.* Washington, DC: National Academies Press; 2006.

[21] Emanuel, E. J., Fuchs, V. R. Shortening medical training by 30%. *JAMA* 2012, 307, 1143-1144.

[22] Boodman, S. G. Should medical school be shortened to three years? Some programs try fast tracking [online]. *Washington Post,* January 13, 2014. [cited 2014 May 21] Available at: http://www.washingtonpost.com/national/health-science/medical-school-done-faster/2014/01/13/4b6d9e54-5c40-11e3-be07-006c776266ed_story.html.

[23] Goldfarb, S., Morrison, G. The 3-year medical school - change or shortchange? *N. Engl. J. Med.* 2013, 369, 1087-1089.

[24] Dornan, T., Littlewood, S., Margolis, S. A., Scherpbier, A., Spencer, J., Ypinazar, V. How can experience in clinical and community settings contribute to early medical education? A BEME systematic review. *Medical Teacher,* 2006, 28, 3-18.

[25] Rabinowitz, H. K., Diamond, J. J., Markham, F. W., Wortman, J. R. Medical school programs to increase the rural physician supply: a systematic review and projected impact of widespread replication. *Academic Medicine,* 2008, 83, 235-243.

[26] Eley, D., Baker, P. Does recruitment lead to retention? Rural clinical school training experiences and subsequent intern choices. *Rural Remote Health,* 2006, Jan.-Mar.; 6(1), 511; Epub. 2006 Feb. 3.

[27] Hurt, M. M., Harris, J. O. Founding a new college of medicine at Florida State University. *Academic Medicine,* 2005, 80, 973-979.

[28] *Home page of the Asklepios Campus Hamburg.* [cited 2013 June 15] Available at: http://www.asklepios.com/ams_Unsere_Klinik.Asklepios?ActiveID=3503.

[29] *Home page of the Ochsner-Queensland Clinical School.* [cited 2013 June 15] Available at: http://academics.ochsner.org/queensland.aspx.

[30] *Home pages of the Joint Medical Program on University of Newcastle and University of New England websites* [cited 2013 June 15] Available at: http://www.newcastle.edu. au/joint-medical-program; http://www.une.edu.au/about-une/academic-schools/school-of-rural-medicine/about-us.

[31] *Home page of the Cleveland Clinic Lerner College of Medicine of Case Western Reserve University.* [cited 2014 May 21] Available at: http://portals.clevelandclinic. org/cclcm/CollegeHome/tabid/7343/Default.aspx.

[32] Josiah Macy Foundation. Transforming patient care: aligning interprofessional education with clinical practice redesign. *Conference Recommendations, January 17-20, 2013, Atlanta Georgia [online].* [cited 2013 May 15]. Available at: http://macy foundation.org/publications/publication/aligning-interprofessional-education.

[33] Pelling, S., Kalen, A., Hammar, M., Wahlström, O. Preparation for becoming members of health care teams: findings from a 5-year evaluation of a student interprofessional training ward. *Journal of Interprofessional Care,* 2011, 25, 328-332.

[34] Interprofessional Education Collaborative Expert Panel. *Core Competencies for Interprofessional Collaborative Practice: Report of an Expert Panel.* Washington, DC: Interprofessional Education Collaborative; 2011.

[35] Gilbert, J. H. Interprofessional learning and higher education structural barriers. *Journal of Interprofessional Care,* May 2005, Supplement 1, 87-106.

[36] Mies van der Rohe, L. *Speech to architecture students.* Armour Institute, Chicago 1938. [Online]. [Cited 2012 June 27] Available at: http://www.scribd.com/doc/91739267/ Mies-speech-to-architecture-students-IIT-1938.

[37] Aretz, H. T., Armstrong, E. L. Undergraduate Education. In: Walsh, K. (ed.) *The Oxford Textbook of Medical Education.* Oxford University Press, Oxford, UK; 2013; 325-339.

[38] Bass, E. B. Step 1: Problem Identification and General Needs Assessment. In: Kern, D. E., Thomas, P. A., Hughes, M. Y. (Editors). *Curriculum Development for Medical Education. A Six-Step Approach.* (Second edition). Baltimore: The Johns Hopkins Press; 2009; pp. 10-26.

[39] Hughes, M. T. Step 2: Targeted Needs Assessment. In: Kern, D. E., Thomas, P. A., Hughes, M. Y. (editors). *Curriculum Development for Medical Education. A Six-Step Approach.* (Second edition). Baltimore: The Johns Hopkins Press; 2009; pp. 27-42.

[40] Boggis, P., Trafford, D. How operating principles can make strategies meaningful. [Online] *Formicio Insight September 2013* [cited 2014 May 25]. Available at: http:// formicio.com/wp-content/uploads/2013/08/Formicio-Insight-Article_How-Operating-Principles-Can-Make-Strategy-Meaningful.pdf.

[41] Hayes, R. H., Wheelwright, S. C., Clark, K. B. *Dynamic Manufacturing*. New York: The Free Press, 1988, p. 279.

[42] Clark, K. B., Wheelwright, S. C. Organizing and leading "heavyweight" development teams. *California Management Review,* Spring 1992, 9-28.

[43] Biggs, J. S., Wells, R. W. The social mission of Australian medical schools in a time of expansion. *Australian Health Review,* 2011, 35, 424-429.

[44] Gano-Phillips, S., Barnett, R. W. Against all odds. Transforming institutional culture. *Liberal Education*, Spring 2008, 36-41 [cited 2014 May 21]. Available at: http://www. uwosh.edu/grants/cetl/archive/general-education-best-practice-resources/documents/ Against-All-Odds-Transforming-Institutional-Culture.pdf.

[45] Committee on the Health Professions Education Summit. Greiner, A. C., Knebel, E. (Editors). Institute of Medicine of the National Academies. *Health Profession Education: A Bridge to Quality.* Washington, DC: The National Academies Press; 2003.

[46] Core Committee, Institute for International Medical Education. *Global minimum essential requirements in medical education [Online].* Institute for International Medical Education, White Plains, New York, US. [cited 2014 May 11], Available at: http://www.iime.org/documents/gmer.htm.

[47] Pruitt, S. D., Epping-Jordan, J., Preparing the 21st century global healthcare workforce. *BMJ* 2005, 330, 637-639.

[48] *Mercer University School of Medicine.* [Online] 2002, [Cited 2012 May 17] Available at: http://medicine.mercer.edu/about/mission/

[49] Mercer University School of Medicine. *Medical Student handbook 2011-2012*, pp. 52-55. [Online] [Cited 2012 May 17] Available at: http://medicine.mercer.edu/mu-medicine/academics/catalogs/upload/studenthandbook.pdf.

[50] Moore, D. E., Green, J. S., Gallis, H. A. Achieving desired results and improved outcomes: integrating planning and assessment throughout learning activities. *J. Contin. Educ. Health Prof.*, 2009, 29 (1), 1-15.

[51] WFME Global Standards for Quality Improvement in Medical Education. European Specifications. [Online]. *Medine – The Thematic Network on Medical Education in Europe. 2007* [cited 2014 January 12]. Available at: http://www.amse-med.eu/files/ europeanspecifications.pdf.

[52] Sparrow, B., Liu, J., Wener, D. M. Google effects on memory: cognitive consequences of having information at our fingertips. [Online] *Sciencexpress*; 14 July 2011, 10.1126/ science.1207745, pp. 1-4 [cited 2011 July 22] Available at: http://www.sciencemag. org/content/333/6043/776.abstract.

[53] Shaw, T., Long, A., Chopra, S., Kerfoot, B. P. Impact on clinical behavior of face-to-face continuing medical education blended with online spaced education: a randomized trial. *J. Cont. Educ. Health Professions,* 2011, 31, 103-108.

[54] Friedlander, M. J., Andrews, L., Armstrong, E. G., et al. What can medical education learn from the neurobiology of learning? *Academic Medicine,* 2011, 86, 415-420.

[55] Wetzel, M., Reid, L. *The multistation exercise: accessible, adaptable active-learning.* Presented at the Association of American Medical Colleges National Meeting; 1991; Washington, DC.

[56] Zimmerman, R. K. *Facilitator's guide to the multistation clinical teaching scenarios (MCTS) method and the TIME project.* [online] Centers for Disease Control and

Prevention. 20 June 2008 [cited 2014 June 2]. Available at: http://stacks.cdc.gov/view/cdc/23159.

[57] Bowe, C. M., Voss, J., Aretz, H. T. Case method teaching: An effective approach to integrate the basic and clinical sciences in the preclinical medical curriculum. *Medical Teacher,* 2009, 31, 834-841.

[58] Ten Cate, O., Snell, L., Mann, K., Vermunt, J. Orienting teaching toward the learning process. *Academic Medicine* 2004, 79, 219-228.

[59] Weber, R. A., Aretz, H. T. Climbing the ladder from novice to expert plastic surgeon. *Plast. Reconstr. Surg.,* 2012, 129, 1191-1197.

[60] Sullivan, G., Simpson, D., Cooney, T., Beresin, E. A milestone in the milestones movement: the JGME Milestones Supplement. *J. Graduate Med. Educ.* 2013, 5 (1), 1-4 Available at: http://www.jgme.org/doi/pdf/10.4300/JGME-05-01s1-08.

[61] Furman, R. Reinventing the one-room schoolhouse. [Online] *Huffington Post,* 6 January 2014, updated 8 March 2014. [cited 2014 June 2]; Available at: http://www.huffingtonpost.com/rob-furman/reinventing-the-one-room-_b_4545983.html.

[62] Barrett, D. A curriculum for the selfie generation. *The Chronicle of Higher Education.* [online], 2 June 2014 [cited 2014 June 2] Available at: http://chronicle.com/article/A-Curriculum-for-the-Selfie/146873/

[63] Prober, C. G., Khan, S. Medical education reimagined: a call to action. *Academic Medicine,* 2013, 88, 1407-1410.

[64] Mehta, N. B., Hull, A. L., Young, J. B., Stoller, J. K. Just imagine: new paradigms for medical education. *Academic Medicine,* 2013, 88, 1418-1423.

[65] Ho, A. D., Reich, J., Nesterko, S. O., et al. Harvard X and MITx: the first year of open courses, fall 2013 - summer 2013. *Social Science Research Network* [Online] 21 January 2014. [cited 2014 June 2] Available at: http://papers.ssrn.com/sol3/papers.cfm?abstract_id=2381263.

[66] Useem, J. Business School, disrupted. *New York Times,* 1 June 2014. [cited 2 June 2014] Available at: http://www.nytimes.com/2014/06/01/business/business-school-disrupted.html?_r=2.

[67] Waldrop, M. M. The virtual lab. *Nature,* 2013, 499, 268-270.

[68] Sallie, E. *Total Quality Management in Education.* (Third Edition), London, UK: Kogan Press; 2002.

[69] Armstrong, E. G., Mackey, M., Spear, S. Medical education as a process management problem. *Academic Medicine,* 2004, 79, 721-728.

[70] Dalt, L. D., Callegaro, S., Mazzi, A., et al. A model of quality assurance and quality improvement for post-graduate medical education in Europe. *Medical Teacher* 2010, 32, e57-e64.

[71] Goldman, E. F., Swayze, S. S., Swinehart, S. E., Schroth, W. S. Effecting curricular change through comprehensive course assessment: using structure and process to change outcomes. *Academic Medicine ,* 2012, 87, 300-7.

[72] Stratton, T. D., Rudy, D. W., Sauer, M. J., Perman, J. A., Jennings, C. D. Lessons from industry: one school's transformation toward "lean" curricular governance. *Academic Medicine,* 2007, 82, 331-40.

[73] World Federation for Medical Education. *Standards.* [Online] [cited 2014 June 2] Available at: http://www.wfme.org/standards.

[74] Loewenberg, S. *Mumbai: learning form failure.* [Online] Pulitzer Center on Crisis Reporting, 5 February 2013; [cited 2013 May 2] Available at: http://pulitzercenter. org/reporting/urban-health-development-maternal-newborn-aid-development-india-research.

In: Health and Disease   ISBN: 978-1-63463-052-8
Editor: Paul Ganguly   © 2015 Nova Science Publishers, Inc.

Chapter 4

INTEGRATION IS THE KEY

Sabri Kemahli [*]

Professor of Pediatrics (Pediatric Hematology),
Alfaisal University, Riyadh, Kingdom of Saudi Arabia

ABSTRACT

Integration is one of the six principles of medical education that are summarised with the acronym 'SPICES' (student-centred, problem-based, integrated, community-based, electives and systematic) and probably is the most important of them. Many developments and changes have taken place in medical education since the beginning of 20th century and the majority of these changes are aimed to achieve a full integration. Integration can simply be classified as horizontal and vertical. Another classification is based on the 11 steps described by Ronald Harden, where each further step aims for more integrated learning. Although most of the integration focuses on the first 2-3 years of medical curriculum, integration in clinical clerkships should not be neglected. It is a well-known fact that there are always differences between planned, implemented and received (or learned) curricula; and a good assessment system is a must to achieve the desired outcomes. Therefore integration of assessment is another dimension of integration that should always be taken into account.

INTRODUCTION

Integration is perhaps the most important concept that has to be achieved in medical education. When we review the history of medical education we can see that it is in fact a history of integration. Successive steps of development have all been aimed to ensure better and more meaningful integration to help the students see the big picture rather than the details of each individual discipline.

It is sometimes argued that any education system can produce good doctors and those trained in traditional style are given as examples. It is true that the success of individuals rely

---

[*] Corresponding author: E mail address: skemahli@alfaisal.edu.

on their personal motivation and self-study. Various strategies help to motivate students to study more and in a more meaningful way. Studying the connections between different disciplines and relevance of each other is the ultimate aim. It is a well-known fact that knowledge is gained and retained if acquired and organized in a meaningful context. Integration and integrated curricula help the students to achieve this concept. On the other hand the exponential increase in the body of knowledge to be covered during a limited time necessitates more productive strategies. It is impossible to deliver all required content in 4 or 6 years of medical education by traditional methods and strategies. Thus new methods and strategies are continuously being developed.

History

How Did Our Current Concept of Integration Develop over Time?

Medical school curricula started as apprenticeship model from early ages. As there have been advances in the medical sciences the necessity has risen that the students should be exposed to various clinical disciplines. This trend has started earlier in Europe than North America. In the late 19th century most medical schools in Europe had discipline-based curricula but the disciplines involved were mostly clinical ones. Basic sciences received little attention during this time and the emphasis was on content deemed to have practical, clinical value. The first year was followed by one- to three-year apprenticeship near a private practitioner. Anatomy and physiology were taught in the first year(s) of the training, which were followed by exposure to clinical areas of internal medicine, surgery, obstetrics-gynaecology and paediatrics. In North America the curriculum consisted of a total of 500 hours of lectures in anatomy, physiology, pathology, chemistry, surgery, medicine, pharmacology, obstetrics-gynaecology and paediatrics in one semester, which were repeated in the second semester [1, 2]. During those years many students travelled to European countries, mostly to England, France and Germany, to study medicine and have later tried to implement a similar system in USA [3]. Flexner report in 1910 has changed the medical education in North America with solid recommendations to have 2 years of basic science and 2 years of clinical science training. This curriculum structure was later adopted by all North American medical schools. This has resulted in more structured discipline-based curricula in medical schools that survived after Flexner report. [1, 4]

In discipline-based curricula the students are expected to integrate the acquired knowledge after finishing all courses. As there is no planned connection and no relevance is sought between two or more disciplines the knowledge acquired remains to be isolated. It is evident that learning the function (physiology) of any system is very difficult (almost impossible) without having a sound knowledge about the structure (anatomy and histology). Another problem caused by this structure was that students were expected to remember and apply all these facts by the time they started clinical clerkships. This system was criticised for exposing the students to subjects that were "unnecessarily disjointed, repetitive and undesirable for this level of details" [1, 5]. In order to address this problem a new curriculum structure was suggested.

The first effort for integration was to teach all relevant topics of an organ-system during the same time period. This 'temporal coordination' was perhaps one of the first implemented types of integration. Although discipline-based structure continued the sequence of topics was planned and coordinated in such a way that all disciplines covered the same organ-system simultaneously.

It was only in 1950s that 'integration' was mentioned for the first time. This was later called 'organ-system based integration' and it continues to be the most widely used integration [1]. Departmental barriers were removed and all curricular content was overseen by "topic committees" with representatives from relevant departments.

Organ-system based integration is based on the principle that the structure and function is best understood when learned simultaneously. It first started at Western Reserve School of Medicine. However each topic was still presented separately and thus the information was perceived as disjointed. Despite being a major change, organ-system-based model had some problems: the "integrated" curriculum did not necessarily lead to integration within learners' minds and it did not enable the students to do differential diagnosis. The main reason for these seemed to be due to the fact that the information was not delivered in a clinical context. It is a well-known educational and cognitive science principle that the knowledge is best acquired and retained if learned, practiced and assessed in the context in which it will be used [4]. However organ-system-based model with no or little clinical content failed to achieve this. This problem was partly corrected by creation of basic science groups for team-teaching of certain topics. Later clinical case encounters (clinical correlates) were introduced to show the clinical relevance of basic science topics [1].

There were further trials to find ways to integrate, not only among the courses during a single year but also among courses and phases that were traditionally delivered in different years and among different areas such as behaviour, ethics, society. So the idea of 'vertical integration' rose. How could this be achieved? The students were studying the basic science concepts and disciplines during the first 2-3 years of medical schools with no or little clinical knowledge and no relevance being sought. The challenge was to teach basic sciences in a relevant clinical context. This has led to the 'revolution' of problem-based learning (PBL). The ultimate goal was to teach basic science with relevance to clinical, behavioural, societal, ethical issues. Structure, function and clinical problems had to be perceived in a holistic way. With this holistic approach patients are seen as individuals with social environment, behavioural and mental issues, not as organ systems only. This approach is in line with the definition of health according to World Health Organization, which states: "Health is a state of complete physical, mental and social well-being and not merely the absence of disease or infirmity". (http://www.who.int/about/definition/en/print.html)

In PBL the students are presented with a problem that they try to solve by group work and self-study. The learners are expected to recognize their knowledge deficits and study these in turn. By synthesizing their previous knowledge, presented patient information and newly acquired knowledge they proceed to solve the problem and eventually learn the required pre-defined objectives. The cases may lead to learning objectives in various areas such as clinical, basic, behavioural sciences, ethics, public health or societal issues [6]. The clinical problems presented are actually learning opportunities to integrate basic and clinical sciences in a meaningful context. As it has been put by Neufeld and Barrows "*since the problems encountered in medicine are primarily those of individual patients most problem situations presented to the student relate to an individual case*" [6]. Scenarios that address problems in a society (such as an epidemic), groups or sometimes families (diseases of different family members and/or interpersonal relationships) are also used. It was soon appreciated that despite all these developments the students still were experiencing difficulty in performing clinical work during clinical clerkships. In order to understand the meaning of clinical information the learners needed to start practicing on patients earlier. However it was not until 1980s that structured clinical skills training started for undergraduate medical students. Training for clinical skills was later seen as an integral part of the first years of medical education. Early clinical exposure included clinical information with relevant basic sciences and clinical skills training. This approach has helped the students appreciate different aspects of medical sciences and clinical practice and prepared them for clinical clerkships. Increased motivation has been another gain from these sessions. Thus students started clinical clerkships with clinical skills they needed and some clinical knowledge.

Medical education necessitates the acquisition of knowledge, skills and attitudes by prospective physicians in a limited time frame. So the specifications of the graduates had to be clearly defined. The "end product" had to be specified in order to define what has to be learned/taught. At this stage the "outcomes" were defined and medical education reached a new phase: outcome-based education [7]. General competencies and outcomes are defined at different levels in a number of documents, such as Scottish Doctor, Tomorrow's Doctors, CanMeds, MEDINE and WFME standards [8-12]. So medical education is now shaped as based on the expected outcomes and this has necessitated integrated learning starting from day 1 of medical training.

In summary, medical education evolved from an apprenticeship and clinical-practice-only model to a structured model defining clear lines between basic and clinical sciences that were later replaced by organ-system-based integration. The following phase has been integration of knowledge and clinical skills in a meaningful manner starting on individual cases as in PBL curricula. This was followed by the era of outcome-based education.

Many Facets of Integration

Is There Only One Type or Way of Integration?

Although we are talking of integration as a single concept there are many different ways and types of integration.

Integration can be classified as horizontal and vertical in the simplest way. When courses in the same phase or year are coordinated or integrated it is called horizontal integration. There is however a strict boundary between pre-clinical or basic science and clinical years. Vertical integration, on the other hand, means integrating courses and themes across years and phases. In other words, addressing and learning basic sciences and relevant clinical topics at the same time period means vertical integration. Vertical integration has also changed the traditional two separate phases of basic science-clinical years divide. Clinical content starts from the first year and gradually increases reaching a maximum in clinical clerkships phase. Similarly basic science content decreases over the course of years but never drops to zero. This can be illustrated as a transition from an H-shaped curriculum where basic science and clinical phases are strictly separated, to a Z-shape where basic sciences decrease and clinical sciences increase over time. However neither is zero at any time (Figure 1).

Harden has described various integration models as a road from a completely disintegrated curriculum to fully integrated programmes in 11 steps [7]:

- **Isolation** – Each department prepares its own syllabus on its own with no reference to other disciplines
- **Awareness**- Each department plans its own programme but they are aware of what is being covered by other departments
- **Harmonization** – Departments consult and communicate about their individual courses
- **Nesting** – Content from another course is inserted to enrich the teaching.
- **Temporal co-ordination** – Discipline-based teaching where related or similar topics within the subjects are scheduled at the same time. Most programmes called as "integrated teaching" are often temporally coordinated programmes.
- **Sharing**- Two departments agree to plan and implement a programme jointly.
- **Correlation**- While the emphasis remains on subject-based teaching some integrated sessions correlating different disciplines take place.
- **Complementary**- There are integrated and subject-based teaching sessions. Integrated sessions run over a topic or a theme, to which relevant disciplines contribute, but there are some subject-based teaching sessions too.
- **Multi-disciplinary**- A number of disciplines are brought together with themes, problems, topics or issues as the focus for the learning. The theme transcends subject boundaries but disciplines preserve their identity with the theme seen through the lens of each one of them. Each department contributes to the theme by its own view.
- **Inter-disciplinary**-There is a further shift to emphasise the themes and there is usually no reference to individual disciplines. Disciplines are not identified as departments in the timetable.
- **Trans-disciplinary**-Here the curriculum transcends individual disciplines as in the previous step. The focus however is on real-world situations, not on themes. Students work on real patients' problems or tasks not necessarily being attached to certain clinical departments.

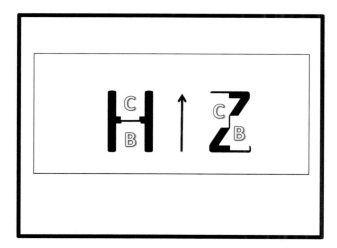

Figure 1. H-shaped curriculum with distinct divide between basic science (B) and clinical clerkship (C) phases and Z-shaped curriculum where basic and clinical sciences co-exist from the beginning till the end.

As one moves up the ladder, there is less emphasis on the role of disciplines, an increasing requirement for a central curriculum, organizational structure and a requirement for greater participation by staff in curriculum discussions and planning. There is increased coordination and collaboration between departments at every further step compared with the previous one [7].

Integration and Teaching/Learning Strategies

Are Learning Methods and Strategies Important to Achieve Integration?

It is evident from the preceding discussion that as curricula evolved from discipline-based to integrated types changes and innovations in the teaching and learning strategies and methods were inevitable. It was impossible to deliver curricula, that no longer evolve around disciplines but themes, by traditional lectures only. Teaching in large groups or lectures has been enriched by interactive techniques. PBL is a revolutionary strategy by itself and is a perfect tool for integrated learning. Team-based learning is another interactive educational strategy used in larger groups. Task-based learning is being used as a tool for integrated learning in real-life situations, i.e. for trans-disciplinary integrated programmes. Thus progress towards integrated curricula also defined the way it is delivered. With time, even more traditional or discipline-based programmes started using these interactive techniques. While PBL curricula had started as pure-PBL, with no lectures, by time there was a change to hybrid curricula, where PBL is enriched with lectures and other activities.

Using multiple modes of teaching/learning methods is an important requisite of an integrated curriculum. While lectures, PBL, team-based- and task-based-learning, various small group techniques are being used, the ever increasing usage of internet- and computer-based learning/teaching methods constitute another important mode of information transfer. It should always be kept in mind that the learning objectives of all these different modes of learning and teaching should not overlap but instead complement each other. For example learning objectives of PBL and lectures should not be the same, otherwise the interest in one of these will fade away.

Outcomes and Integration

What Is the Relevance between Outcomes, Outcome-Based Learning and Integration?

Medical education has reached a new stage by defining learning outcomes and has emphasised importance of integration more clearly. Since basic sciences, clinical sciences, clinical experiences, social and behavioural aspects, as well as ethical issues have interactions with each other "holistic approach" is perhaps another key word for this new era.

Any of the learning outcomes necessitates knowledge and skills that encompass different disciplines, ranging from normal structure and function, disorders of structure and the mechanisms that lead to disease and clinical manifestations, social implications and ethical and even economic issues. The learning outcome of "planning the management of diseases" can be given as an example. In order to manage a disease, such as an HIV infection, oneshould have the knowledge about immune system (structure, physiology, immunological

be a discipline-based learning, although the curriculum or the programme was intended to be an integrated one.

The best way to overcome this obstacle and ensure integration in assessment and evaluation is having groups of teachers (faculty members) to come together and write integrated questions. It is not an easy task, especially in medical school where most faculty members are trained in a traditional way. However faculty development activities focusing on integrated assessment can help.

Planning for an integrated course or curriculum necessitates planning for an integrated assessment as well. It is always much easier for the content- or discipline-experts to write questions or OSCE/OSPE stations in a single discipline. In order to achieve integrated assessment, experts or faculty members from different areas should come together and plan an integrated assessment tool. Good integrated MCQs can be written in such a way that, for example, in order to answer a clinical question the student should have a good knowledge about the underlying pathophysiological mechanism or the mode of action of a drug. Integrated questions should be written in such a way that they should not point to a certain department as the origin. If questions can easily be recognized as by the origin of them (department, discipline) assessment is not integrated. OSPEs can be prepared in the same way, asking not only about an anatomical structure but the function of that structure and radiology as well [25]. OSCE stations should be designed that address not only certain physical examination skills but clinical reasoning, communication, professionalism and ethical approach as well. Even, concepts or knowledge addressed in separate sessions can be questioned in a single MCQ. Similar to using a multitude of methods in teaching and learning, use of multiple valid and reliable tools in assessment and evaluation is also a must.

SUMMARY

The developments in medical education have taken place due to the need of more integration among different disciplines and phases. Integration is an ever-evolving concept and it is never complete. Keeping in mind that there is never a complete overlap among planned, implemented and received curricula, complete integration can only be achieved if the students perceive it as integrated. In addition to vertical and horizontal integration we can add a third dimension as "integration in assessment". If the assessment supports and encourages integrated learning ideal integration is much easier to reach.

REFERENCES

[1] Papa, FJ; Harasym, PH. Medical curriculum reform in North America, 1765 to the present: A cognitive science perspective. *Academic Medicine*, 1999, 74, 154-164.

[2] Fulton, JF. History of medical education. *British Medical Journal*, 1953 Aug 289, 2(4834), 457-461.

[3] Baron, JH. American medical students in 19th century Europe. *The Mount Sinai Journal of Medicine*, 2005, 72, 270-273.

[4]   Cooke, M; Irby, DM; Sullivan, W; Ludmerer, KM. American medical education 100 years after Flexner report. *N Eng J Med*, 2006, 355 (13), 1339-1344.

[5]   Harden, RM: The integration ladder: a tool for curriculum planning and evaluation. *Medical Education*, 2000, 34, 551-557.

[6]   Neufeld, VR; Barrows, HS. The "McMaster Philosophy": An approach to medical education. *The Journal of Medical Education*, 1974, 49, 1040-1050.

[7]   Harden, RM. Learning outcomes and instructional objectives: is there a difference? *Medical Teacher*, 2002, 24, 151-155.

[8]   General Medical Council: Tomorrow's Doctors, 2009. http://www.gmc-uk.org/Tomorrow_s_Doctors_0414.pdf_48905759.pdf (accessed 19 June, 2014)

[9]   Scottish Doctor. http://www.scottishdoctor.org/ (accessed 19 June, 2014)

[10]   The CanMeds framework. http://www.royalcollege.ca/portal/page/portal/rc/canmeds/framework (accessed 19 June, 2014)

[11]   Cumming, A; Ross, M. On behalf of the Tuning Project (Medicine) Steering Group and Task Force 1 of the MEDINE Thematic Network.: Tuning : Competencies of European Medical Graduates. http://medine2.com/archive/medine1/docs/competences.pdf (accessed 19 June, 2014)

[12]   MEDINE: The Thematic Network on Medical Education in Europe. WFME Global Standards for Quality Improvement in Medical Education. European Specifications. http://www.wfme.org/standards/european-specifications (accessed 19 June, 2014)

[13]   Worley, P; Silagy, C; Prideaux, D; Newble, D; Jones, A. The parallel rural community curriculum: in integrated clinical curriculum based in rural general practice. *Medical Education*, 2000, 34, 558-565.

[14]   Ogur, B; Hirsh, D; Krupat, E; Bor, D. The Harvard Medical School-Cambridfge Integrated clerkship: an innovative model of clinical education. *Academic Medicine*, 2007, 82, 397-404.

[15]   Bell, SK; Krupat, E; Fazio, SB; Roberts, DH; Schwartzstein, RM. Longitudinal pedagogy: a successful response to the fragmentation of the third-year medical student clerkship experience. *Academic Medicine*, 2008, 83, 467-475.

[16]   Norris, TE; Schaad, DC; DeWitt, D; Ogur, B; Hunt, DD. Longitudinal integrated clerkships for medical students: an innovation adopted by medical schools in Australia, Canada, South Africa and the United States. *Academic Medicine*, 2009, 84, 902-907.

[17]   Poncelet, A; Bokser, S; Calton, B; Hauer, K; Kirsch, H; Jones, T; Lai, CJ; Mazotti, L; Shore, W; Teherani, A; Tong, L; Wamsley, M; Robertson, P. Development of a longitudinal integrated clerkship at an academic medical center. *Medical Education Online*, 2011, 16, 5939-DOI: 10, 3402/meo.v16i0.5939.

[18]   Dahle, LO; Brynhildsen, J; Behrbohm Fallsberg, M; Rundquist, I. Pros and cons of vertical integration between clinical medicine and basic science within a problem-based undergraduate medical curriculum: examples and experiences from Linköping, Sweden. *Medical Teacher*, 2002, 24, 280-285.

[19]   Richards, J; Schwartzstein, R; Irish, J; Almeida, J. Roberts. Clinical physiology grand rounds. *Clinical Teacher*, 2013, 10, 88-93. doi: 10.1111/j.1743-498X.2012.00614.x.

[20]   Abu-Hijleh, MF; Chakravarty, M; Al-Shboul, Q; Kasaab, S; Hamdy, H. Integrating applied anatomy in surgical clerkship in a problem-based learning curriculum. *Surg Radiol Anat*, 2005, 27, 152-157.

[21] Wendelberger, KJ; Burke, R; Haas, AL; Harenwattananon, M; Simpson, D. Identifying Opportunities for Vertical Integration of Biochemistry and Clinical Medicine. *Adv Health Sci Educ Theory Pract*, 1998, 3, 157-164

[22] Sakles, JC; Maldonado, RJ; Kumari, VG. Integration of basic sciences and clinical sciences in a clerkship: a pilot study. *JIAMSE*, 2006, 16, 4-9.

[23] Beech, DJ; Domer, FR. Utiity of case-method approach for the integration of clinical and basic science in surgical education. *Journal of Cancer Education*, 2002, 17(3), 161-164).

[24] O'Neill, PA. The role of basic sciences in a problem-based learning clinical curriculum. *Medical Education*, 2000, 34, 608-613.

[25] Yaqinuddin, A; Zafar, M; Ikram, MF. Ganguly: What is an objective structured practical examination in anatomy? *Anatomical Sciences Education.*, 2013, 6, 125-133.

In: Health and Disease

Editor: Paul Ganguly

ISBN: 978-1-63463-052-8

© 2015 Nova Science Publishers, Inc.

Chapter 5

CURRICULUM MAPPING IN THE DISEASE PATHWAY

Shabih H. Zaidi *

American University of Barbados, School of Medicine, Christchurch, Barbados

ABSTRACT

Curriculum is a dynamic exercise which lacks a precise definition. Perhaps it can be best described as a planned academic activity. In actual fact it is a sophisticated blend of the educational activity encompassing many items like, 'the course content, learning outcomes, educational experiences, educational environment, an individual students' learning style, personal timetable and programme of work' (AMEE Guide no. 21: 2001). It is a process which involves many steps; in fact six in all, which are generally considered to be almost gold standard (Grant, J. 2010). An important concept in the context of curriculum is that of curriculum mapping which, as the name indicates, plans out the academic activities related to the delivery of a curriculum.

INTRODUCTION

Syllabus is its main component. Teaching or instructional strategy is another; and then of course the all important element of assessment and evaluation, without which the process of education remains incomplete.

Modern medical education has benefitted a great deal through the efforts of general educationists such as Knowles, who developed the theories and principles of learning, and Bloom for his taxonomy based upon the detailed analysis of human mind, the cognitive and psychomotor domains etc.

Flexner was a pioneering educationist. He is credited with the development of the traditional curriculum. His immense knowledge of the process of teaching and learning made him the best choice in those early days by the Carnegie foundation to conduct research and design a curriculum. Obviously he did an excellent job in the light of Terms of Reference

---

* Corresponding author: Shabih H. Zaidi. E-mail address: shabih514@gmail.com, shzaidi@hotmail.co.uk.

given to him. He developed a curriculum which would serve a doctor in good stead in all and sundry circumstances that existed in the early days of the nineteenth century.

Much criticism has been directed towards the traditional curriculum by the modern educationists calling it an overloaded, overbearing, subject centred and out dated. Suffice it to say that despite all those negative comments it is still going strong in many parts of the world.

One must however agree with McMaster philosophy which challenged the traditional curriculum, giving an alternate approach to medical education, using it in their school of nursing in 1972 (Baker 2000). It was called the Problem Based Learning, (Barrows, 1998) which actually originated at the Case Western Reserve University in mid 1950s (Baker 2000, Kelly et al., 2005). Since those early days much water has flown under the bridge. Innovative techniques, and fresh curricula are now in practice in many institutions.

University of Dundee has played a major role in developing highly exciting strategies, since 1970s. A name emerged on the horizon of medical education, which has been shining since then. Ronald Harden is globally acknowledged to be a great medical educationist. Along with Laidlow and others he has written a vast number of papers, chapters and books on various subjects in the field of medical education.

Dundee also introduced the Spiral curriculum and the SPICES model (Harden, RM; Stamper, N; 1999). Horizontal and vertical integration of curriculum has been the major contribution of many educationists, but mainly Harden. It is now customary throughout the world to teach medicine through an integrated curriculum.

Another major contribution made by Harden is the introduction of Curriculum Mapping to modern education. He calls it 'Today's agenda'.

Curriculum mapping is not new. Its application, however, in contemporary medical education is innovative and exciting. It can help both, the students and the faculty by displaying all key elements of a curriculum, and relationship between those activities. It may include (1) the expected learning outcomes (2) curriculum content or areas of expertise covered (3) student assessment (4) learning opportunities (5) learning location (6) learning resources (timetable (7) staff (9) curriculum management (9) students. Nine steps are described in the development of a curriculum map in this historical document (AAME Guide. 21; 2001).

Darzi et al. (2008) identified and mapped the decisions made in the patient care with gallstone disease. They interpreted the competency and noted that every procedure in surgical care should include the individual's ability to make appropriate and timely decisions in surgical care. It is a fine illustration of curriculum mapping in the pathway of a disease.

In the autumn meeting of the Royal College of Physicians, a poster was presented, (Hermione Price, 2012) showing the role of mapping in a disease pathway. The meeting also contained a report duly highlighting the role of mapping an Endocrinology and Diabetes Mellitus Curriculum. The authors believe that curriculum mapping is a formative process for trainees and their supervisors, developing the curriculum and employing the learning facilities, identifying the learning objectives and identifying the available resources, making each item more transparent. In return, they believe, it allows the programme director, to ensure deficiencies, which can then be compensated for by the targeted the training or indeed planned teaching (Schofileld, Younis, Baker, 2012).

Concerns were raised by the patients and professional bodies in the UK on the poor standard of teaching about allergy in the medical schools. So Shehta and colleagues (2006) investigated the role of mapping and assessment of an undergraduate curriculum. They undertook a systematic analysis of learning objectives of modules taught during the five years of undergraduate teaching at the Edinburgh University.

This chapter illustrates a few examples of employing curriculum mapping in the disease pathways.

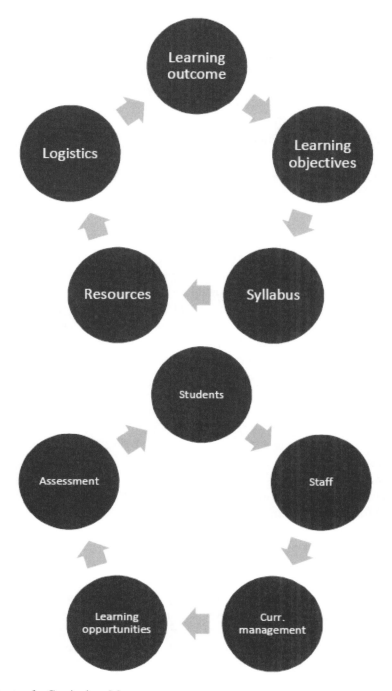

Figure 1. Contents of a Curriculum Map.

Every traveller knows that a map along with other accessories is an essential content of the backpack. Before the advent of the GPS and Sat Navs, we all relied on the road maps to go from point A to point B. In fact the history of Seafaring is inundated with stories of sailors who used the maps to circumnavigate the world on their sojourns.

One such seafarer however, lost his way, possibly didn't have the right map. His name was Christopher Columbus. He inadvertently discovered America, who many generations later gave the world Harvard and legends like Flexner.

A curriculum map is akin to a flight plan, often seen in a travel agent's office or in an inflight magazine. It informs the onlooker about all those destinations a certain air lines would take you. It is also an indicator of many destinations in the region or stop over on the way to a destination. It is also a good way of tracking your journey if you want to change your flight and wish to go to a different location.

If you travel on the London underground, or the Metro in Paris, Toronto or elsewhere, you need to check your destination on a map. It is usually colour coded and allows you to look at different stops that your train would stop on your way to a given destination. If you decide to change your track and catch a different train on a different pathway, the map would guide you to change at a junction, and so forth. So the beneficiary in both these scenarios namely the airlines and the train journey is you i.e. the customer or the client.

How does it help the air lines or the traffic controller on a railway station? Well the answer is simple. He just follows the track and traces the train or the plane by looking at the map and monitoring its progress along the journey. If a flight or a train is delayed, he can immediately check it by looking at the map and locate it.

The company owners benefit with a map of an airline or train by keeping the records of their activities under control and active monitoring. They can plan the journey, further progress, investments, cutbacks etc., by following the progress of a given route. If the passengers or the clients are lagging behind or the particular branch of the journey is losing customers, they can investigate the cause and attend to it. So a map is an absolutely essential arsenal in many fields.

Medical education is a long and tortuous journey. It is a marathon race. The process may take the participant through flat lands, green pastures, prairies, hills and mountains, vales and dales before reaching the winning pole. So there must be road map in medical education akin to the maps needed for another journey, comprising of a matrix of topics under various specialities/themes and corresponding educational hours.

A curriculum map is an educational tool that combines what is taught, how it is taught, when it is taught, and the measures used to assess if the teaching has successfully occurred. (Harden RM, AMEE Guide no. 21: Curriculum mapping: a tool for transparent and authentic teaching and learning. Medical teacher, 2001, 23(2):123-37, 39(3):154-61.

Roger Wong and Mark Robert (2007) carried out a study of the development of a curriculum map for the academic half days (AHD) in a core internal medicine residency program. They created a 3 year cyclical curriculum map based upon the educational tools, combining the content, methodology, and time tabling.

A curriculum map is indeed that and much more. Surprisingly enough it has not yet reached its due zenith nor indeed reached its full utilization in the vast field of medical education. Perhaps it is an under rated and even less understood entity. In due course of time it is bound to gain a position in the hierarchy of education that it richly deserves.

A curriculum map can be used in many ways and for many beneficiaries.

So let us look at its utility in modern medical education.

CURRICULUM MAPPING

Here are a few illustrations of Curriculum mapping employed in an integrated curriculum.

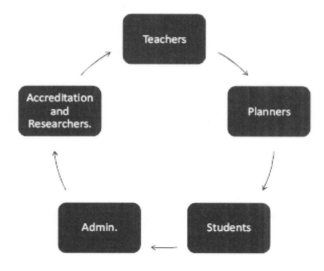

Students

Faculty

Administration

Beneficiaries

University

Government

Funding agencies.

Figure 2. Showing a List of Beneficiaries.

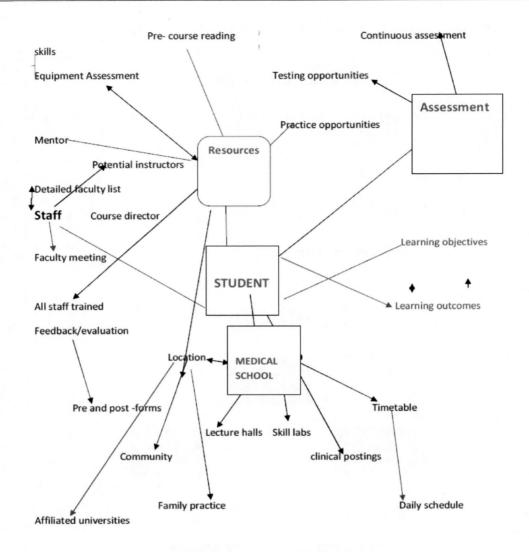

Clinical Scenario

A young man was brought to the A and E with a stab wound in the left side of his neck. He was conscious but disorientated. His pulse was 120 bpm and thready. His BP was 80/50 mm Hg. He was profusely sweating despite a freezing February weather in West Midlands. He was receiving IV fluids and blood had been sent for to be transfused. His breathing was shallow, and respiratory rate was 18/m.

Clinical Scenario

A 60 year old man presented with shortness of breath on exertion, missing heartbeat, light headedness, fatigue and general tiredness. He had no history of diabetes, or an Angina.

He was a non-smoker professional, enjoying an otherwise good health. He could walk and work albeit have those symptoms from time to time. His primary physician had arranged for detailed haematological investigation which was normal, except for a mild B 12 deficiency. He had recently had an EKG, which showed a Wenkebach phenomenon (2nd Degree heart block).

Themes in Curriculum Mapping

Besides mapping specific clinical conditions like Diabetes, or MI, Themes like Pain, Shock, Dizziness, and Headache etc. can also be mapped. They are basically manifest symptoms of an underlying pathology. So in order to teach undergraduates through an integrated curriculum, such themes can function as the Trigger points to cultivate, develop and formulate a debate. Thus they can be extremely potent means of imparting education. Here are a couple of illustrations of curriculum mapping based upon couple of common Themes.

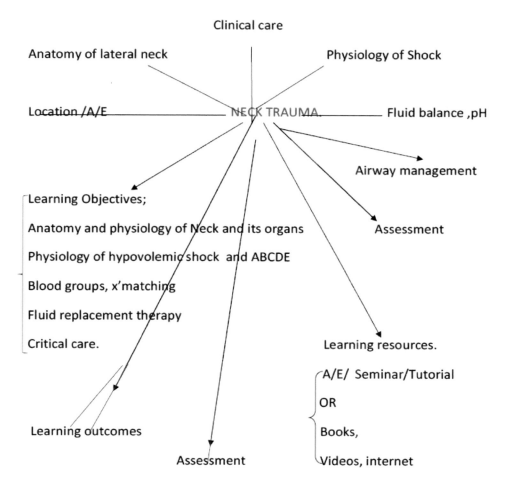

Integration of Basic and Clinical sciences.

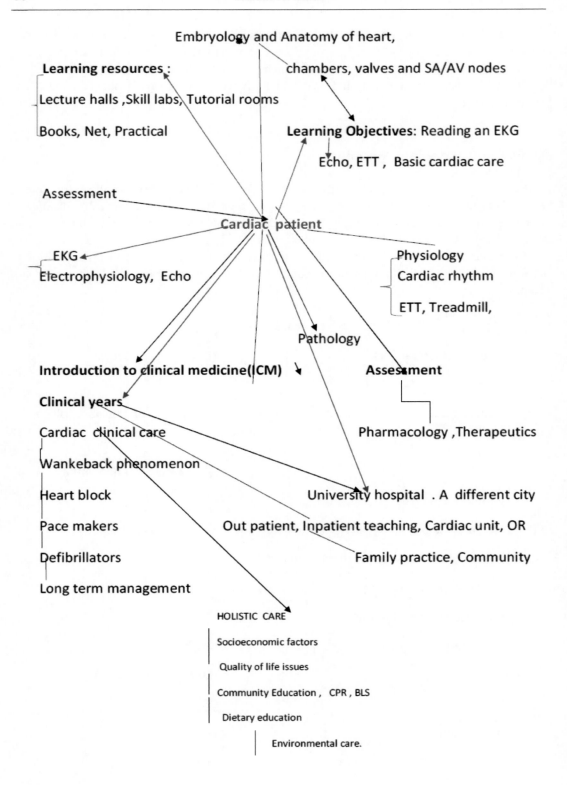

Embryology and Anatomy of heart,

chambers, valves and SA/AV nodes

Learning resources :

Lecture halls ,Skill labs, Tutorial rooms

Books, Net, Practical

Learning Objectives: Reading an EKG

Echo, ETT , Basic cardiac care

Assessment

Cardiac patient

EKG

Electrophysiology, Echo

Physiology

Cardiac rhythm

ETT, Treadmill,

Pathology

Introduction to clinical medicine(ICM)

Assessment

Clinical years

Cardiac clinical care

Wankeback phenomenon

Heart block

Pace makers

Defibrillators

Long term management

Pharmacology ,Therapeutics

University hospital . A different city

Out patient, Inpatient teaching, Cardiac unit, OR

Family practice, Community

HOLISTIC CARE

Socioeconomic factors

Quality of life issues

Community Education ,   CPR , BLS

Dietary education

Environmental care.

Scenario

A 30 year old woman presented in the Headache clinic with a history of frequent headaches for last several years. The attack was often initiated with tiredness, lack of sleep or stress at home or work place. She denied any history of depression, grief, medication or a metabolic disease. She had often noticed that the attack was often related to her periods. She also had a history of irregular cycles, photophobia, sickness and fatigue.

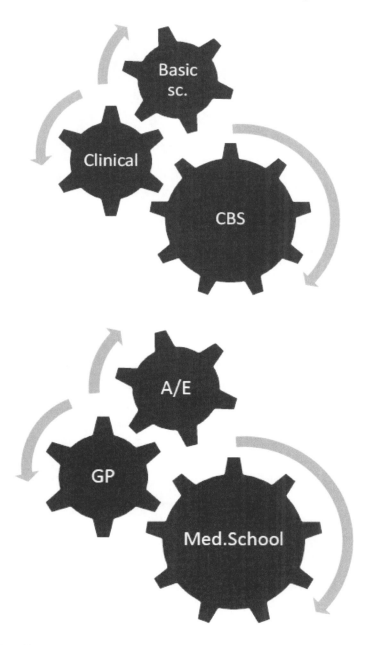

Figure 3. (Continued).

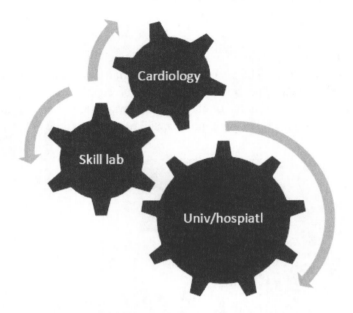

Figure 3. Inter- service dialogue. The activities may be spread out but can be esailly mapped out.

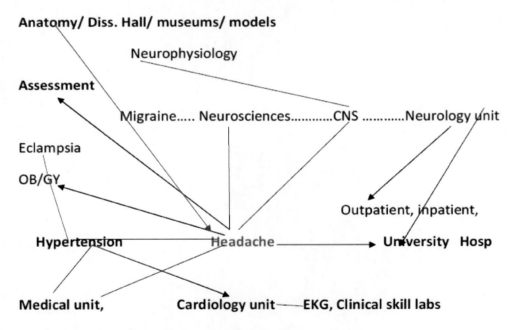

Here is an illustration of mapping the activities of a module on neurology employing a CBD. One may teach headache in targeting the basic sciences such as Neuro-Anatomy, Neurophysiology, Pain pathways, tracts etc. The Skill labs can be used for demonstration of certain elements like transmission of pain through different cranial nerves etc. Likewise the teacher may talk of patho- physiology of possible underlying causes, pharmacology etc. Clinical work up could be integrated by a visit to the neurology unit, cardiology unit, a family practice, a community health centre or a specialised headache unit in teaching hospital.

All activities such as teaching material, instructional strategies, logistics, and resources etc., can be mapped out in the department of medical education or the Dean's office to keep a track of academic activities.

CONCLUSION

The triangle of education is formed of Knowledge, Skill and Attitude. They must complement each other to achieve a given outcome. All three elements are contained in a package called Curriculum. The curriculum has many contents such as Syllabus, teaching strategies, and evaluation/assessment etc.

A curriculum may be taught at different locations of a university, as indeed contain a plethora of subjects to be delivered to a student. So, besides many others, if the student is the main beneficiary, the best way to keep a track of all academic activities is through Curriculum mapping. This chapter describes many ways in which a curriculum map can be highly productive in the process of medical education in 21st century. It duly emphasizes the role of mapping in the disease pathway, which may be specific clinical scenario like a Coronary Artery Disease or indeed a theme like Pain or Shock.

REFERENCES

AMEE Guide no. 21: (2001). Curriculum mapping: a tool for transparent teaching and learning. *RM Harden, Medical teacher*, Vol. 23: 123-137.

Baker, C. M. (2000). PBL for nursing: integrating lessons from other disciplines with nursing experience. *Journal of professional nursing*. 16(5), 258-266.

Barrows, H. S. (1998). The essentials of PBL. *Journal of dental education*. 62(9), 630-633.

Grant, J., (2010). Principles of curriculum design. In: Swanwick, T. (ed.). *Understanding medical education, Evidence, Theory and Practice.* Wiley-Blackwell, Chichester. 'A description of the steps in curriculum design'.

Harden, R. M., Stamper, N., (1999). What is a spiral curriculum? *Med. Teacher* 21, 141-143.

Jacklin, R., Sevdalis, N., Drazi, A., Vincent, C., (2008) Mapping surgical practice decision making: an interview study to evaluate decisions in surgical care. *The American Journal of Surgery,* May 2008, vol. 195(5) 689-696.

Mapping the Endocrinology and Diabetes Mellitus Curriculum (2012) (Jonathan Schofileld, Naveed Younis, Paul Baker, North West Deanery).

Saver and Duffy, Zavery, J. R., Duffy, T. M. (1996). *PBL, an instructional model and its constructive framework in B.* Wilson 9 ed.; pp. 135-148.

Spiral curriculum, in the Al Faisal University Riadh, Saudi Arabia. (*Personal interview with Paul Ganguly, Chair Anatomy, Jan., 2014*).

The autumn meeting of the Royal College of Physicians held a meeting on 9th Nov. 2012. In a poster, (Hermione Price, 2012).

Wong, Y. R., Roberts, J. M., (2007) Real time curriculum map for internal medicine residency. *BMC Medical Education*, 2007, 7:42.

Yasser Shehata, Michael Ross, Aziz Sheikh. (2006) Undergraduate allergy teaching in a UK medical school: mapping and assessment of an undergraduate curriculum. *Primary Care Respiratory Journal*, June 2006, vol. 15(3) 173-8.

Zaidi, S., Nasir, M., *Teaching and Learning methods in Medicine*. (2014), Under publication by Springer. Medicine. General. Springer.com.

In: Health and Disease
Editor: Paul Ganguly

ISBN: 978-1-63463-052-8
© 2015 Nova Science Publishers, Inc.

Chapter 6

INTERPROFESSIONAL EDUCATION (IPE): THE NEXT CHAPTER IN HEALTH PROFESSIONS EDUCATION

N. Lynn Eckhert[*]

Director of Academic Programs, Partners HealthCare International, Boston, MA, US

ABSTRACT

A new wave of education is sweeping the health professions in the 21st century, inter professional education (IPE). Prompted by a global shortage of health professionals and a need to reform health care delivery systems to be more responsive to populations needs, there exists a growing international recognition that training across various health professions offers value for trainees and for health care. (IEPC 2011), MACY (2010), WHO (2013) Proponents of IPE advocate such collaborative training will promote a better understanding of one's own and other professions, encourage interprofessional collaborative practice (IPC), enhance health care systems and improve health outcomes of patients and of populations. In an effort to integrate IPE into the foundation of learning of their students, health professions programs are working collectively to create curricula which bring students of multiple professions to learn together for the purpose of improving the care of patients.

This chapter will define IPE and the parameters of collaborative practice, discuss the value of IPE to the community, patients and families, students and the faculty. Successful models and national endeavors will be presented, as well as, how programs are implemented, and ongoing IPE experiences. The author will present outcomes expected of IPE, how achievements may be measured and what research endeavors and networks are underway. The challenges of IPE will be considered and the possible next steps for this new way of teaching.

[*] Corresponding author: N. Lynn Eckhert, M.D., MPH, DrPH. E-mail address: LECKHERT@PARTNERS.ORG.

INTRODUCTION

Although for generations a mainstay of education in schools of public health brought students from various health professions together to learn, IPE encompasses a more in depth educational process deliberately emphasizing cooperation, collaboration, communication and experiential learning among the professions. IPE calls attention to students from different disciplines, helps them learn about their own health profession, recognizes the strengths and boundaries of their own profession and how their profession integrates into the health care team and the overall health care delivery system. At the same time the student gains knowledge of the roles and responsibilities of other health professionals, their capabilities and boundaries and how health professionals can work together. By learning side by side students can recognize the gaps and the redundancies in the delivery of services and how the health professions can collaborate to find the solutions which reduce inefficiencies and fill deficiencies in order to improve the health outcomes of the patients.

IPE may be directed toward both the prelicensure/preregistraion level and/or the post licensure/post registration level. While both are valuable this chapter addresses IPE for prelicensure/preregistration students who have chosen a health profession but are early in their development and not yet fully acculturated into their roles. Presumably early exposure to IPE may prepare students to envision their roles as part of a team of health care providers who are interdependent upon one another for improving health care delivery and health outcomes. While much of learning will still occur in the silos of the individual professions learning together underscores the value of numerous health professions in providing patient centered care. The movement toward IPE calls for the health professions to agree upon a set of definitions which allow for common understanding. This chapter will utilize the commonly accepted definitions as defined by WHO (2010); Interprofessional education (IPE) an educational experience which "occurs when students from two or more professions learn about, from and with each other." Collaborative practice ready health worker- "A health professional who has learned how to work in an interprofessional team and is competent to do so." Interprofessional collaborative practice (IPC)- "When multiple health workers from different professional backgrounds work together with patients, families, carers[sic], and communities to deliver the highest quality of care."

In addition, the Robert Wood Johnson Foundation publication (2011) defines Interprofessional team-based care as care delivered by intentionally created, usually relatively small work groups in health care, who are recognized by others as well as by themselves as having a collective identity and shared responsibility for a patient or group of patients e.g., rapid response team, palliative care team, primary care team, operating room team.

In addition, D'Amour and Oandasam (2005) described a new term, Interprofessionality as "the process by which professionals reflect on and develop ways of practicing that provide an integrated and cohesive answer to the needs of the client/family/population.

RATIONALE FOR IPE

Numerous changes in worldwide demographics, patterns of illness, new health professions and the delivery of health services contribute to the movement toward team based care and thus the value of training health professionals together. Aging populations face more chronic conditions, cancers and co morbidities which call for a broader array of services at home, in ambulatory and community settings and in hospitals. Furthermore, the availability of new technologies spawned the development of numerous new health professions with specialized skills to provide care to patients e.g. physician assistants, respiratory therapists, imaging technicians. At the same time inpatient hospital care became increasingly complex requiring more specialized care by a team of highly trained health professionals in a variety of disciplines. At the same time, economic imperatives prompted shortened hospital stays and the discharge of sicker patients with greater health service needs to be provided in home by families and visiting health professionals. As the systems became more complex, the value of greater collaboration and communication among health professionals and with patients becomes more apparent. Moreover, it became evident that a single practitioner could not provide the breadth of care needed by the patient or the population. As the complexity of care required by patients with multiple chronic conditions escalated, patients relied on numerous care givers but lamented the fragmentation of services and the difficulty of anyone being in charge and coordinating their care. While an overall shortage of physicians is evident it is also the paucity of primary care practitioners which underscores the need for more coordinated and team based care. In the United States given the dynamic and competitive health environment a marketing strategy of health delivery systems is to highlight their capability to provide patient centered care over the entire lifetime of the patient.

To provide such comprehensive services encompassing the full range of preventive, curative, rehabilitative and palliative care requires a broad array of caregivers with different skills, attitudes and competencies. To bring these services together IPE creates the learning environment at both the prelicenusre and postlicensure levels to align these services in the best interest of the patients.

BACKGROUND

Faced with a shortage of 4.3 million health workers (Frenk 2010) the World Health Organization eager to rapidly scale up the production of the health professions workforce established a WHO Study Group on Interprofessional Education (IPE) and Collaborative Practice (CP). (WHO 2013) Nations around the world were seeking solutions to their own health care worker shortages and ways of transforming ineffective fragmented health systems that not only fell short of meeting the needs of their populations, but also required increasing fiscal resources. An apparent solution could be found in the interwoven concepts of IPE and collaborative practice which are thought to be an innovative strategy to meet the growing crisis of the global workforce shortage of health professionals and at the same time a mechanism to strengthen health systems. In an effort to promote IPE and CP the WHO study group was tasked with producing an action framework that would provide communication tools, guidelines and resources for both developing and developed countries. Equipped with the IPE and CP tools health care providers could influence national health policy and transform the poorly functioning health care delivery systems. The WHO Study Group conducted an international environmental scan of IPE practices to determine the current status of IPE around the globe, to identify best practices and to provide examples of IPE successes and concerns. The breadth of learners of IPE was extensive representing the full scope of practice of allied health, nursing, medicine, pharmacy, psychology and social work. The report covering nearly 50 years of experience points out the benefits of IPE as it enables collaborative practice in improving access and coordination of services, improves satisfaction of both patients and health professionals and improves health outcomes. Furthermore, the report brings together the data which support the value of collaborative practice in decreasing hospital admissions, length of stay, clinical errors and mortality rates. The framework stresses the importance of training of the health professions to be "collaborative practice ready" not to practice their individual skills in parallel but to work together to create mechanisms whereby health professions working together are complementary to each other and are capable of transforming health systems. The WHO report calls for nations to take action and in a summary framework identifies mechanisms to shape IPE and IPC that can be adapted by various health systems around the world. The WHO Framework for Action in figure 1 illustrates the role of interprofessional education as a key step at the local level in developing health professionals who are ready for collaborative practice. Theoretically, once practice ready in IPC the health professionals will create policies and pathways to strength the fragmented health system which should result in improvements in health outcomes.

While the WHO Report provides an overview of the possibilities and potentials of IPE and IPC many individual nations also acknowledged that health care reform was needed and that the current health workforce could not meet the health needs of the population going forward thereby prompting an acceleration in the movement toward IPE.

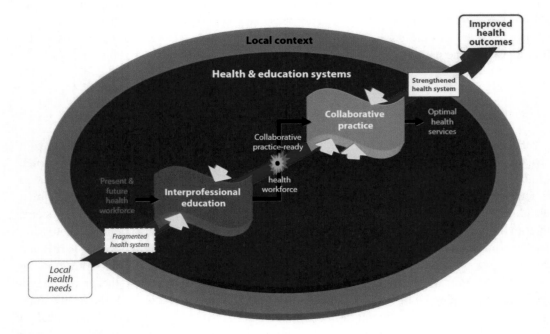

Figure 1. Describes the interprofessional education.

To develop IPE programs requires the creation of an environment that supports innovation in learning and practices and enables the transformation of the educational curriculum as well as health care practice. Ho and colleagues (Ho 2008) advocate for academic institutions and their faculties to be the institutional vehicles which can promote the changes necessary for success.

In an analysis of five successful IPE programs in Canada Ho identified five key factors needed for IPE implementation; 1. champions of IPE at the leadership and practice levels 2. a common vision, values and goal sharing 3. development of faculty and staff participating in IPE 4. opportunities for collaborative work in learning and practice 5. consideration of sustainability. Numerous national and international efforts supporting the concept of IPE and promoting collaborative practice and research and the exchange of ideas began to take shape around the globe.

Australia

In 2013 Australia published Curriculum Renewal for Interprofessional Education in Health (Australia 2013) a product of a two year study of IPE in nine Australian Universities, two government agencies and one non governmental organization. The report highlights five recommendations which enhance the movement toward IPE; develop national leadership in the development of IPE across higher education, health, the profession and the government, develop a nationally coordinated IPE curriculum and faculty development, incorporate IPE into accreditation standards of all health profession, promote research and develop a virtual knowledge repository.

Canada

Recognizing the importance of promoting IPE as a way to strengthen health care systems in 2007 Health Canada funded the Accreditation of Interprofessional Health Education Initiative (AIPHE) which brought together eight organizations responsible for accreditation of prelicensure education for six health and social service professions; medicine, nursing, pharmacy, physiotherapy, occupational therapy and social work. Since accreditation standards guide educational programs, the purpose of AIPHE was to ensure that the principles of IPE were integrated into the accreditation standards of each of the professions. Through the Canadian Interprofessional Health Collaborative (CIHC), a national organization, the health professions have access to resources to facilitate IPE and collaborative practice (CIHC 2011).

Several networks of likeminded health professionals promoting IPE are in effect. The Canadian Interprofessional Health Collaborative Research Net is a national network in Canada designed to foster interprofessional collaborations among students, faculty, practitioners and organizations who are involved in interprofessional research studies.

Besides promoting research collaborative efforts the network wishes to develop evidenced based best practices in IPE and collaborative practice and disseminate these studies to a wider audience of health professionals.

Japan

In 2008 ten Japanese universities implementing IPE in their health professions education programs established JIPWEN, the Japan Inter Professional Working and Education Network a network to advocate and strengthen IPE.

JIPWEN a member of the Global Health Workforce Alliance publicizes Japanese IPE case studies in English and seeks advice and criticism on these programs. The two key roles JIPWEN has crafted to promote and improve IPE are an ongoing interaction of the network with international academics and promotion of IPE to the government health policy planners.

Singapore

While Western nations have placed significant emphasis on IPE learning, little has been known as to the readiness of Asian students for IPE. A study of the first year healthcare undergraduates at the National University of Singapore was conducted to determine the readiness of first year dentistry, nursing, medical and pharmacy students for interprofessional education. Utilizing the Readiness for Interprofessional Learning Scale (RIPLS), IPE readiness was found to be high but the readiness of pharmacy and dentistry lagged behind those of medicine suggesting a need to enhance students' awareness of their role in collaborative practice (Ahmad, Chan et al.).

As these various efforts move forward and collaboration within and among nations flourishes the discipline of IPE and IPC will be enhanced by the sharing of knowledge and the establishment of research projects to determine the best practices.

United Kingdom

The United Kingdom based Centre for the Advancement of Interprofessional Education (CAIPE) developed a guide for authorities responsible for commissioning and regulating IPE for medicine, health, social care and related fields. The guide develops the case for well planned interactive learning which will promote patient centered cost effective care by team members who are supportive and adaptable to the changing needs in the health care system.

The set of principles addressing the development of IPE outlined in the report can readily be applied to learning in a variety of educational, health service, governmental and private settings.

The United Kingdom IPE agenda goes beyond the development of educational programs to modification of the policies of the regulatory bodies. IPE requirements are embedded into health care delivery through the National Health Service regulations, into improving care by the Quality Assurance Agency regulations and into the accrediting standards for the health professions. In an effort to improve collaborative practice in the NHS, IPE is required during pre registration education of health professions. Recognizing the value of learning across the health professions in the setting of future practice, the Department of Health funds joint programs in IPE among the institutions of higher education and the NHS. The Quality Assurance Agency encourages IPE by emphasizing the importance of meeting the patients' needs through effective teams, interprofessional and interagency care.

The United Kingdom regulatory bodies overseeing medicine, nursing and midwifery, allied health professions and social work all underscore the assurance that students work with and learn from other health and social services professions and their students by requiring IPE as elements of the standards of accreditation.

US

Sparked by several Institute of Medicine reports on safety, quality and health professions education in which interdisciplinary education had yet to become the norm in health professions education (IOM 2003) in the United States an expert panel, the Interprofessional Education Collaborative (IPEC) was conveyed. Endorsed by six health professions; dentistry, nursing, medicine, osteopathy, pharmacy and public health and sponsored by three private foundations and the US Health Resources and Services Administration the panel was committed to preparing students to work together in a deliberative fashion.

Two reports were produced. The first report, Core Competencies for Interprofessional Collaborative Practice (RWJ) identified four domains to be addressed in IPE; values/ethics for interprofessional practice, roles/responsibilities, interprofessional communication and teams and teamwork.

The second, Team-Based Competencies Building a Shared Foundation for Education and Clinical Practice building on the four domains developed core competencies and strategies for implementation for IPE (RWJ).

The accreditation organization of US and Canadian medical schools the Liaison Council on Medical Education (LCME) recently added an accreditation requirement that the core curriculum of medical education must prepare medical students to function collaboratively on health care teams that include other health professional (LCME 2013).

Thus in the US,

IPE is a growing concept in medical education, the percentage of medical schools requiring interprofessional education as part of t.(a curriculum increased from 44% to 76% in 2011-2012 (AAMC 2014).

A greater in depth analysis of IPE examples at the University of Toronto and the University of Minnesota will be illustrative of the strategic role of the academic institutions in formulating IPE programs.

The Toronto Model of IPE and Overview of IPE (Nelson 2014)

Since 2000 the University of Toronto has been a leader in IPE bringing together eleven health professions and forty-nine teaching hospitals in the creation of an Interprofessional Education and Care (IPE/C) program. Prompted by a desire to best serve the needs of complex patients, to improve health outcomes and quality and to increase patient safety a consortium of University of Toronto health professions educators and teaching hospitals came together to co- develop the curriculum and learning activities. The curriculum was designed to provide health professionals with the core competencies to enable practitioners to provide evidenced based collaborative care in a team based practice. Table 1 illustrates elements of success for IPE with highlights from the Toronto Model and concepts to consider.

Beyond the elements highlighted in Table 1 is the role IPE and its champions played on the national stage as Canada formulated new guidelines of accreditation for the health disciplines. The faculty of the University of Toronto were engaged in the ongoing work of the Accreditation of Interprofessional Health Education Initiative (AIPHE) as standards of IPE were incorporated into the accreditation standards of the six member organizations; medicine, nursing, physiotherapy, occupational therapy, social work and pharmacy.

Table 1. Elements and concepts of success for IPE

Element	Toronto Model Highlights	Concepts to Consider
Human Resources Commitment	• By Deans of Schools involved in IPE • By Chief Executive Officers of the teaching hospitals • By a cadre of champions in university and health centers where teaching and practice will occur	• **Commitment by the upper leadership** is complemented by the buy in, enthusiasm, and energy of educators and clinicians at multiple levels and sites who are directly involved in IPE and IPC • **Faculty and staff development** are necessary for learning about IPE and IPC. Ongoing faculty development and engagement can enhance continued interest.
Governance	• Toronto Health Science Network has an overlapping structure of the university and the teaching hospital network which enabled collaboration	• Assuring a **governance** structure that allows for collaboration and supports creativity in formulating IPE programs and IPC practice
Shared Vision	• Leadership developed and shared a common vision for education and practice.	• A **shared vision**, values and expected outcomes sets the stage for moving the program forward. • **Building on strengths** already in place can serve as a foundation for the IPE program
Curriculum	• The IPE curriculum is based on the core competency framework of three key constructs; communication, collaboration and values and ethics which move across the span of the students experience of exposure, immersion and competence. Major challenges existed in integrating IPE and in finding time in packed curricula of the various schools.	• A **curriculum** specific to IPE must be developed collaboratively offering both required and elective experiences. • **Faculty experienced** in their own discipline benefit from faculty working together in creating an IPE transformative curriculum. • The IPE curriculum is integrated into the overall curriculum
Practice Sites	• A scan was conducted of what IPE activities were in place before beginning the program allowed for inclusion in the program and served as models for other practice sites. • Clinical placements sites needed to be identified, prepared and staff needed coaching in IPE.	• **Clinical placements** require identification and nurturing of the sites and accommodation of them to IPE teaching. • **The changing educational program** in IPE will alter the expectation of practice by the students and may stimulate changes in practice which should be encouraged and supported.
Assessment	• There are various opinions on how best to assess IPE. A key question maybe assessment by the measurement of patient outcomes.	• In health professions schools students are most frequently assessed on their individual performance. The introduction of IPE/IPC challenges the development of assessment tools that assess the individual as a team member and the team as a whole. • In addition methods of assessment of the overall program are important as are the feedback loops to implement improvements.
Quality	• To ensure consistency of learning experiences in both content and process a quality framework, Points for Interprofessional Education Systems(PIPES) was created.	• **Underscoring all activities** is a continuous commitment to quality, its measurement and the how the results are used to improve IPE.

More information on the Toronto Model can be obtained from a recent *publication Creating the Health Care Team of the Future, The Toronto Model for Interprofessional Education and Practice* by Sioban Nelson, Maria Tassone and Brian D. Hodges.

University of Minnesota a Model of Shared Resources (University of Minnesota 2014)

Building on creative work in IPE initially funded by a US Federal grant from the Health Resources and Service Administration several private foundations, the Robert Wood Johnson Foundation, the Josiah Macy, Jr. Foundation the Gordon and Betty Moore Foundation and the John A Hartford Foundation have added their support for the development of the National Center for Interprofessional Practice and Education at the University of Minnesota. This center, a public-private partnership, promotes IPE and collaborative practice with a goal of transforming the health care system so as to improve health outcomes and patient care while controlling health care costs. The work of the center focuses on five key core domains: leadership; collaborative practice and health system transformation; education and training; research, evaluation and scholarship; and innovative and novel models. Serving as a resource for IPE a Nexus has been created to encourage ongoing conversations on transforming education and practice within the IPE community and among educators and practitioners. The organization can be an excellent resource for all faculty interested in IPE as it provides a wealth of articles and has established advisory groups to share experiences and move the IPE agenda forward.

Value

A common denominator of the recommendations for IPE is the underlying value of IPE as a tool to achieve several key goals; better systems of care, better patient centered care, more efficient and affordable care and improved education of health care professions together.

The premise of IPE is that care of patients will be improved if health professionals function as a team providing coordinated care. In order to provide comprehensive services each profession needs an understanding of its own roles, responsibilities and limitations, as well as, those of the other health care providers. Communication is a critical element in inter professional care and in itself may result in improved care by a reduction of medical errors. (IOM 1999) The Joint Commission Center for Transforming Health Care (Joint Commission 2014) estimates that 80% of medical errors involve miscommunication when care givers are hand off patients from one caregiver to another.

Patients with multiple and complex medical needs must rely on a variety of health professionals. Unfortunately too often their experiences have been less than satisfactory as patients complain of fragmented care and seek ombudsmen to organize, coordinate and interpret their care. Collaborative practice provided by a team can be expected to improve both the quality of care and rein in costs as teams can oversee care, improve efficiency and effectiveness by recognizing and filling the gaps and eliminating and reducing the redundancies that may occur. Although much of education of the health professions is discipline specific and will continue to occur in a silo format; i.e. nursing students training with nursing students, pharmacy with pharmacy and medicine with medicine a careful analysis of the curriculum of the health professions recognizes specific areas where efficiency and effectiveness could be improved.

As one example, all health professions have some exposure to anatomy which may be taught in labs, lectures, seminars and by electronic methods. At the same time student learning is enhanced by peer teaching which under the IPE system could be strengthened by teaching across disciplines as one could foresee physiotherapy and medical students teaching each other musculoskeletal anatomy. Furthermore, costly, highly technical anatomy labs commonly are underutilized for much of the day, but could be set up with demonstrations for nursing or other health professions students.

In clinical scenarios many simulation centers train teams of health care professions together for high intensive care as in multidisciplinary teams for advanced life support or emergency trauma.

Nonetheless, there are numerous less intensive scenarios that could support IPE. As an example various health professions learn to do the same skills in the simulation lab; measuring of vital signs, drawing blood, inserting a foley catheter thereby setting in place the opportunity for IPE. In other simulated scenarios a single procedure requires the skills of more than one profession. As an example a lumbar puncture may be performed by a physician but the role of the nurse clearly is essential. Opportunities to train together in the simulation centers can more closely resemble the real life scenario if health professionals learn procedures together and familiarize themselves with their roles as well as those of the team. Joint learning through IPE can improve the efficiency of the teaching staff and the facility potentially improving utilization and reducing cost while at the same time representing a more realistic scenario.

In 2010 the Commission on Education of Health Professions for the 21st Century (Frenk) illustrated the interdependence of the health systems and the education systems. The new educational and service delivery models call on greater accountability to population health needs while breaking down the professional silos and hierarchical relationships harmful to collaborative practice.

CHALLENGES TO INTERPROFESSIONAL EDUCATION

To bring learners together from various health professions for interprofessional learning may be challenging as barriers may be significant. From the onset to reduce the tendency of thinking only within one's own profession a culture of sharing and collaboration must be shaped in which faculty from two or more health professions are identified for their commitment to IPE, their respect for and fluency in understanding the role of the other collaborating health professions and their shared vision of striving to improve health outcomes and patient care through teams by training health professionals together. Since IPE is a relatively recent model of teaching, faculty albeit experienced in working in high functioning teams, nevertheless have little if any expertise in teaching multiple health professions together.

Thus faculty development addressing collaborative teaching becomes a critical necessity whereby IPE educators come together to learn how to write objectives, create a curriculum, determine methods of teaching and develop new teaching materials emphasizing IPE.

In addition IPE brings new challenges to methods of assessment requiring new thinking as to how to measure competency of working in teams both for individual team members and the team as a whole.

Numerous logistic challenges also must be overcome; bringing together busy clinically active faculty with competing demands, finding or reallocating time in a tight curriculum, securing adequate and appropriate learning spaces and synchronizing sessions for joint learning initiatives for students from different schools.

Furthermore, the cost of having multiple faculty teaching together at one time may require negotiation with concerned academic administrators.

POTENTIAL BENEFITS OF IPE AND COLLABORATIVE PRACTICE

IPE can offer trainees with a better understanding of the parameters of their own role, responsibilities, limitations and manner in which each profession working collaboratively can complement other health professions. In a broad sense learners can gain an appreciation of the roles of other health professions. The opportunity to work as a team to improve effectiveness and efficiency provides learners with the prospect to improve communication not only with other team members, but also with the patient and the family. If students see themselves as essential members of a team there is greater satisfaction both as individuals and as a team. The most important benefit is to the patient who becomes integrated in the decision and who may move toward better health outcomes.

CONCLUSION AND WHAT IS NEXT?

Around the globe the need for more health professionals is critical as is the need to develop more reliable and effective systems to deliver health care. In the United States the passage of the Patient Protection and Affordable Care Act of 2010 placed greater emphasis on improving outcomes in primary care and the redesign of care to create "medical homes" with interprofessional teams to provide comprehensive care of patients over a life time and across chronic diseases.

If we continue to train health professional students only in silos we cannot expect they will be "collaborative practice ready". If health professionals are expected to work together in teams in a reformed health care system, it is reasonable that their training should be modified to reflect a collaborative environment. Working in teams the next generation of health professionals could be prepared to work together in meaningful and productive ways.

It is encouraging that efforts are underway to reform practice models to enhance collaborative practice while at the same time health professions programs and schools are striving to establish the principles of IPE, to define the competences of IPE and to write the objectives for the educational programs to train students from various disciplines. Models and methods of teaching are being tested to determine what works best in which type of settings. External support for IPE by private foundations encourages the development of pilot practice and educational programs and brings together the community of practitioners and scholars who are striving to define the discipline, create a network of interested parties and test what works well and what is not successful.

Since health systems differ around the global we can anticipate that one size will not fit all and that there will be lessons that can be modified and tested in various health systems. IPE and collaborative practice are evolving concepts that hopefully will streamline health care delivery and improve the health outcomes of populations.

REFERENCES

AAMC. (aamc.org/initiatives/cir/311972/interprofessionaleducation.html0.

Australia Curriculum Review for 2013 (www.ipehelath.edu.au).

Canadian Interprofessional Health Collaborative, A National Interprofessional Competency Framework February 2011. (http://www.cihc.ca/files/Synopsis%20of%20CIHC-Research Net,%20Revised%20Jan%2025th,%202011.pdf).

D'Amour, D. and Oandasan, I. (2005). Interprofessionality as the field of interprofessional practice and interprofessional education: An emerging concept. *Journal of Interprofessional Care,* 19 (Supplement 1), 8-20.

Frenk, J., Chen, L., Bhutta, Z. A., Cohen, J., Crisp, N., Evans, T., Fineberg, H., et al. Health Professionals for a new century: transforming education to strengthen health systems in an interdependent world. *The Lancet* 2010; 376(9756): 1923-58.

Ho, K., Jarvis-Selinger, S., Borduas, F., et al. Making Interprofessional Education Work: The Strategic roles of the academy. *Academic medicine* 2008; 83: 934-40.

Institute of Medicine (1999), *To Err Is Human: Building a Safer Health System.* Ed. L. T., J. M. Corrigan and M. S. Donaldson Washington DC.

Institute of Medicine (2003) *Health Professions Education: A Bridge to Quality.* Washington DC: National Academy of Sciences. http://www.iom.edu/Reports/2003Health-Professions-Education-A-Bridge_to Quality. aspx. Accessed June 10, 2014.

Interprofessional Education Collaborative Expert Panel. (2011). *Core competencies for interprofessional collaborative practice: Report of an expert panel.* Washington, DC: Interprofessional Education Collaborative.

Joint Commission Center for Transforming Health Care http://www.centerfortransforming healthcare.org/assets/4/6/CTH_HOC_Fact_Sheet.pdf Accessed June 7, 2014.

Josiah Macy Jr. Foundation (2010) *Educating Nurses and Physicians: Toward New Horizons Conference Summary.* Accessed June 10 2014. http://www.macyfoundation.org/docs/macy_pubs/JMF_Carneige_Summary_WebVersion_3.pdf.

Proposed Accreditation Standards 19-A Liaison Committee on Medical Education http://www.lcme.org/new_standard_ed-19-a.htm Accessed June 10, 2014.

Nelson, S., Tassone, M. and Hodges, B. D. *Creating the Health Care Team of the Future, The Toronto Model for Intrprofessional Education and Practice.* ILR Press an imprint of Cornell University Press, Ithaca, 2014.

Interprofessional Education Collaborative Expert Panel. (2011). *Core competencies for interprofessional collaborative practice: Report of an expert panel.* Washington, DC: Interprofessional Education Collaborative. https://www.aamc.org/download/186750/data/core_competencies.pdf. Accessed June 10, 2014.

RIPLS:Readiness for Interprofessional Learning Scale, 2009 https://nexusipe.org/resource-exchange/ripls-readiness-interprofessional-learning-scale Accessed August 18, 2014

Robert Wood Johnson Foundation Team - Based Competencies Building A Shared Foundation for Education and Practice. *Confeence Proceedings February 16-17, 2011,* Washington, DC.

Rodger, S., Hoffman, S. on behalf of the World Health Organization Study Group on Interprofessional Education and Collaborative Practice. Where in the world is interprofessional education? A global environmental scan. *Journal of Interprofessional Care* 2010;24(5):479-491.

University of Minnesota National Center for Interprofessional Practice and Education http://www.ahceducation.umn.edu/national-center-for-interprofessional-practice-and-education/Accessed June 7,2014.

University of Toronto Interprofessional Education Curriculum. http://www.ipe.utoronto.ca/sites/default/files/Interprofessional%20Education%20Curriculum%20Brochure_0.pdf Accessed June 10, 2014.

World Health Organization (2010) *Framework for Action on Interprofessional Education and Collaborative Practice.* Geneva, Switzerland: World Health Organization; 2010. http://www.who.int/hrh/framework_action/en/index. html. Accessed June 10, 2014.

World Health Organization (2013). *Transforming and scaling up health professionals' education and training: WHO Guideline 2013.* Geneva, Switzerland.

In: Health and Disease
Editor: Paul Ganguly

ISBN: 978-1-63463-052-8
© 2015 Nova Science Publishers, Inc.

Chapter 7

MOLECULAR MEDICINE IS WHERE CHRONIC DISEASES, NUTRITION AND PHYSICAL ACTIVITY INTERSECT: A SUGGESTION ON HOW TO DEAL CHRONIC DISEASES IN THE BIOMEDICAL CURRICULUM

Bernhard H. J. Juurlink, [1,2,*] *and Abdulhadi A. Al-Amodi* [1,3,†]

[1]College of Medicine, Alfaisal University, Riyadh, Kingdom of Saudi Arabia
[2]College of Medicine, University of Saskatchewan, Saskatoon, Saskatchewan, Canada
[3]School of Graduate Studies in the Health Sciences, University of Mississippi Medical Center, Jackson, Mississippi, US

ABSTRACT

Chronic diseases that become more common with aging impose an increasingly large burden on the health care system and on society in general yet chronic diseases are poorly dealt with in the medical curriculum, in both the basic biomedical sciences and the clinical sciences. The drivers of chronic diseases are oxidative stress and generalized non-infectious inflammation, topics that are poorly dealt with in the medical education but are critical in understanding chronic diseases. In this chapter we outline a series of concepts, in a specific sequence, that should enable students to develop fundamental concepts that are critical in understanding the basic biomedical sciences behind the disruptions of cellular signaling and metabolism that underlie oxidative stress and non-infectious inflammation. Such an understanding should enable the future physician to better advise on life style changes that might prevent, or at least ameliorate, chronic diseases and give the tools for most effective treatment.

* Bernhard H. J. Juurlink, PhD. E-mail address: Bernhard.juurlink@usask.ca or jbernhard@alfaisal.edu.
† Abdulhadi A. AlAmodi, MBBS. E-mail address: aalamodi@umc.ed.

INTRODUCTION

A major problem in any area of education is the development of skills allowing one to integrate information from divers sources and to become life-long learners. This is a particular problem in medical education where there is an exponential increase in biomedical information but the time allocated for basic biomedical medical education is limited to about two years or less. The solution is to develop effective conceptual frameworks: this can only be done where additional information can be related to a pre-existing 'cognitive framework' [1]. Effective teachers enable students to want to develop such conceptual frameworks. They also promote a deep strategy of learning that supports application to real life scenarios.

One area that is particularly poorly dealt with in medical education is chronic diseases. Knowledge about chronic diseases is "primarily attained through disparate lectures in the epidemiology, pathophysiology, and pharmacology during the preclinical years." [2]. Holman also has pointed out that medical education does not prepare physicians well with dealing with the most prevalent problem in healthcare today, chronic diseases [3]. Chronic diseases that become more common with aging tend to be treated as unrelated disease entities. Holman was concerned with clinical education; however, equally problematic is that there is a lack of education in the basic biomedical sciences, with each chronic disease usually taught in isolation. Yet there are many commonalities in causal factors involved in the development of these chronic diseases. A better understanding of these factors will lead to better preventive strategies as well as better treatment regimens. All chronic diseases that become more common with age have underlying oxidative stress and inflammatory components to them. These diseases include atherosclerosis [4] and attendant problems of hypoperfusion, non-Alzheimer's dementia [5], Alzheimer's disease [6], myocardial infarction [7], hemorrhagic and thrombotic stroke [8]; hypertension [9] and attendant problems of vascular dementia [10] and thrombotic as well as hemorrhagic stroke [11, 12]; Alzheimer's disease [13]; type 2 diabetes [14]; dyslipidemia [15]; chronic kidney disease [16]; osteoporosis [17] and obesity [18]. Although, these are being commonly treated as isolated diseases, there clearly are physiological interconnections amongst these disorders; indeed, there is now some recognition that a number of these diseases can be grouped into a disorder known as metabolic syndrome. Metabolic syndrome is a major health problem in the developed and the developing world. The World Health Organization (WHO) defines metabolic syndrome as characterized by high fasting glucose, impaired glucose tolerance or frank type 2 diabetes (all associated with insulin resistance) as well as at least two of the following: obesity, lowered serum high density lipoprotein (HDL), increased serum triglycerides, microalbuminuria (indicative of kidney damage) and hypertension [19]. Although atherosclerosis is not a component of metabolic syndrome, it clearly is related. The metabolic syndrome incidence is rapidly rising around the world affecting younger and younger individuals, for example, 25% of adult Canadians [20] and adult Latin Americans [21] are now diagnosed with the syndrome and even higher incidence levels in places like India [22]. As with the individual components, what drives metabolic syndrome is low-grade tissue inflammation [23, 24]. Reaven has suggested that metabolic syndrome be replaced with insulin resistance syndrome [25].

More recently it has been proposed that a terminology that better describes this syndrome is "chronic systemic low-grade inflammation induced energy reallocation syndrome" [26] since there is an underlying inflammatory component and changes in metabolism associated with metabolic syndrome. An understanding of this inflammation-driven energy reallocation syndrome necessitates an integration of metabolism, cellular signaling, gene expression and the influences of diet and physical activity on these processes.

Since one is not born with chronic low-grade inflammation, one can deduce that epigenetic changes are associated with the development of this inflammation. One of us had previously argued that cell biology/ histology can be a facilitator for integrating biomedical sciences in the medical curriculum [27], but perhaps the theme of low-grade inflammation should form the corner stone around which molecular medicine is organized.

The questions is how to design a conceptual map framework and fit such a map into the curriculum. It is important that the conceptual maps being developed be incremental and reflexive. It is also important in the development of conceptual maps that an easily understood example or two, but not more than two, be given to reify the concept.

Chronic diseases involve disturbances in redox states. Although oxidative stress is a very commonly used term, it is poorly understood by most physicians and, indeed, by most life scientists. Oxidant production and inactivation is a topic that should play a central role in biomedical education since it is oxidative stress or its associated low-grade chronic inflammation that drives most chronic diseases that are related to aging.

Below is a suggested sequence of concept maps that ought to enable students to better integrate topics that are normally treated separately in biochemistry, physiology, pharmacology and pathology. These concepts should be covered during the biomedical sciences component of the curriculum. Many of the components of the concepts listed below, if taught, are taught by biochemists, but this is not necessary, and perhaps not even desirable.

If biochemists are teaching many of the concepts they should be reminded that they are teaching essential concepts for future medical practitioners, not biochemistry graduate students. In what courses or in what manner these topics are covered is not important. It is important, though, that there be a coordinator ensuring topics are covered in in a certain order and in not too great detail since once the students understand the basics they can readily get the details on their own. Essential concepts are best delivered in didactic sessions that promote active learning and reinforced through a problem-based learning sessions.

CONCEPT MAPS

1. Electrons and Energy States

Following a consideration of the fundamental molecules of life the curriculum should soon deal with the concept that the energy that sustains life is harvested from electrons in the foods we eat. They should become very familiar with oxidation (loss of electrons) and reduction (gain of electrons) reactions.

This should be dealt with in a very simple manner by pointing out that that like in a fire where the products of combustion are carbon dioxide and water plus free (or Gibbs) energy, combustion of foods results in the production of carbon dioxide and water plus free energy.

Whereas in fire, the free energy is released as heat, with our foods, a significant fraction of the free energy is temporarily stored in molecules such as adenosine triphosphate (ATP).

The students should develop the concept that the free or Gibbs energy is derived from the difference in the energy states of the electrons involved in the various chemical bonds of the food molecules versus the chemical bonds in water and carbon dioxide. As an example, Table 1 illustrates the approximate energy required to break the bonds in glucose and oxygen (bond energy or bond enthalpy) during glucose oxidation as well as the energy required to break the bonds in the combustion products carbon dioxide and water. More energy is required to break the bonds of the combustion products than the combustants. This difference (i.e., ΔG) of ~ - 2700 kilojoules/mole is what is available for work – note there is some uncertainty since glucose can exist in the open or closed molecular form – the above calculation is for the closed ring form of glucose. There is no need for the students to memorize these values.

One might point out that this combustion of glucose in the cell occurs over a number of steps with about 40% of the energy being ultimately stored in the molecule adenosine triphosphate (ATP), the remaining released as heat.

The students should also have the concept that the hydrolysis of the phosphate bonds of ATP releases energy available for work (mechanical such as muscle contraction or ion movement across membranes or for synthesis of compounds). Students should be introduced to the concept that cells harvest this energy from foodstuffs and ultimately store much of it in the form of ATP in an orderly manner that requires temporary electron storage reservoirs such as flavin adenine dinucleotide ($FADH_2$), nicotinamide adenine dinucleotide (NADH) and nicotinamide adenine dinucleotide phosphate (NADPH) (Figure 1).

2. Mitochondrial Electron Transport Chain - ATP and Oxidant Production

Once the students have the concept that usable energy can be obtained from changes in chemical bond states and that much of this usable energy can be temporarily stored in reduced nucleotides such as $FADH_2$ and NADH, then students should be exposed to the of the mitochondrial electron transport chain (Figure 2) and the chemiosmiotic theory of mitochondrial ATP synthesis. Here one should also introduce the topic of oxidative stress - it should be pointed out how saturation of the electron carriers promote the formation of superoxide anions (Figure 3) that in turn can be converted to hydrogen peroxide [28], since this is one link between have greater caloric intake than caloric expenditure and a link to low-grade inflammation. Not many details should be given at this point. The key to developing conceptual maps is to slowly establish such maps using a reflexive approach.

Table 1A. Bond Energies for Combustants: Glucose and Molecular Oxygen

Bond Type	Quantity	Bond Energy (kJ/mol)	Total Bond Energy
C-C	5	346	1730
O-H	5	464	2320
C-H	7	414	2898
C-O	5	358	1790
C=O	1	799	799
O=O	6	494	2964
			12501

Table 1B. Bond Energies for Combustion Products: Carbon Dioxide and Water

Bond Type	Quantity	Bond Energy (kJ/mol)	Total Bond Energy
O-H	12	464	5568
C=O	12	799	9588
			15156

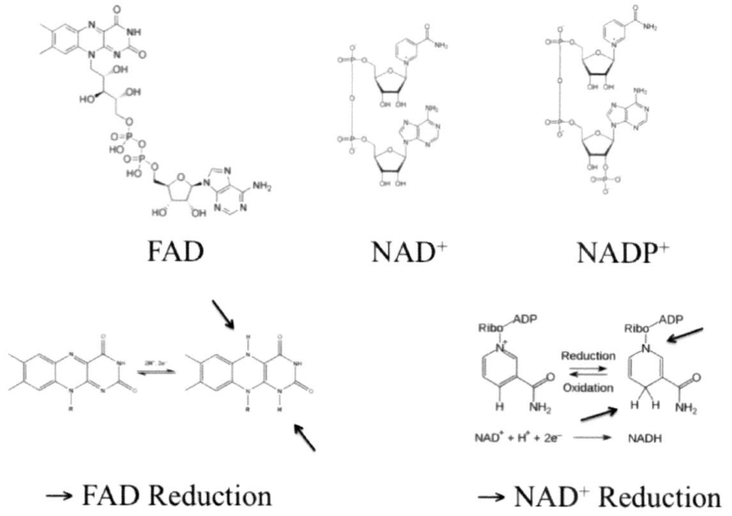

FAD   NAD⁺   NADP⁺

→ FAD Reduction   → NAD⁺ Reduction

The images are taken from the Wikimedia Commons and are in the public domain. The authors are Edgar181 (FAD) and NEUROtiker6 (NAD⁺ and NADP⁺). Websites are: http://en.wikipedia.org/ wiki/Flavin_adenine_dinucleotide;http://commons.wikimedia.org/wiki/File:NAD%2B_phys.svg; http://en.wikipedia.org/wiki/Nicotinamide_adenine_dinucleotide_phosphate.

Figure 1. On the top are chemical diagrams of the electron-storing nucleotides FAD, NAD⁺ and NADP⁺. Below the direction of the arrow shows the reduction of FAD (author is DMACK) and NAD⁺ (NADP⁺ reduction is similar to NAD⁺ reduction: author is Fvasconcellos). Arrows indicate the molecular sites where electrons (with or without accompanying hydrogen atoms) have been gained.

3. Introduction to the Citric Acid Cycle

Once students have a good grasp of the function of the mitochondrial electron transport system, one should start with considering the role of the citric acid (Kreb's) cycle (Figure 4) in converting the usable energy in the acetate of acetyl-CoA into the electron energy storage forms of $FADH_2$ and NADH. What should be emphasized at this point is that the cycle starts off with a 6-carbon molecule (citrate) and ends with a 4-carbon molecule (oxaloacetate) with the release of two carbon dioxide molecules and that one FAD molecule and two NAD⁺ molecules are reduced with each turn of the cycle as well as the synthesis of one ATP-equivalent molecule (GTP). Students should also be introduced to the concept that a 2-carbon acetate moiety derived from acetyl-Coenzyme A (acetyl-CoA) is attached to oxaloacetate to regenerate citric acid allowing the cycle to turn again. This is the essential information necessary at this stage of learning.

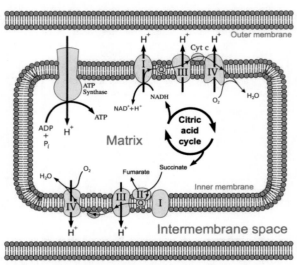

Image taken from the Wikimedia Commons and is in the public domain. Author is Fvasconcellos. Website is: http://en.wikipedia.org/wiki/File:Mitochondrial_electron_transport_chain—Etc4.svg.

Figure 2. Mitochondrial electron transport chain demonstrating the flow of electrons from $FADH_2$ and NADPH to the electron carriers ultimately reducing oxygen to water. The energy given up by the electrons as they move from carrier to carrier is used to pump protons from the mitochondrial matrix to the intermembranous space setting up a proton and electrical gradient that is used by complex V (ATP synthase) to attach a phosphate to adenosine diphosphate (ADP) forming ATP.

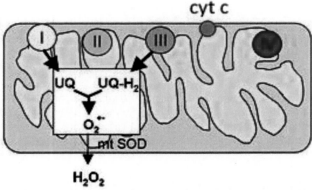

Original image is taken from Figure 2 in: Major cellular sources of ROS in living cells. Novo and Parola Fibrogenesis and Tissue Repair 2008 1:5 doi:10.1186/1755-1536-1-5. Website is: http://en.wikipedia.org/wiki/Reactive_oxygen_species.

Figure 3. Diagram illustrating formation of superoxide anion and thence hydrogen peroxide when electron the mitochondrial electron carriers are saturated when electrons encounter oxygen before reaching complex IV. Image taken from Wikimedia Commons and is in the public domain. Authors are Erica Novo and Maurizio Parola.

It is essential that students are not introduced to too many concepts at once since this will greatly interfere with the establishments of conceptual maps; hence, later in the curriculum students can be introduced to other concepts involving the citric acid cycle such as the production of intermediates for synthetic purposes, anaplerotic reactions, etc.

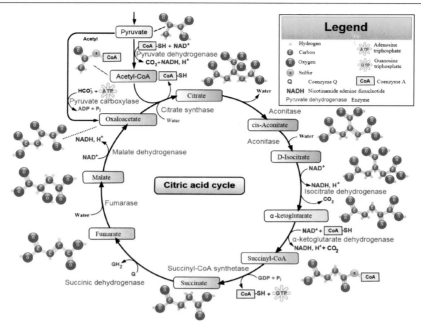

Author is Daniel Ramsköld. Website is: http://commons.wikimedia.org/wiki/File:Citric_acid_cycle_with_aconitate_2.svg.

Figure 4. Citric acid cycle. Image taken from the Wikimedia Commons and is in the public domain.

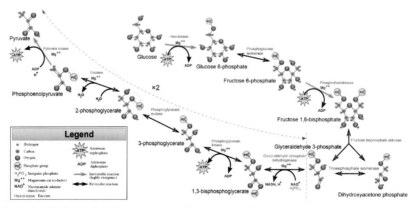

Image taken from the Wikimedia Commons and is in the public domain. Author is Johny Abb. Website is: http://en.wikipedia.org/wiki/File:Glycolysis2.svg.

Figure 5. Glycolysis.

4. Introduction to Glycolysis

At this point students should be eager to learn the source of acetyl-CoA and this is the opportune time to consider how glycolysis feeds into the Kreb cycle as well as provide the reducing equivalents in the form of NADH. Again, at this stage it is essential that not too many details are introduced. For example, for glycolysis (Figure 5) one should point out that one starts with a 6-carbon glucose molecule and ends with two 3-carbon pyruvic acids.

At this point students should also know: 1) that glycolysis results in the net synthesis of 2 ATP and reduction of 2 NAD^+ molecules, 2) that the conversion of glyceraldehyde-3-phosphate to 1,3-biphosphoglycerate requires the reduction of NAD^+ and this step is feedback-inhibited by NADH - this latter will set the stage for future understanding of the necessity of anaerobic glycolysis.

In addition, students should learn that pyruvic acid is acted upon by pyruvate dehydrogenase to form a carbon dioxide molecule and the 2-carbon acetate in the form of acetyl-CoA and that this activity is associated with the reduction of NAD^+.

Later one can introduce more details, for example, when gluconeogenesis is considered one can consider which reactions are reversible and which are not.

5. Beta Oxidation of Free Fatty Acids

Glycolysis can be followed by mitochondrial beta oxidation of medium (fatty acids shorter than 20 carbons) and short chain fatty acids resulting in the formation of acetyl-CoA and the reduction of NAD^+ and FAD. At this point in the curriculum students need only be concerned with the mechanisms of fatty acid transport into mitochondria and subsequent beta oxidation of even-numbered saturated fatty acids. The essentials the student needs to know at this time is that cleavage of each two-carbon residue from the acyl-CoA forms one acetyl-CoA as well as one molecule each of NAD^+ and FAD are reduced (Figure 6). Students should be reminded again that the energy captured from the carbon skeleton of our foodstuffs mainly funnel to the reduction of NAD^+ and FAD. Later in the curriculum students can deal with the metabolism of odd-number fatty acids, unsaturated fatty acids and branched fatty acids.

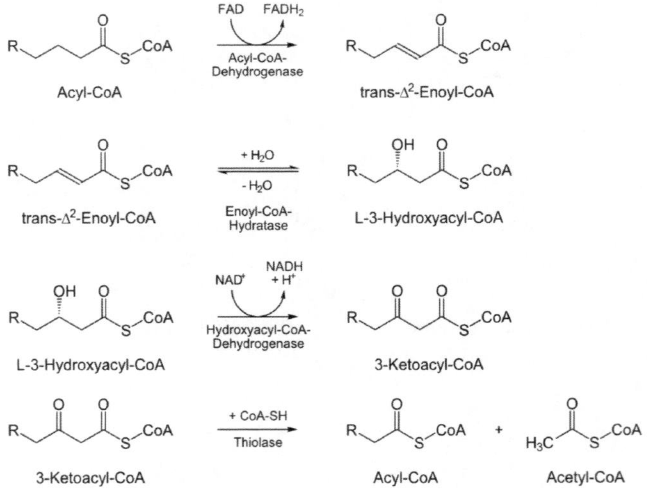

Diagram taken from the Wikimedia Commons and is in the public domain. Author is NEUROtiker. Website is: http://en.wikipedia.org/wiki/Beta_oxidation.

Figure 6. Critical reactions in beta oxidation of medium and short chain fatty acids. Students should note that oxidation of every two carbons of the fatty acid results in the reduction of one molecule of FAD and one molecule of NAD^+ as well as the formation of one acetyl-CoA.

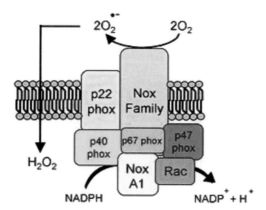

Authors are Erica Novo and Maurizio Parola. Original image is taken from Figure 2 in: Major cellular
    sources of ROS in living cells. Novo and Parola Fibrogenesis and Tissue Repair 2008 1:5
    doi:10.1186/1755-1536-1-5. Wiki site is: http://en.wikipedia.org/wiki/Reactive_oxygen_species.

Figure 7. Diagram of NAD(P)H oxidase localized in the plasmalemma of cells. Activation of this
enzyme complex results in the transfer of electrons from either NADH or NADPH to molecular oxygen
resulting in the formation of superoxide anions that in turn are converted to hydrogen peroxide. Image
is taken from the Wikimedia Commons and is in the public domain.

6. Oxidant Production

Oxidant production by the mitochondrial respiratory chain should be reviewed. Introduce
the student to the concept that one of the functions of peroxisomes is to convert very long
chain fatty acids (20 carbons or longer) to short chain fatty acids that then are exported to
mitochondria. Beta oxidation reactions in peroxisomes is similar to that in mitochondria with
one major difference in that in the first step of the process the electrons are donated to
molecular oxygen rather than FAD – this results in the formation of superoxide anions that
are dismutated by superoxide dismutase to hydrogen peroxide.

Other oxidases are also present in peroxisomes with the result that peroxisomes can be a
significant source of oxidants. Students can also be introduced to the concept that the
plasmalemma can contain NAD(P)H oxidase, an enzyme whose function is to transfer
electrons from either NADH or NADPH to molecular oxygen, thus producing superoxide
anions (Figure 7). Students now have the fundamental concept that three cellular organelles,
with specific spatial localization, can be sources of strong oxidants.

7. Oxidant Scavenging Pathways

This is an opportune time in the curriculum to introduce students to the major oxidant
scavenging pathways (Figure 8) and the necessity to scavenge superoxide anions and their
hydrogen peroxide products. Critical concepts include: 1) Conversion of superoxide anion to
hydrogen peroxide by mitochondrial Mn superoxide dismutase (Mn-SOD) and the cytosolic
and extracellular isoforms of Cu-Zn-SOD (equation i). The ability of transition metal ions to
convert hydrogen peroxide to the hydroxyl free radical, a very powerful oxidant (equation ii).

(i) $O_2^{\cdot-} + O_2^{\cdot-} + 2H^+ \rightarrow H_2O_2 + O_2$

(ii) $H_2O_2 + Fe^{2+} (or\ Cu^+) \rightarrow OH^- + OH^{\cdot} + Fe^{3-} (or\ Cu^{2+})$

(iii) $2H_2O_2 \rightarrow 2H_2O + O_2$

(iv) $2GSH + H_2O_2 \rightarrow GSSG + 2H_2O$

(v) $2GSH + LOOH \rightarrow GSSG + LOH + H_2O$

(vi) GSH +

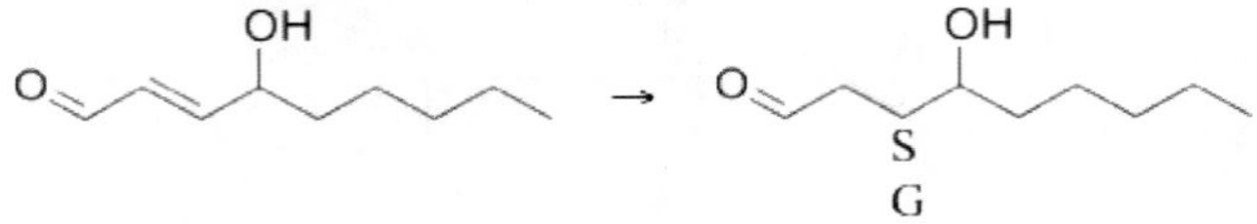

Figure 8. The following equations demonstrate: i) Conversion of superoxide anions into hydrogen peroxide by the superoxide dismutase family. ii) The ability of transition metal ions to convert the relatively innocuous hydrogen peroxide into the hydroxyl radical, a free radical with strong oxidizing ability. iii) The reduction of hydrogen peroxide to water and molecular oxygen by catalase. iv) The reduction of hydrogen peroxide to water by glutathione peroxidases, an enzymatic reaction that oxidizes glutathione (GSH) to GSSG. v) The reduction of organic hydroperoxides to alcohols and water by glutathione peroxidases with the oxidation of GSH to GSSG. vi) The inactivation of organic oxidants (e.g., 4-hydroxynonenal) by formation of glutathiyl adducts by the enzyme family glutathione S-transferases.

The ability of catalase, localized mainly in peroxisomes, to convert hydrogen peroxide to water and molecular oxygen (equation iii). It should be pointed out that although catalase has a high capacity for this catalysis, it has a low affinity for hydrogen peroxide with a K_m around 40 mM. Glutathione peroxidases (equation iv) can also scavenge hydrogen resulting in the formation of water. Glutathione peroxidases have a lower capacity for reducing hydrogen peroxide than catalase but have a higher affinity with a Km in the low micromolar range. This reduction of hydrogen peroxide by glutathione peroxidases requires glutathione (GSH) as an electron donor. In addition to being able to bring hydrogen peroxide to lower concentrations than catalase, glutathione peroxidases can also reduce organic peroxides (equation v).

The final scavenging pathways that should be considered are those dependent upon glutathione S-transferases (equation vi) where glutathiyl adducts are formed to inactivate organic oxidants. At this point students should be introduced to the general idea that oxidants can oxidize macromolecules and, thus, interfere with their function.

8. Cellular Redox State and Thiols

The concept of reduction:oxidation (redox) state should be introduced. The common oxidant scavenging pathways should be reviewed (Figure 8). A critical concept to be learned is that many thiols, particularly when they are deprotonated to form thiolates, are readily oxidized to disulfides or to sulfenic residues (Figure 9).

Sulfenic acid residues are readily reduced and, thereby, act as redox switches. Under conditions of extreme oxidative stress the sulfenic acid residues can be oxidized to sulfinic acid residues and even to sulfonic acid residues. There are no known cellular mechanisms to reduce sulfonic acid residues and only a few mechanisms to reduce sulfinic acid residues.

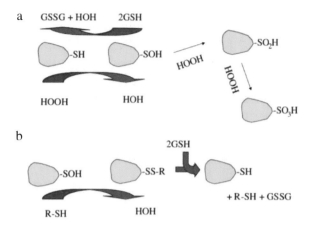

Figure 9. A: Diagram illustrating the oxidation of thiol groups by hydrogen peroxide giving rise to sulfenic (-SOH) that in turn can be oxidized to sulfinic acid (-SO₂H) that in turn can be oxidized to sulfonic acid (-SO₃H). Sulfenic acid can be reduced directly (A) or indirectly (B) by GSH.

The roles of thioredoxin, glutaredoxin and glutathione should be reviewed in the reduction of sulfenic acid and disulfides should be reviewed.

Students should appreciate that under conditions of extreme oxidative stress many of the cellular thiolates can be oxidized to sulfinic and sulfonate acid residues, thereby inactivating the functions of the proteins involved.

9. Introduction to Cellular Signaling Pathways

Students should be introduced to the general concept of intracellular signaling: the distinction between hydrophobic molecule signaling via nuclear receptors that results in alterations of gene expression and hydrophilic signaling via membrane-associated receptors linked to intracellular signaling pathways that can alter metabolism as well as influence gene expression.

10. Post-Translational Modifications That Alter Protein Function

A brief overview of post-translational modifications with emphasis on thiol modification and phosphorylation of amino acid residues should be given.

One should point out that forming disulfide bonds or oxidizing thiolates to sulfenic acid residues alters protein charge distribution and therefore morphology and function.

Furthermore, phosphorylating tyrosine, serine and threonine residues of proteins will also alter charge and thereby morphology and function.

General principles should be emphasized such as the proteins affected by post-translational modifications may include ion pumps, carrier proteins, signaling proteins, transcription factors, etc.

11. Kinase-Mediated Signaling

Students should be introduced to the concept of kinase signaling, in particular protein kinase A (PKA), protein kinase G (PKG), protein kinase C (PKC), calcium-calmodulin kinase (CaM kinase). Students should be introduced to the concept that protein kinases may influence metabolism by influencing the functional state of specific enzymes. An example should be given that students have already encountered.

For example, the phosphorylation of glycogen phosphorylase, thereby activating it, by PKA or inhibition of glycogen synthase by PKA-mediated phosphorylation.

Too many examples will lead to confusion. What is essential is that all students grasp the concept that phosphorylation of specific amino acid residues will result in changes of protein charge, morphology and thereby function.

Kinase signaling may also result in changes in gene expression. A good example to give is the phosphorylation of the transcription factors, Cyclic AMP-Response Element Binding (CREB) protein, by kinases such as PKA or CaM Kinase. One of the target genes of CREB is phosphoenolpyruvate carboxykinase, an important gluconeogenic gene.

Parenthetically, one can point out the role of PKA in integrating metabolism with gene expression in that decreasing glycogen synthase activity, increasing phosphorylase activity as well as increasing gluconeogenesis results in increased availability of glucose to tissues.

12. Guanosine (G) Protein-Coupled Signaling Pathways

Students are now ready to consider the common G protein-coupled signaling pathways. This will give them a perspective on PKA and CaM kinase signaling. In brief, students should develop the concepts that there are several different Gαs: Gα stimulatory (G$_s$) that activates adenylate cyclase resulting in cAMP formation thereby promoting the activation of PKA; Gα inhibitory (G$_i$) that inhibits adenylate cyclase thereby decreasing cAMP levels and thereby decreasing PKA activity; and, G$_q$ that activates phospholipase C that acts on the membrane phospholipid phosphatidylinositol-4,5-bisphosphate resulting in the release of inositol-3,4,5-triphosphate (IP$_3$) and diacylglycerol.

Students should also learn that IP$_3$ induces release of Ca^{2+} from the endoplasmic reticular stores and one of the consequences is Ca^{2+} binding to calmodulin and thereby activating CaM kinase. If students have taken, or are taking, the cardiovascular system one can examine G protein-coupled signaling in the context of alpha and beta adrenergic signaling as well as angiotensin II signaling on vascular smooth muscle.

13. Other Signaling Pathways

Once the students are familiar with G protein-coupled signaling they should be introduced to the idea of other major signaling pathways such as receptor tyrosine kinases and mitogen-activated protein kinase cascades. They should be introduced to the concept that many of these signaling pathways converge onto intracellular kinase cascades known as mitogen-activated protein (MAP) kinases (Figure 10).

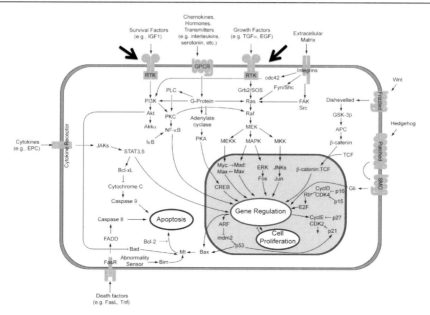

Image is in the public domain and taken from the Wikimedia Commons (http://en.wikipedia.org/wiki/ Cell_signaling). Author is Roadnottaken.

Figure 10. Diagram illustrating a number of signaling pathways. Students should focus on: i) receptor tyrosine kinase (RTK) family indicated by the arrow heads and ii) how many of the signaling pathways converge (indicated by yellow square) onto mitogen-activated protein (MAP) kinase pathways (represented in this diagram by ERK and JNKs). The MAP kinases ERK and Jun as well as p38 MAP kinase (not represented in this diagram) are regulated by upstream kinases as shown in Figure 14.

Students should be introduced to the concept that kinase signaling pathways occur in relatively localized areas of the cell. Students should be introduced to the concept that protein tyrosine kinases act as an off-on switch that involve the binding of adaptor proteins allowing interaction with other intracellular signaling pathways.

A consideration of insulin signaling [29] is a clinically relevant way to introduce the concepts of receptor tyrosine kinase and MAP kinase signaling (Figure 11). The concepts to be introduced include: ligand binding results in receptor dimerization followed by autophosphorylation of the intracellular domains that allows the subsequent phosphorylation and binding of adaptor proteins such as the insulin receptor substrate (IRS) proteins.

Activation of IRS results in activation of phosphoinositide-3-phosphate kinase (PI_3K). PI_3K then phosphorylates phosphatidylinositol-4,5-phosphate (PIP2) to phosphatidylinositol-3,4,5-phosphate (PIP3).

Amongst other actions, PIP3 results in activation of protein kinase B (PKB, also known as AKT). One of the results of PKB activation is movement of the glucose transporter-4 (Glut4) from endoplasmic reticular stores to the plasmalemma, hence promoting movement of glucose from extracellular fluids into skeletal muscle cells and adipocytes.

Another consequence of PKB activation is decreased gluconeogenesis that results in reduced glucose efflux from liver. Activated IRS will also interact with adaptor proteins that activate MAP kinase pathways that ultimately will influence transcription factor phosphorylation status and, thereby, gene transcription.

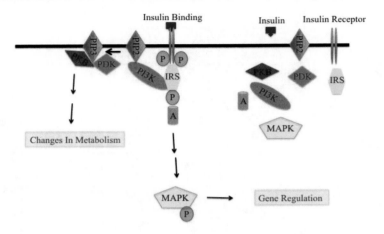

Figure 11. Schematic outlining several aspects of insulin signaling. To the right are some of the molecular players that include the dimeric insulin receptor, insulin, phosphatidylinositol-4,5-phosphate (PIP2), insulin receptor substrate protein (IRS), phosphoinositide-3-phosphate kinase (PI3K), phosphoinositide-dependent protein kinase (PDK), protein kinase B (PKB), any of a number of adapter proteins (A) and mitogen-activated protein kinase (MAPK). On the left is a demonstration that when insulin binds to its receptor it results in receptor autophosphorylation and subsequent phosphorylation and binding of IRS. The phosphorylated IRS binds and activates PI3K resulting in formation of PIP3 that leads to activation of PDK and PKB. Activation of PKB results in signaling cascades that results in changes in metabolism. Phosphorylated IRS also interacts with a variety of adaptor proteins (A) some of which will initiate a signaling cascade that activates MAP kinases that in turn alters the phosphorylation of transcription factors that will influence gene expression.

14. Kinase Actions Are Countered by Phosphatase Actions

The students should be introduced to the concept that kinase activities on tyrosine, serine and threonine are countered by phosphatase activities. Hence, the length of time insulin signaling occurs is dependent upon not only the spatiotemporal pattern of PI3 kinase and MAP kinase activities but also upon the spatiotemporal patterns of the corresponding phosphatase activities.

The simplest would be to build on previous examples and focus on the lipid phosphatase known as phosphatase and tensin homologue (PTEN) that converts PIP3 back to PIP2 and the protein tyrosine phosphatase PTB1B that dephosphorylates the insulin receptor and the insulin substrate proteins [30], thereby inhibiting insulin signaling.

The students should be made aware that at all levels of kinase cascades one has phosphatases countering the actions of kinases. Furthermore, phosphatases can be divided into two broad groups based upon their catalytic sites: the dimetal-based (Fe^{2+}, Mn^{2+} and/or Mg^{2+}) serine/threonine phosphatases [31] and the larger group of cysteine-based phosphatases [32, 33]. Both groups can be oxidized resulting in inactivation of their catalytic activities [33].

Students should be reminded that the initial oxidation of cysteine residues results in the formation of sulfenic acid residues that can be readily reduced back to thiols. The focus should be on the cysteine-based phosphatases involved in critical aspects of insulin signaling, PTEN and PTB1B.

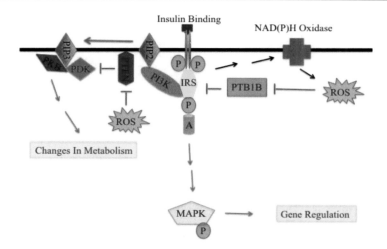

Figure 12. Protein phosphatases involved in the insulin signaling pathways include the lipid phosphatase PTEN that converts PIP3 back to PIP2, PTP1B that dephosphorylates the insulin receptor and IRS proteins as well as phosphatases that act downstream of PKB and the MAP kinase cascades (not shown). These phosphatases can be inactivated by oxidants. Also shown in this diagram is NAD(P)H oxidase that is activated in some yet unknown manner by insulin signaling. Activation of NAD(P)H oxidase results in oxidant production that prolongs the insulin signaling.

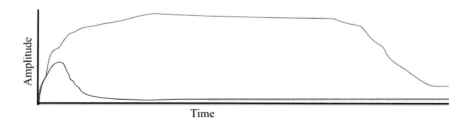

Figure 13. Influence of oxidative stress on kinase-dependent signaling. Increased oxidative stress converts normal signaling (black line) into an abnormal prolonged signaling with increased amplitude and with increased basal signaling activity (red line).

15. Oxidants and Insulin Signaling

Activation of the insulin receptor is linked in a yet unknown manner with activation of NAD(P)H oxidase [29, 34] resulting in localized production of superoxide anion that is dismutated to hydrogen peroxide (Figure 12).

Consequences of this include oxidation of critical thiolates in PTEN and PTB1B to sulfenic acid residues, thereby inactivating these phosphatases until their sulfenic acid residues are reduced back to thiolates. The inactivation of the phosphatases results in a prolongation of insulin signaling [29]. Concepts that should be emphasized include that signaling pathways such as the insulin pathways have both spatial and temporal localization. This should be followed by a discussion that an increase in oxidant production by the cell, or decreases in the capacity to scavenge oxidants, will distort signaling pathways that involve kinases as demonstrated in Figure (Figure 13).

Another possible consequence of increased oxidants is the oxidation of thiols in IRS resulting in the blocking of the insulin signaling pathways, perhaps the main mechanism whereby oxidative stress results in insulin resistance.

16. Oxidants and Non-Infectious Inflammation

The heterotrimeric transcription factor complex nuclear factor kappa B (NFκB) drives many of the inflammatory mechanisms [35]. It is activated, normally in response to signaling cascades (Figure 14), by phosphorylation of the inhibitory kappa B (IκB) subunit that then is polyubiquinated and proteasomally degraded allowing nuclear translocation of the p50/p65 heterodimer to the nucleus. The p50/p65 heterodimer binds to kappa B elements promoting transcription of the associated genes, mainly pro-inflammatory genes. Examples of pro-inflammatory genes include cell adhesion molecules that promote movement of leukocytes from blood into tissues, cytokines, chemokines, cyclooxygenase-2 (COX2) and inducible nitric oxide synthase (iNOS). The signaling cascades that can activate NFκB typically are initiated by Toll-like receptors or by cytokine receptors. Toll-like receptors interact with specific microorganismal macromolecules (e.g., lipopolysaccharide, double-stranded RNA) or with specific cell breakdown products; hence, Toll-like receptors are involved in the signaling associated with both infectious and non-infectious inflammation (e.g., after tissue damage). This is an appropriate time in the curriculum to introduce the concepts of innate immunity and non-infectious inflammation. One can introduce the concept that oxidants also cause activation of NFκB [36], likely through inactivation of phosphatases in the signaling cascades that result in phosphorylating IκB. What should be emphasized is that oxidative stress lowers the set-point at which NFκB pathway is activated.

NFκB Is Central In Inflammation

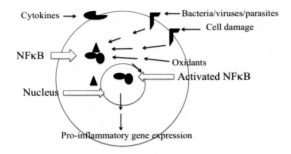

Figure 14. The heterotrimeric nuclear Factor kappa B (NFκB) plays a central role in inflammation. Activation of NFκB is initiated by phosphorylation of the I kappa B (IκB) member of the heterotrimer resulting in polyubiquination and degradation of IκB allowing the p50/p65 heterodimer to translocate to the nucleus promoting the expression of genes with kappa B elements in their promoter regions - these are mostly pro-inflammatory genes. Normally, NFκB is activated in response to Toll-like receptor activation by microorganism macromolecules and/or cell damage products or by cytokine receptor activation. However, oxidative stress, likely by inactivating protein phosphatases, can also activate NFκB.

17. Eicosanoids and Inflammation

A brief overview should be given of eicosanoids (Figure 15) that can be produced through the action of enzyme on prostaglandin H_2 (PGH$_2$) [37]. It should be pointed out that the receptors for eicosanoids are G-protein coupled and that the consequences of activation of such receptors are context-dependent; however, very often activation of eicosanoid receptors promotes inflammation.

It should also be pointed out that eicosanoids are important in certain non-inflammatory contexts. A good example to give is the effect of PGE$_2$ in promoting mucin production by stomach enterocytes. Critical concept to put across in the formation of eicosanoids is the release of arachidonic acid from the SN-2 position of membrane phospholipids by the calcium-dependent phospholipase A$_2$ (PLA$_2$). Arachidonic acid is then acted upon by cyclooxygenase (Cox) 1 or 2 to form PGH$_2$. One mechanism whereby glucocorticoids have a potent anti-inflammatory action is through promotion of expression of lipocortin-1 that inhibits the activity of PLA$_2$. The major action of non-steroidal anti-inflammatory drugs (NSAIDs) is to block Cox activity. It should be pointed out to students that although Cox2 is inducible in response to NFκB activation, it is constitutively expressed in a few locations, e.g., the macula densa of the kidney. It should become apparent to students that blocking Cox1 activity through the use of NSAIDs may have untoward effects on the stomach and that blocking Cox2 activity may have untoward effects on blood pressure.

18. Xenobiotic Metabolism

This may be an opportune time in the curriculum to consider essential aspects of xenobiotic metabolism where students consider how the body deals with the myriad of complex chemicals that we consume, particularly phytochemicals and how the body deals with prescribed and non-prescribed drugs that are taken in. Although this is a complex topic, at this stage in the curriculum one must strive to keep it simple.

Students should realize by now that hydrophilic compounds are simply excreted by the kidneys whilst it is a more complicated matter to deal with the majority of xenobiotics that are hydrophobic. The essential concept to be grasped is that somehow the hydrophobic compound must be made hydrophilic so that they can be excreted by the kidneys. Students should be introduced to the concept of phase 1 enzymes (mainly cytochrome P450s) that convert hydrophobic compounds into either electrophilic or nucleophilic reactive forms and phase 2 enzymes that convert the reactive compounds into an innocuous water soluble form by forming glutathiyl, acetyl, glucoronosyl or sulfate adducts (Figure 15).

19. Nuclear Factor (Erythroid-Derived 2)-Like-2 (Nrf2) and the Anti-Oxidant Defense System

The Nrf2 signalling system plays an important role in health. Students should now be introduced to the concept that the phase 2 enzymes involved in xenobiotic metabolism have an anti-oxidant response element (ARE) in their promoter regions.

Synthesis of Prostanoids

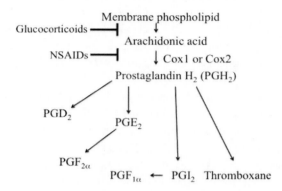

Figure 14. Schematic of eicosanoid synthesis. This pathway starts off by the release of arachidonic acid from the SN-2 position of membrane phospholipids through the action of the calcium-dependent phospholipase A_2 (PLA$_2$). The released arachidonic acid is then acted upon by cyclooxygenase 1 or 2 (Cox1 or Cox2) to give rise to prostaglandin H_2 (PGH$_2$) that in turn is acted upon by downstream enzymes to give rise to a number of eicosanoids, many of which promote inflammation. Which specific eicosanoids are synthesized is dependent upon the enzymes present in the cell. The anti-inflammatory action of glucocorticoids are mediated to a great extent through inhibition of release of arachidonic acid while the non-steroidal anti-inflammatory drugs act mainly by inhibiting the activity of Cox1 and Cox2.

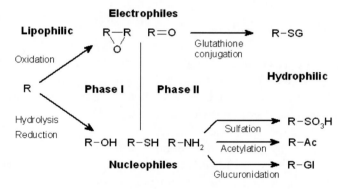

The author is TimVickers. Website is: http://en.wikipedia.org/wiki/Drug_metabolism.

Figure 15. Diagram illustrating the two phases of xenobiotic metabolism. This diagram is taken from the Wikimedia Commons and is in the public domain.

Binding of AREs by the transcription factor complex comprised of Nrf2 and small Maf proteins promotes transcription of the involved genes [38].

Nrf2 is normally bound by Kelch-like ECH protein 1 (Keap1) to the actin cytoskeleton. Oxidation of Keap1 thiols results in release of Nrf2 allowing translocation to the nucleus where it heterodimerizes with small Maf proteins resulting in binding to AREs (Figure 16).

A large number of genes contain AREs – for references see [39]. These include both the regulatory and catalytic subunits of γ-glutamylcysteine ligase (GCL), the rate-limiting enzyme for GSH synthesis. Other GSH-related genes also contain AREs in their promoter regions: these include: the cystine-glutamate antiporter that is the main mechanism taking up cystine into cells (cystine is then reduced to cysteine, the rate-limiting amino acid in GSH synthesis); glutathione reductase that reduces oxidized-glutathione back to GSH; glucose-6-phosphate dehydrogenase that provides the NADPH necessary for glutathione reductase action; the glutathione S-transferases that inactivate a variety of electrophiles by forming glutathiyl adducts; the selenoprotein glutathione peroxidase-2 that uses GSH as an electron donor to convert the reactive hydroperoxides to inactive alcohols or water and molecular oxygen in the case of hydrogen peroxide; and peroxiredoxin-1, 3 and 5 that are GSH-dependent enzymes that convert alkylhydroperoxides to inactive alcohols.

AREs are also found in ferritin H and L chains that sequester redox-active iron as Fe^{3+}; metallothioneins that sequester other redox active metal ions such as copper; and thioredoxin reductases, important in regulating protein thiol redox status.

Students should now appreciate the commonalities in how the cells deal with xenobiotics and oxidants and that activation of Nrf2 will decrease oxidative stress via many endogenous mechanisms [40]. The concept that should be emphasized is that most protein products of genes that have an ARE in their promoter site either promote scavenging of oxidants or decrease the likelihood of oxidant formation; hence, activation of Nrf2 leads to a reduction in oxidative stress.

20. Aging Is Associated with a Decline in the Anti-Oxidant Defense System

Students should be introduced to the concept that the GSH-dependent anti-oxidant defense system normally declines with age (Figure 17), references in [39]. This appears, to a great extent, to be due to decreased activation of Nrf2 [41].

This decline is associated with increased oxidative stress and generalized inflammation and, thus, associated health problems. Students should be introduced to the concept that decreasing oxidative stress and inflammation will lead to healthier aging.

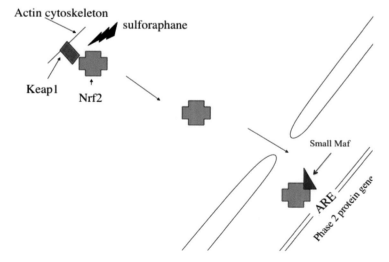

Figure 16. Cartoon showing how compounds such as sulforaphane cause oxidation of Keap1 thiols allowing translocation of Nr2 to the nucleus where it can dimerize with small Maf proteins, thereby promoting expression of genes with AREs in their promoter regions.

Relationships Amongst GSH, Oxistress & Age

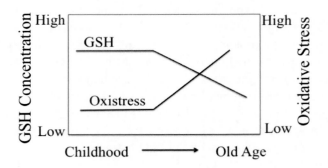

Figure 17. Graph schematically representing the typical decline in the average person of tissue GSH levels from around the forties onwards and the associated increase in oxidative stress.

21. The Lipid Peroxidation Cascade

Students should be introduced to the concept that one of the consequences of oxidative stress is a lipid peroxidation cascade whereby polyunsaturated fatty acids in membrane phospholipids are oxidized forming lipid hydroperoxides (Figure 18). This is initiated by the presence of a strong oxidant such as the hydroxyl radical and requires molecular oxygen. It should be pointed out to students that free transition metal ions such as Fe^{2+} will be localized at anionic sites such as the phosphate groups of phospholipids, i.e., where the most damage can be done when forming the hydroxyl radical from hydrogen peroxide. Lipid peroxidation increases membrane permeability, inactivates critical membrane proteins and results in the formation of strong lipid oxidants and pro-inflammatory lipid molecules. The roles of vitamin C, vitamin E and glutathione-dependent processes in preventing lipid peroxidation should be reviewed [40] – see Figure 18.

22. Adipose Tissue Is an Endocrine Gland

Students should be introduced to the concepts of brown and white adipose tissues and that adipose, particularly white, tissue is an endocrine gland [42]. A brief review of the known roles of adipokines should be given: The role of leptin in appetite control, adiponectin on insulin sensitivity and resistin in the promotion of inflammation [43].

This should be followed by a brief discussion on body mass index (BMI) [44] and the physiological differences between visceral fat as opposed to subcutaneous fat. Larger adipocytes secrete more pro-inflammatory cytokines than smaller adipocytes [45] and visceral fat tissues secretes significantly more adipokines as well as cytokines such as interleukin 6 (IL6) than somatic fat and, thus, increased fat deposition, particularly in visceral adipose tissue, promotes generalized inflammation [46] as well as insulin resistance [47].

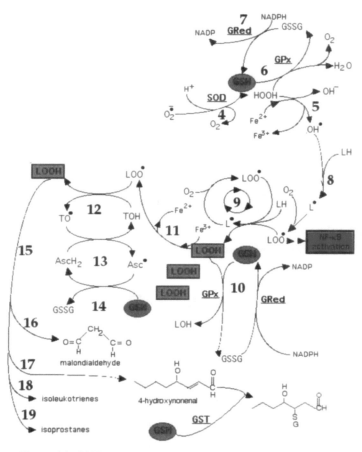

Figure adapted from Figure 1 in [40].

Figure 18. Lipid peroxidation is initiated in the presence of a strong oxidant like the hydroxyl radical (step 8) and once initiated continues as long is there is molecular oxygen and unsaturated fatty acids (LH) forming lipid hydroperoxides (LOOH). The lipid hydroperoxides formed can break down to other oxidants as well as pro-inflammatory lipid molecules. Vitamin E (TOH) plays an important role in inactivating the lipid peroxyl radicals (LOO·) formed (step 12) and ascorbic acid ($AscH_2$) reduces the oxidized vitamin E (step 13) while GSH reduces the oxidized ascorbate (step 14). It is clear from these sets of reactions that vitamins E and C play important but limited roles in inhibiting lipid peroxidation. As important is the scavenging of the lipid hydroperoxides by glutathione peroxidase and peroxiredoxins (step 10). Also included in this diagram are the roles of superoxide dismutases (step 4), glutathione reductase (steps 7 and 10) in these oxidant scavenging processes.

23. Excessive Caloric Intake Is Associated with Oxidative Stress and Inflammation As Well As Obesity

Students should be reminded that much of the energy captured from foodstuffs is funneled mainly to the reduction of NAD^+ and FAD (Figure 19). An important concept is that one consequence in having a larger caloric intake than output is that an increased proportion of NAD^+ and FAD is in the reduced form resulting in a saturation of the mitochondrial electron transport carriers resulting in increased superoxide production [28].

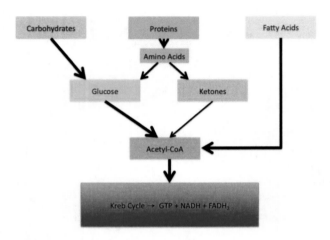

Figure 19. Much of the energy captured from foodstuffs is funneled mainly to the reduction of NAD^+ and FAD.

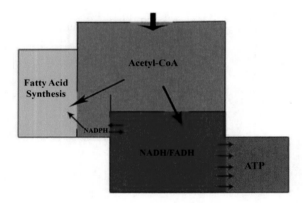

Figure 20. Cartoon depicting, in the presence of energy-providing nutrients, how when cellular levels of ATP levels are high acetyl-CoA levels rise and the electrons present in NADH are used to reduce $NADP^+$ resulting in high levels of NADPH. High levels of NADPH and high levels of acetyl-CoA promote fat synthesis in liver and fat tissue.

This increased oxidative stress promotes inflammation through a number of mechanisms including activation of NFκB.

Another consequence of the increased proportion reducing equivalents is that transhydrogenases will promote increased reduction of $NADP^+$ that in turn promotes lipid synthesis (Figure 20), thereby, promoting obesity. This is an opportune time in the curriculum to consider essential aspects of fatty acid synthesis.

As noted previously, adipose tissue, particularly visceral adipose tissue, drives inflammation and insulin resistance through the secretion of pro-inflammatory cytokines.

24. Hyperglycemia, Oxidative Stress and Inflammation

At some point the students should be introduced to the concept that carbonyls are reactive groups and that carbonyls are found in aldose and ketose sugars. Since many organs are very dependent upon glucose for a energy source, the body has an interesting problem since glucose must attain a certain level in the blood to adequately supply organs mainly dependent upon glucose but not so high as to exacerbate the problem of carbonyls reacting with other macromolecules, particularly proteins. This is an opportune time in the curriculum to consider glucose transport and the type of transporters required if glucose is to be taken up against its concentration gradient or down its concentration gradient. The formation of advanced glycation endproducts (AGEs) by glucose and derivatives should also be considered.

Formation of AGEs results in inactivation of the proteins involved and, as well, the AGEs form ligands for the receptor for advanced glycation endproducts (RAGE) [48]. Activation of RAGE activates NAD(P)H oxidase resulting in increased oxidative stress (Figure 21).

Increased oxidative stress promotes the formation of dicarbonyls (α-oxoaldehydes) from glucose and other sugars [49]. Dicarbonyls are powerful oxidants that increase the amount of oxidative damage including increased formation of AGEs. Students should be beginning to appreciate that there are many positive feedback loops involving oxidative stress and inflammation. Dicarbonyls are scavenged using the GSH-dependent glyoxalase system [50]. Students should be introduced to the concept that measuring the percentage of hemoglobin glycated (HbA1c) is a good index of blood glucose control history with normal levels being between 4 and 5.9%.

25. Plasma Glucose Homeostasis and Carbohydrate Digestion

Students now appreciate that plasma glucose levels should be maintained around 5 mM allowing a sufficient concentration gradient to allow flow into cells but not much higher since this increases AGE formation. Glucose levels are determined by glucose inflow into the plasma via gluconeogenesis and uptake from the gut versus outflow to cells (Figure 22).

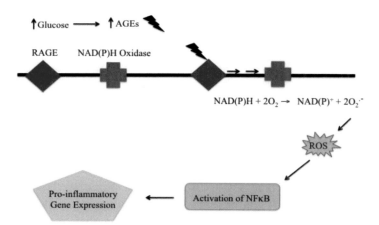

Figure 21. Diagram illustrating the relationship between the Receptor of Advanced Glycation Endproducts (RAGE) and NAD(P)H oxidase. Increasing glucose concentration increases the formation of Advanced Glycation Endproducts (AGEs). AGEs form ligands for RAGE and activation of RAGE results in activation of NAD(P)H oxidase resulting in the formation of superoxide anions that dismutate to other reactive oxygen species (ROS). Amongst the consequences of the increase in oxidative stress is the activation of NFκB that increases pro-inflammatory gene expression.

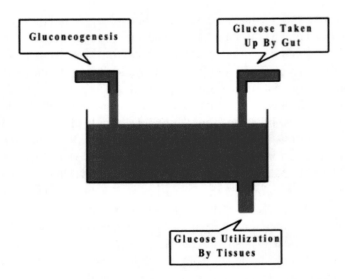

Figure 22. Cartoon illustrating the major components that determine blood glucose levels: these are glucose entry into the blood and glucose exit from the blood. Glucose enters either as newly formed glucose (either via phosphorylase activity or gluconeogenesis) from liver and kidneys or from glucose absorbed by the small intestine. Glucose leaves the blood to enter tissues and this is driven by tissue glucose utilization. In healthy persons glucose entry into and exit from the blood is well balanced.

This is an opportune time in the curriculum to consider gluconeogenesis and the role of the pancreatic islet cells in plasma glucose homeostasis. Students should be reminded of how oxidative stress disrupts insulin signaling and the consequences on plasma glucose control. It is also a good time in the curriculum to consider how carbohydrate intake and digestion influences postprandial blood glucose levels. In particular the role of soluble fibres on chyme viscosity and how this influences digestion and movement of small nutrients to the apical surface of the enterocytes. Furthermore, there should be some emphasis on the fact that the unbranched amylose starch is much more slowly digested than the branched amylopectin starch and that simple sugars such as sucrose are quickly digested and taken up. There should be some discussion on glycemic index and glycemic loads [51], and their significance in chronic diseases. There should be some discussion on the low glycemic index of legumes [52] due to their high amylose contents as well as their content of α-amylase inhibitors.

26. Regulators of Appetite

Excessive caloric intake increases oxidative stress directly though mitochondrial superoxide formation or indirectly via increases in fat tissue, particularly visceral fat tissue. Excessive adipose tissue increases generalized inflammation that is also associated with increased oxidant production. A balance between caloric intake and caloric output is determined by the nature of the foods taken in, the quantity of foods taken in (governed by appetite) and by energy utilization, mainly through physical activity. For most people the regulation of appetite plays a more important role than physical activity in balancing caloric intake versus caloric output. Knowledge of the regulators of appetite [53] should form a very important part of the medical curriculum. Specifically, the role of the appetite suppressants including the adipokine leptin and the intestinal peptides cholycystokinin, pancreatic polypeptide, peptide tyrosine-tyrosine, glucagon-like peptide-1 (GLP1) both through a direct CNS effect and through ileal braking and oxyntomodulin. All these are peptides are released by the presence of small nutrients from different regions of the gut. The appetite stimulant ghrelin released in response to lack of gastrin inhibiting signals. Gastrin secretion is stimulated by distension of the stomach and by the presence of amino acids and peptides in the stomach. The key to decreasing food intake is to consume foods that are slowly digested since this allows longer release of appetite suppressors. Students should be introduced to the glycemic index and glycemic load of commonly consumed foods [54].

There should be a review of other factors that influence the rate of digestions. For example, intake of insoluble fibres decreases nutrient concentrations thereby decreasing the rate of digestion; soluble fibres increase viscosity, again decreasing the rate of digestions and uptake of nutrients (as well as promote the presence of beneficial gut bacteria); and increased consumption of amylose starch relative to amylopectin starch. Such a diet not only prolongs the feelings of satiety but also decreases the postprandial plasma glucose spikes.

27. Dietary Nrf2 Activators to Decrease Oxidative Stress and Inflammation

In *Section 26* students have already begun to consider aspects of diet that prolong feelings of satiety and thus decrease the probability of obesity. They have also considered how such changes to diet decrease the postprandial glucose spikes. They have also considered the role of Nrf2 in regulating the endogenous anti-oxidant defense systems. There should be some consideration given to dietary sources of Nrf2 activators and how diet can promote the expression of endogenous anti-oxidant defense systems and thereby decreases oxidative stress and inflammation [38-40]. The effect of dietary Nrf2 activators is conceptually illustrated in Figure 23.

28. Increasing Consumption of Omega-3 Polyunsaturated Fatty Acids to Decrease the Inflammatory Environment

Students are already familiar with the roles of PLA_2 and COX enzymatic activity in inflammation. They should be introduced to the idea that increased consumption of omega-3 polyunsaturated fatty acids (PUFAs) will decrease generalized inflammation [55]. This is an opportune moment to consider the incorporation of fatty acids into phospholipids, with the SN-1 position typically occupied by a saturated fatty acid residue while the SN-2 position is typically occupied by an unsaturated fatty acid residue.

Which fatty acid gets incorporated is very dependent upon the cellular fatty acid profile that in turn is very dependent upon dietary intake of fatty acids. Hence, the SN-2 position although commonly occupied by an omega-6 PUFA (e.g., the 20-carbon arachidonic acid), may also be occupied by an omega-3 PUFA (e.g., the 20-carbon eicosapentaenoic acid [EPA] or the 22-carbon docosahexaenoic acid [DHA]).

The typical Western diet has a dietary intake ratio of omega-6 to omega-3 of around 15:1 whereas the ideal ratio should be 1:1 [56].

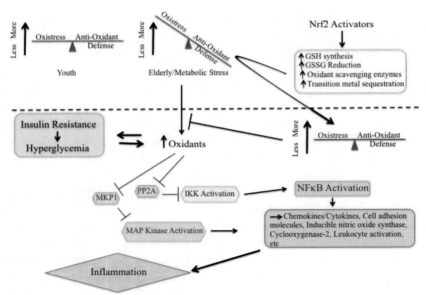

This diagram is modified from Figure 1 in [39].

Figure 23. Diagram illustrating how consumption of dietary Nrf2 activators by promoting the endogenous anti-oxidant defense systems can decrease oxidative stress and thereby decrease insulin resistance and generalized inflammation. PP2A and MKP1 are protein phosphatases. Phosphorylation of IKK (I kappa B kinase) results in IKK phosphorylating I kappa B, thus activating NFκB.

COX will also act upon omega-3 PUFAs and the resulting eicosanoids produced, termed resolvins, have anti-inflammatory properties [57]. Decreasing the ratio of omega-6 to omega-3 at the SN-2 position will decrease the probability of the development of generalized inflammation in response to stimuli that result in the activation of PLA_2. Furthermore, omega-3 fatty acids will also bind and activate the G protein-coupled receptor GPR120 resulting in anti-inflammatory and insulin-sensitizing actions [58].

Hence, an important part of the curriculum should be a review of the common dietary sources of omega-6 PUFAs and omega-3 PUFAs as well as the conversion of the 18-carbon omega-6 linoleic acid into arachidonic acid as well as the 18-carbon α-linolenic omega-6 into EPA and DHA. There should be some consideration given to dietary sources of omega-3 and omega-6 PUFAs [59].

29. Increasing Physical Exercise to Decrease Oxidative Stress and Inflammation

Even 15 minutes per day of moderate physical activity increases lifespan by 3 years [60], emphasizing the importance of physical activity. There is an abundance of evidence demonstrating that exercise improves insulin sensitivity and decreases the probability of developing type 2 diabetes [61] as well as other health effects, including improving blood pressure. There also is an abundance of literature demonstrating that exercise decreases generalized inflammation associated with aging [62]. Why exercise decreases generalized inflammation and improves insulin sensitivity is likely multifactorial.

One obvious factor is that exercise has the potential to decrease adipose tissue; however, actively working muscle also release factors that play a role in this. Indeed there is considerable evidence that muscle secretes a variety of factors, both when inactive and when active [63]. Such factors have been termed myokines.

One of the factors is interleukin-6 (IL6). IL6 normally is thought of as an inflammatory cytokines. This is an opportune time to discuss that active muscle secretes elevated levels of IL6 that improves insulin sensitivity but results in low plasma levels of IL6 - that reduces generalized inflammation - when muscles are at rest. Why IL6 has differing effects depending upon plasma concentration is not known but may be due to interacting with receptors of differing affinities.

This is also an opportune time to review adipokines and the role that adiponectin secreted by small adipocytes plays in promoting insulin sensitivity. What is most important is that students realize that skeletal muscle, whether inactive or active, secretes factors that influence the metabolism and gene expression of non-muscle tissues and that active muscles promote health, this is particularly important in this age when most activities are sedentary.

FINAL COMMENTS

What one must strive for in the medical curriculum is the development of independent learners. In any curriculum it is critically important to actively engage the student's minds. Although didactic lectures are an efficient way to transfer information it can too easily become mind numbing. It is important that problems are posed and questions asked to keep the students' minds active.

It is also important for the student to become engaged from the beginning in solving clinically-relevant problems, ideally in small group settings that facilitate discussions amongst the group. This engagement of the students with the topics being covered will lead not only to a curiosity about how the body and mind functions but also to a realization that although much is still unknown, they (the students) have the intellectual ability to add to our body of knowledge. When nurtured, this realization is quickly followed by a desire to contribute to our body of knowledge.

In the College of Medicine at Alfaisal University - through the promotion of active learning involving solving clinically-relevant problems, introduction to research and by promoting a research atmosphere - the majority of our medical students have developed the desire to make a contribution to our body of knowledge. The students have taken an active role in promoting research and with assistance from faculty have developed a student-run Undergraduate Research Committee that runs several programs including the Summer Program for International Research and Training or SPIRIT, Local Research Training Program, Knowledge Dissemination Program, Assessment and Development Program and a Recognition and Awarding Program [64]. The Undergraduate Research Committee not only identifies possible summer research positions locally as well as abroad, it also und raises to give some financial support for students going abroad to carry our research. The ability to add to our body of knowledge is not only most satisfying to the student but this experience further promotes the integration of concepts and stimulates the development of critical thinking skills [65] that are necessary to become effective physicians.

CONCLUSION

In the development of concepts it is important that students are given problems whereby they must use the knowledge that they are gaining. The topics listed above ought to better prepare students for the biomedical bases of chronic diseases. Undoubtedly, the list and sequence of topics can be improved. There are many topics that have not been covered, for example the role of stress in increasing plasma cortisol concentrations [66, 67] and that increased cortisol promotes gluconeogenesis [68] that, in turn, can increase plasma glucose levels, thereby increasing AGE formation and resultant oxidative stress. Nor have the mutations that involve glucose-6-phosphate dehydrogenase been considered and how such mutations influence the ability to cope with oxidative stress and how this may influence malarial infections. Nor the fact that there are likely epigenetic changes underlying chronic diseases and that such epigenetic changes may be reversed through alterations in diet [69].

Nevertheless, students that have developed the above concepts ought to readily learn additional concepts when clinically-relevant problems arise.

ACKNOWLEDGMENTS

The challenges of starting a new medical school with only a few faculty in the beginning results in one (BHJJ) teaching many new topics, resulting in new and broader perspectives. Furthermore, the development of a curriculum *de novo* and the discussions involved in this activity causes one to reflect more deeply on the essential biomedical information a student should encounter. In the development of the curriculum it became obvious that the commonalities in the drivers of chronic diseases are typically poorly dealt with. BHJJ thank the medical students at Alfaisal University for allowing me to develop ideas on how to introduce fundamental concepts in the medical curriculum that will better enable students to understand and treat chronic diseases. I have never encountered students that were so keen to make a contribution to our body of knowledge through research and publication.

REFERENCES

[1]   Torre, D. M., Durning, S. J., Daley, B. J. Twelve tips for teaching with concept maps in medical education. *Medical teacher*. 2013;35:201-8.

[2]   Mayer, R. S., Shah, A. A., de Lateur, B. J., Thomas, P. A. Chronic disease and disability for medical students. In: Kern, D. E., Thomas, P. A., Hughes, M. T., editors. *Curriculum Development for Medical Education A Six-Step Approach*. Baltimore, MD: Johns Hopkins University Press; 2009. p. 184-200.

[3]   Holman, H. Chronic disease--the need for a new clinical education. *JAMA: the journal of the American Medical Association*. 2004;292:1057-9.

[4]   Libby, P. Inflammation in atherosclerosis. *Arteriosclerosis, thrombosis, and vascular biology*. 2012;32:2045-51.

[5]   Dolan, H., Crain, B., Troncoso, J., Resnick, S. M., Zonderman, A. B., Obrien, R. J. Atherosclerosis, dementia, and Alzheimer disease in the Baltimore Longitudinal Study of Aging cohort. *Annals of neurology.* 2010;68:231-40.

[6]   Roher, A. E., Tyas, S. L., Maarouf, C. L., Daugs, I. D., Kokjohn, T. A., Emmerling, M. R., et al. Intracranial atherosclerosis as a contributing factor to Alzheimer's disease dementia. *Alzheimer's and dementia: the journal of the Alzheimer's Association.* 2011; 7:436-44.

[7]   Hald, E. M., Lijfering, W. M., Mathiesen, E. B., Johnsen, S. H., Lochen, M. L., Njolstad, I., et al. Carotid atherosclerosis predicts future myocardial infarction but not venous thromboembolism: the Tromso study. *Arteriosclerosis, thrombosis, and vascular biology.* 2014;34:226-30.

[8]   Ohira, T., Shahar, E., Iso, H., Chambless, L. E., Rosamond, W. D., Sharrett, A. R., et al. Carotid artery wall thickness and risk of stroke subtypes: the atherosclerosis risk in communities study. *Stroke; a journal of cerebral circulation.* 2011;42:397-403.

[9]   Androulakis, E., Tousoulis, D., Papageorgiou, N., Latsios, G., Siasos, G., Tsioufis, C., et al. Inflammation in hypertension: current therapeutic approaches. *Current pharmaceutical design.* 2011;17:4121-31.

[10]   Sharp, S. I., Aarsland, D., Day, S., Sonnesyn, H., Alzheimer's Society Vascular Dementia Systematic Review G, Ballard C. Hypertension is a potential risk factor for vascular dementia: systematic review. *International journal of geriatric psychiatry.* 2011;26:661-9.

[11]   Chen, Y. C., Sun, C. A., Yang, T., Chu, C. H., Bai, C. H., You, S. L., et al. Impact of metabolic syndrome components on incident stroke subtypes: a Chinese cohort study. *Journal of human hypertension.* 2014.

[12]   Feldstein, C. A. Early treatment of hypertension in acute ischemic and intracerebral hemorrhagic stroke: Progress achieved, challenges, and perspectives. *Journal of the American Society of Hypertension: JASH.* 2014;8:192-202.

[13]   Serpente, M., Bonsi, R., Scarpini, E., Galimberti, D. Innate immune system and inflammation in Alzheimer's disease: from pathogenesis to treatment. *Neuroimmunomodulation.* 2014;21:79-87.

[14]   Eguchi, K., Manabe, I. Macrophages and islet inflammation in type 2 diabetes. *Diabetes, obesity and metabolism.* 2013;15 Suppl. 3:152-8.

[15]   Esteve, E., Ricart, W., Fernandez-Real, J. M. Dyslipidemia and inflammation: an evolutionary conserved mechanism. *Clinical nutrition.* 2005;24:16-31.

[16]   Ruiz, S., Pergola, P. E., Zager, R. A., Vaziri, N. D. Targeting the transcription factor Nrf2 to ameliorate oxidative stress and inflammation in chronic kidney disease. *Kidney international.* 2013;83:1029-41.

[17]   McLean, R. R. Proinflammatory cytokines and osteoporosis. *Current osteoporosis reports.* 2009;7:134-9.

[18]   Xu, H. Obesity and metabolic inflammation. *Drug discovery today Disease mechanisms.* 2013;10.

[19]   Potenza, M. V., Mechanick, J. I. The metabolic syndrome: definition, global impact, and pathophysiology. *Nutr. Clin. Pract.* 2009;24:560-77.

[20]   Riediger, N. D., Clara, I. Prevalence of metabolic syndrome in the Canadian adult population. *CMAJ.* 2011;183:E1127-34.

[21]   Marquez-Sandoval, F., Macedo-Ojeda, G., Viramontes-Horner, D., Fernandez Ballart, J. D., Salas Salvado, J., Vizmanos, B. The prevalence of metabolic syndrome in Latin America: a systematic review. *Public Health Nutr*. 2011;14:1702-13.

[22]   Ravikiran, M., Bhansali, A., Ravikumar, P., Bhansali, S., Dutta, P., Thakur, J. S., et al. Prevalence and risk factors of metabolic syndrome among Asian Indians: a community survey. *Diabetes Res. Clin. Pract*. 2010;89:181-8.

[23]   Shah, A., Mehta, N., Reilly, M. P. Adipose inflammation, insulin resistance, and cardiovascular disease. *JPEN J. Parenter Enteral Nutr*. 2008;32:638-44.

[24]   Troseid, M., Seljeflot, I., Arnesen, H. The role of interleukin-18 in the metabolic syndrome. *Cardiovasc. Diabetol*. 2010;9:11.

[25]   Reaven, G. M. The insulin resistance syndrome: definition and dietary approaches to treatment. *Annual review of nutrition*. 2005;25:391-406.

[26]   Ruiz-Nunez, B., Pruimboom, L., Dijck-Brouwer, D. A., Muskiet, F. A. Lifestyle and nutritional imbalances associated with Western diseases: causes and consequences of chronic systemic low-grade inflammation in an evolutionary context. *The Journal of nutritional biochemistry*. 2013;24:1183-201.

[27]   Juurlink, B. H. J. Cell biology/histology can be the facilitator for integrating biomedical sciences in the medical curriculum. In: Ganguly, P., editor. *Education In Anatomical Sciences*. New York: Nova Science Publishers; 2013. p. 101-12.

[28]   Fisher-Wellman, K. H., Neufer, P. D. Linking mitochondrial bioenergetics to insulin resistance via redox biology. *Trends in endocrinology and metabolism: TEM*. 2012;23: 142-53.

[29]   Bashan, N., Kovsan, J., Kachko, I., Ovadia, H., Rudich, A. Positive and negative regulation of insulin signaling by reactive oxygen and nitrogen species. *Physiological reviews*. 2009;89:27-71.

[30]   Wu, X., Williams, K. J. NOX4 pathway as a source of selective insulin resistance and responsiveness. *Arteriosclerosis, thrombosis, and vascular biology*. 2012;32:1236-45.

[31]   Shi Y. Serine/threonine phosphatases: mechanism through structure. *Cell*. 2009;139: 468-84.

[32]   Tonks, N. K. Protein tyrosine phosphatases--from housekeeping enzymes to master regulators of signal transduction. *The FEBS journal*. 2013;280:346-78.

[33]   Salmeen, A., Barford, D. Functions and mechanisms of redox regulation of cysteine-based phosphatases. *Antioxidants and redox signaling*. 2005;7:560-77.

[34]   Mahadev, K., Motoshima, H., Wu, X., Ruddy, J. M., Arnold, R. S., Cheng, G., et al. The NAD(P)H oxidase homolog Nox4 modulates insulin-stimulated generation of H2O2 and plays an integral role in insulin signal transduction. *Molecular and cellular biology*. 2004;24:1844-54.

[35]   Christman, J. W., Lancaster, L. H., Blackwell, T. S. Nuclear factor kappa B: a pivotal role in the systemic inflammatory response syndrome and new target for therapy. *Intensive care medicine*. 1998;24:1131-8.

[36]   Christman, J. W., Blackwell, T. S., Juurlink, B. H. Redox regulation of nuclear factor kappa B: therapeutic potential for attenuating inflammatory responses. *Brain pathology*. 2000;10:153-62.

[37]   Khanapure, S. P., Garvey, D. S., Janero, D. R., Letts, L. G. Eicosanoids in inflammation: biosynthesis, pharmacology, and therapeutic frontiers. *Current topics in medicinal chemistry*. 2007;7:311-40.

[38] Kensler, T. W., Egner, P. A., Agyeman, A. S., Visvanathan, K., Groopman, J. D., Chen, J. G., et al. Keap1-nrf2 signaling: a target for cancer prevention by sulforaphane. *Topics in current chemistry.* 2013;329:163-77.

[39] Juurlink, B. H. Dietary Nrf2 activators inhibit atherogenic processes. *Atherosclerosis.* 2012;225:29-33.

[40] Juurlink, B. H. Therapeutic potential of dietary phase 2 enzyme inducers in ameliorating diseases that have an underlying inflammatory component. *Canadian journal of physiology and pharmacology.* 2001;79:266-82.

[41] Ungvari, Z., Bailey-Downs, L., Gautam, T., Sosnowska, D., Wang, M., Monticone, R. E., et al. Age-associated vascular oxidative stress, Nrf2 dysfunction, and NF-{kappa}B activation in the nonhuman primate Macaca mulatta. *The journals of gerontology Series A, Biological sciences and medical sciences.* 2011;66:866-75.

[42] Fietta, P., Delsante, G. Focus on adipokines. *Theoretical biology forum.* 2013;106: 103-29.

[43] Jung, U. J., Choi, M. S. Obesity and Its Metabolic Complications: The Role of Adipokines and the Relationship between Obesity, Inflammation, Insulin Resistance, Dyslipidemia and Nonalcoholic Fatty Liver Disease. *International journal of molecular sciences.* 2014;15:6184-223.

[44] Muller, M. J., Lagerpusch, M., Enderle, J., Schautz, B., Heller, M., Bosy-Westphal, A. Beyond the body mass index: tracking body composition in the pathogenesis of obesity and the metabolic syndrome. *Obesity reviews: an official journal of the International Association for the Study of Obesity.* 2012;13 Suppl. 2:6-13.

[45] Tejero, M. E., Proffitt, J. M., Rodriguez, I. P., Hubbard, G., Freeland-Graves, J. H., Peebles, K. W., et al. Adipokine expression is associated with adipocyte volume in baboons. *Cytokine.* 2008;41:150-4.

[46] Fontana, L., Eagon, J. C., Trujillo, M. E., Scherer, P. E., Klein, S. Visceral fat adipokine secretion is associated with systemic inflammation in obese humans. *Diabetes.* 2007;56:1010-3.

[47] Kwon, H., Pessin, J. E. Adipokines mediate inflammation and insulin resistance. *Frontiers in endocrinology.* 2013;4:71.

[48] Ramasamy, R., Yan, S. F., Schmidt, A. M. Advanced glycation endproducts: from precursors to RAGE: round and round we go. *Amino acids.* 2012;42:1151-61.

[49] Abordo, E. A., Minhas, H. S., Thornalley, P. J. Accumulation of alpha-oxoaldehydes during oxidative stress: a role in cytotoxicity. *Biochemical pharmacology.* 1999;58: 641-8.

[50] Thornalley, P. J. Glutathione-dependent detoxification of alpha-oxoaldehydes by the glyoxalase system: involvement in disease mechanisms and antiproliferative activity of glyoxalase I inhibitors. *Chemico-biological interactions.* 1998;111-112:137-51.

[51] Esfahani, A., Wong, J. M., Mirrahimi, A., Srichaikul, K., Jenkins, D. J., Kendall, C. W. The glycemic index: physiological significance. *Journal of the American College of Nutrition.* 2009;28 Suppl.:439S-45S.

[52] Jenkins, D. J., Kendall, C. W., Augustin, L. S., Mitchell, S., Sahye-Pudaruth, S., Blanco Mejia, S., et al. Effect of legumes as part of a low glycemic index diet on glycemic control and cardiovascular risk factors in type 2 diabetes mellitus: a randomized controlled trial. *Archives of internal medicine.* 2012;172:1653-60.

[53] Yu, J. H., Kim, M. S. Molecular mechanisms of appetite regulation. *Diabetes and metabolism journal.* 2012;36:391-8.

[54] Brand-Miller, J. C., Stockmann, K., Atkinson, F., Petocz, P., Denyer, G. Glycemic index, postprandial glycemia, and the shape of the curve in healthy subjects: analysis of a database of more than 1,000 foods. *The American journal of clinical nutrition.* 2009; 89:97-105.

[55] Ebrahimi, M., Ghayour-Mobarhan, M., Rezaiean, S., Hoseini, M., Parizade, S. M., Farhoudi, F., et al. Omega-3 fatty acid supplements improve the cardiovascular risk profile of subjects with metabolic syndrome, including markers of inflammation and auto-immunity. *Acta cardiologica.* 2009;64:321-7.

[56] Simopoulos, A. P. The importance of the ratio of omega-6/omega-3 essential fatty acids. *Biomedicine and pharmacotherapy = Biomedecine and pharmacotherapie.* 2002; 56:365-79.

[57] Zhang, M. J., Spite, M. Resolvins: anti-inflammatory and proresolving mediators derived from omega-3 polyunsaturated fatty acids. *Annual review of nutrition.* 2012; 32:203-27.

[58] Oh, D. Y., Talukdar, S., Bae, E. J., Imamura, T., Morinaga, H., Fan, W., et al. GPR120 is an omega-3 fatty acid receptor mediating potent anti-inflammatory and insulin-sensitizing effects. *Cell.* 2010;142:687-98.

[59] Kris-Etherton, P. M., Taylor, D. S., Yu-Poth, S., Huth, P., Moriarty, K., Fishell, V., et al. Polyunsaturated fatty acids in the food chain in the United States. *The American journal of clinical nutrition.* 2000;71:179S-88S.

[60] Wen, C. P., Wai, J. P., Tsai, M. K., Yang, Y. C., Cheng, T. Y., Lee, M. C., et al. Minimum amount of physical activity for reduced mortality and extended life expectancy: a prospective cohort study. *Lancet.* 2011;378:1244-53.

[61] Conn, V. S., Koopman, R. J., Ruppar, T. M., Phillips, L. J., Mehr, D. R., Hafdahl, A. R. Insulin Sensitivity Following Exercise Interventions: Systematic Review and Meta-Analysis of Outcomes Among Healthy Adults. *Journal of primary care and community health.* 2014;5:211-22.

[62] Woods, J. A., Wilund, K. R., Martin, S. A., Kistler, B. M. Exercise, inflammation and aging. *Aging and disease.* 2012;3:130-40.

[63] Pedersen, B. K., Febbraio, M. A. Muscles, exercise and obesity: skeletal muscle as a secretory organ. *Nature reviews Endocrinology.* 2012;8:457-65.

[64] Alamodi, A. A., Abu-Zaid, A., Anwer, L. A., Khan, T. A., Shareef, M. A., Shamia, A. A., et al. Undergraduate research: an innovative student-centered committee from the Kingdom of Saudi Arabia. *Medical teacher.* 2014;36 Suppl. 1:S36-42.

[65] Alamodi, A. A. Problem-based learning sessions and undergraduate research: a medical student's perspective and experience. *Perspectives on medical education.* 2014;3:56-60.

[66] Fukuda, S., Morimoto, K. Lifestyle, stress and cortisol response: Review II : Lifestyle. *Environmental health and preventive medicine.* 2001;6:15-21.

[67] Fukuda, S., Morimoto, K. Lifestyle, stress and cortisol response: Review I: Mental stress. *Environmental health and preventive medicine.* 2001;6:9-14.

[68] Oh, K. J., Han, H. S., Kim, M. J., Koo, S. H. Transcriptional regulators of hepatic gluconeogenesis. *Archives of pharmacal research.* 2013;36:189-200.

[69] Senanayake, G. V., Banigesh, A., Wu, L., Lee, P., Juurlink, B. H. The dietary phase 2 protein inducer sulforaphane can normalize the kidney epigenome and improve blood pressure in hypertensive rats. *American journal of hypertension.* 2012;25:229-35.

In: Health and Disease
Editor: Paul Ganguly

ISBN: 978-1-63463-052-8
© 2015 Nova Science Publishers, Inc.

Chapter 8

CLINICAL SKILLS: HOW BEST CAN WE DELIVER?

Muhammed Zafar* and Naif Al-Otaibi
Alfaisal University, Riyadh, Kingdom of Saudi Arabia

ABSTRACT

Clinical skills are the foundation elements of clinical method competencies upon which modern day clinical practice is founded. The mastery of clinical skills is crucial in acquiring clinical proficiency among medical students. At Alfaisal University, College of Medicine, we have adopted a PBL-based hybrid curriculum which is taught in three successive phases over the period of five years. Clinical Skills courses are taught in an integrated fashion with ongoing blocks by using Alfaisal model.

The basic clinical skills course covers the clinical manifestations and the patho-physiological bases of common clinical signs and measurement of vital signs and is conducted through interactive lectures, small group sessions, self-study assignments, and practical sessions and is evaluated through written assignments, performance during course and end of course objective structured clinical examination (OSCE).

The integrated Clinical Skills courses are offered simultaneously to male and female medical students studying in semester-4, year-2, and semester-5 and 6, year-3, respectively. Training involves history taking, symptomatology recognition, clinical examination, common diagnostic methods, and the acquisition and deployment of necessary procedural skills related to system blocks. During the semester during alternate weeks, male and female students visit affiliated hospitals followed by an activity in the simulation lab. Students are divided into 2 large groups as A and B (45-50 students/ group) which have a 2-hour session/week at their respective hospital or university campus. Each group is further divided into 4-subgroups (10-12 students) supervised/ facilitated by a clinician, faculty member or an intern. The course is evaluated through observed performance evaluations (OPE) during clinical sessions, clinical MCQs and end of course objective structured clinical examination (OSCE).

---

* Corresponding author: Muhammed Zafar. E-mail address: mzafar@alfaisal.edu.

HOW CAN WE DEFINE CLINICAL SKILL?

The word "clinical" is derived from a Greek word "klinikos" which means "pertaining to or around the sick bed" [1]. The term "clinical skills" refers to clinical examinations (history taking and systemic physical examinations) including but not limited to procedural skills commonly performed in real world clinic training or simulation centres. Clinical skill may be defined as "any discrete and observable act of clinical care" [2]. Therefore, clinical skills are the foundation elements of clinical method competencies upon which modern day clinical practice is founded. During clinical practice, a physician performs an integrated set of skills which includes patient communication within the context of a professional relationship. This relationship mandates that physicians identify the aetiology of patient suffering.

To achieve this mandate, a patient history is obtained, utilizing an internationally recognized structure called Subjective, Objective, Assessment and Plan (SOAP). Physicians then perform an objective systemic or regional physical examination while ruling in or ruling out relevant pertinent positives and negatives. The physician assessment establishes a differential diagnosis and clinical impression with or without interpretation of laboratory results. Lastly, a plan is created concurrently with orders for clinical tests, prescriptive treatment as necessary and thus a decision to perform a procedure is made.

Teaching of clinical skills is effectively the practical application of basic science subjects which supports the assertion, "practical application is the practice of theory". (Goethe) once said, "Knowing is not enough; we must apply. Willing is not enough; we must do" [2]. While Sir William Osler (1849–1919) said, 'Observe, record, tabulate, and communicate. Use your five senses… Learn to see, learn to hear, learn to feel, learn to smell, and know that by practice alone you can become expert' [1].

Teaching of clinical skills is effectively the practical application of basic science subjects which supports the assertion, practical application is the practice of theory.

HOW DID CLINICAL SKILLS EVOLVE?

The history of clinical skills practice is rich [1, 3]. Ancient Egyptians, Traditional Chinese Medicine and Ayurvedic practitioners have practiced clinical skills since before 2000 BC. The concept of history taking was introduced by Galen (200 AD) by means of basic physical examination. These procedures were developed by Hippocrates (450 BC). Over the next 1000 years, the era of great physicians including the area from Middle East is evidenced by Avicenna and Razi. Today's approach of history taking and systemic examination was developed in this period. During the 19th century, there was little change in examination procedures of prior eras. With the advancement of technologies during the last 50 years, society has seen an increased use of clinical procedures and investigations [1].

WHERE ARE CLINICAL SKILLS TAUGHT?

Traditionally clinical skills are taught at the patient's bedside, hospital wards, outpatient departments or other clinical areas [1].

It is supported by small and large group teaching in the classrooms and lecture halls. Clinical environments, medical technology and working practices are constantly evolving.

As a result, use of clinical skills lab and simulation centres have become common place for teaching and training clinical skills to medical students, residents and other health professionals [4].

WHEN ARE CLINICAL SKILLS TAUGHT?

In most medical curricula, clinical skills are taught during the clerkship phase [1, 2]. Clinical teachers often complain that students are not prepared for clinical teaching.

Students in German schools frequently complain that the subject "clinical examination" is not taught in a satisfying manner due to time constraints and lack of personnel.

While standard medical curricula in the United Kingdom (UK) typically provide basic surgical-skills teaching before medical students are introduced into the clinical environment.

A literature review in 1995 concluded that most medical students were deficient in interviewing, history taking, and systemic examination skills [1, 3].

In 1998, a group on Educational Affairs Plenary of the Association of American Medical Colleges also discussed clinical skills deficiencies of medical students [3, 5].

Data collected from recent clinical performance examinations also suggests that current educational methods are not helpful in obtaining the competencies [6].

Despite all the advancement in medical science and technology, clinical skills teaching are important for the following reasons:

- Communication and clinical skill sets assist students to identify tested methods which instruct how to build trust and rapport between clinician and patient, which is vital for history taking and performing physical examinations
- Provides valuable information about the diagnosis, prognosis, and severity of the patient's condition
- Enables the clinician to make a decision regarding suitable investigations and management
- Isolates which investigations should be undertaken to achieve focused, appropriate and cost effective implementation
- Detailed systemic/regional examinations help to narrow or confirm a diagnosis in situations or conditions where obtaining a history is difficult or a patient is presenting with vague and non-specific symptoms
- The process of collecting information about the patient in a structured and comprehensive manor such as SOAP, helps to clarify the patient's clinical presentation and also allows the clinician to predict or gauge the likelihood for success or failure of purposed treatments

DOES EARLY INTRODUCTION OF CLINICAL SKILLS IN THE PRE-CLINICAL PHASE HAVE A POSITIVE IMPACT?

Yes, especially in a problem based learning (PBL) curriculum where integration is the backbone of the curriculum, early introduction of the clinical skills has been found to be beneficial by facilitating the integration of clinical and basic science knowledge [7]. It increases the student's confidence, improves their performance and makes them "feel" like doctors. It also helps to best prepare students for their clerkship phase [8, 9]. In a PBL system, students are provided with a clinical scenario which mainly contains information about the history of the patient, physical examination findings, lab reports etc. These are all clinical skills and if taught simultaneously, students are able to integrate and digest the ongoing activities. Furthermore, there are limited opportunities for medical students to develop their clinical skills due to certain constraints and at times, adverse influences which may be found in clinical environments. These influences may diminish the quality and content of clinical skills education in hospitals [10]. It may be pointed out that introducing clinical skill teaching at the pre-clinical phase requires an involvement of large number of trained clinical teachers, high financial incentives and availability of multiple resources including time, infrastructure, audio-visual aids, simulators etc. It also requires fixed time slots in the weekly schedule which most traditional medical schools find difficult.

HOW CAN WE ASSESS TEACHING-LEARNING OUTCOME OF CLINICAL SKILLS?

Clinical skills can be assessed by various methods each of which has its own strengths and weaknesses [1, 6, 11-15]. A short list of various assessment methods is as follows:

1   The long case
2   The short case
3   OSCE
4   Workplace-based assessment
    √   Mini-CEX (Mini-Clinical Evaluation Exercise)
    √   DoPS (Direct observation of Procedural Skills
    √   MSF (Multi-source feedback)
5   Observed performance evaluations
6   Peer Review
7   Portfolios
8   Written assignments
9   Case report submission

HOW BEST CAN WE DELIVER?

Because of the diversity of clinical skills components which contribute to learning, the answer to this question remains a mystery. Different medical schools have adopted various methods including, lectures, role plays, videos, use of standardized patients, peer-assisted teaching methods, trained clinicians, etc. [1, 3, 5]. George JH, 2001, described a very simple five-step method for teaching clinical skills [16, 17]. His suggested steps are:

1   Provide an overview of the need for the skill and how it is used in patient care.
2   Demonstrate exactly how the skill is performed without commentary.
3   Repeat the procedure, but describe each step.
4   Have student "talk through the skill" by detailing each step.
5   Observe and provide feedback to the student as he performs the skill.

The mastery of clinical skills is crucial in acquiring clinical proficiency among medical students. Improvement in clinical skill teaching in an undergraduate medical curriculum requires more opportunities for students to participate. It can further be enhanced by unique teaching methods such as:

- Clinical skill workshops
- Simulation training (*So far considered as the best way of teaching clinical skills*)
- Role plays
- Portrayed clinical scenarios by standardized patients
- Small group rotations
- Peer-assisted teaching methods

Assessment methods such as OSCE can also help to focus the attention of medical students in their clinical skills education activities [3, 5, 12]. The most important factor for delivering the best clinical skill education in an undergraduate medical curriculum is the provision of appropriate administrative support and enhanced faculty development [2]. Our experience at Alfaisal University suggests the following factors are important:

- Proper organization of the course
- Provision of clear learning objectives
- Integration of professional skills activities with the ongoing systemic block
- Minimum of lectures
- Hands-on opportunities
- Small groups
- Teaching by experienced and trained clinicians
- Teaching by interns (Peer-assisted learning)
- Provision of enough simulators (low, medium and high fidelity)
- Provision of adequate space
- Increased number of sessions in the simulation lab
- Early exposure to real patients for positive findings
- Trained Standardized Patients (SPs)

Since the most important resource used for clinical skill training at Alfaisal University is simulation either by means of standardized patients or manikins, a brief account of the simulation is provided here. Please note: a detailed description on simulation is included in another chapter.

TEACHING AND LEARNING IN SIMULATED ENVIRONMENT: WHAT IS MEDICAL SIMULATION?

Medical simulation is the most important aspect which guides clinical training to a level of clinical skill mastery, which in turn helps to improve patient safety during student clinical rotations and clerkships [18, 19].

Medical simulation companies and researchers have been successful in providing and developing simulators for a wide range of physical examination, and clinical procedures (e.g. CPR, heart sounds, airway insertion, NGT insertion, eye examination... etc.) and these simulators mimic the patient's role in clinical training [20].

Until now, simulation for human verbal, physical and emotional responses which provide the most important practice in clinical skills training (e.g. History taking, communication, complains... etc.) was not possible. For more understanding of simulation, the readers are referred to next chapter. Simulation can be defined as:

"Simulation is a training and feedback method in which learners practice tasks and processes in lifelike circumstances using models or virtual reality, with feedback from observers, peers, actor-patients, and video cameras to assist improvement in skills."

Simulation also "refers to an activity that is designed to help participants acquire insight into the complex relationships and interconnected structures within a particular context. It is a way of preparing for (or reviewing) action in the real world".

"Simulations are created experiences that mimic processes or conditions that cannot or should not be experienced firsthand by a student because of the student's inexperience or the risk to the patient". "A simulator is a training device that closely represents reality but in which the complexity of events can be controlled." Simulations vary in their relation (fidelity) to Real World experience [20].

Low, Medium and High Fidelity Simulators

Yaeger et al. (2004) broke fidelity down into three general classifications: low- medium- and high-fidelity. Their definitions of each stated:

√   Low-fidelity simulators are focused on single skills and permit learners to practice in isolation.
√   Medium-fidelity simulators provide a more realistic representation but lack sufficient cues for the learner to be fully immersed in the situation.
√   High-fidelity simulators provide adequate cues to allow for full immersion and respond to treatment interventions.

Fidelity

"The term 'fidelity' is used to designate how true to life the teaching/evaluating experience must be to accomplish its objectives [20]. Using this definition, fidelity becomes a sliding scale in which given the objectives, a single piece of medical simulation equipment may be able to provide a "high-fidelity" experience for one objective but be "low-fidelity" for another objective." An example would be the insertion of an intravenous (IV) catheter. If the objective were to merely teach the psychomotor skills required for inserting the catheter, a relatively simple and low-tech IV access arm partial-task simulator would suffice and provide a comparatively high-fidelity experience. But if the objective were expanded to include communication with the patient, then the same device would suddenly become low-fidelity, as there is no feedback being delivered with IV catheter insertion and communication with the patient is not possible.

"Fidelity is the extent to which the appearance and behavior of the simulator/simulation match the appearance and behavior of the simulated system [20]. Another component critical in high-fidelity manikin-based simulators is the ability to provide feedback. Feedback comes in two forms. First is the simulator's response to treatment or intervention by the learner. High-fidelity simulators require the simulator to demonstrate appropriate responses to therapeutic interventions. For instance, if a medication is given to increase the heart rate, then the simulator should respond accordingly with a faster pulse. Conversely, if an intervention is provided that is not indicated and is potentially harmful, the simulator should respond with the physiological changes appropriate for this therapeutic misadventure. A second form of feedback is the ability to provide objective feedback for participant review in the post-simulation setting. At the instructor's command, during or at the end of the training run, the computer will type out in detail a timed, chronological summary of all of the events of the exercise. This printout includes all of the student's manipulations of the simulator, the drugs given (their dosages and when they were given), and the occurrences of any other events [20].

Aside from high-fidelity manikin-based patient simulators, there are many others types of simulation used in healthcare provider education and training. Their compiled list includes:

1   Animal Models
2   Human Cadavers
3   Standardized patients
4   Written Scenarios
5   Computer based simulations
6   Audio-simulations
7   Video-based simulations
8   Three dimensional or static models
9   Task-specific simulators
10 Virtual reality simulation

WHY USE SIMULATORS?

The reasons behind the increased use for patient simulation are many and include:

1   the growth of medical knowledge,
2   changes in medical education,
3   patient safety,
4   improved realism of simulation devices,

5   availability of patients,

6   new demands on student availability,

7   And the ability of simulation to provide standardization and replication.

ADVANTAGES OF SIMULATORS

1   Unlike patients, simulators do not become embarrassed or stressed;

2   have predictable behavior;

3   are available at any time to fit the curriculum needs;

4   can be programmed to simulate selected findings, conditions, situations, and complications;

5   allow standardized experience for all trainees;

6   can be used repeatedly with fidelity and reproducibility;

7   can be used to train both for procedures and difficult management situations

LIMITATIONS OF SIMULATION

1   While realism has been achieved in many areas of patient simulation, there are still many other areas of patient anatomy and physiology that have yet to be realized.

2   "The major hurdles facing medical education are to expand the fidelity of the modeling and to create a business case for simulation centers."

3   Others have also commented on the lack of realism in some areas, including the feel of the skin, skin color, and skin temperature

4   The lack of realism may not just apply to the simulation device.

5   The fast-paced, high- stress environment of a critical care unit is difficult to simulate.

6   As a result, there is no assurance that the learner will make a smooth transition of knowledge from the simulated situation to the actual clinical environment.

Since simulation plays an important role in the better delivery of professional skill course, Alfaisal University has designed an extensive Standardized patient (SP) programme.

Standardized Patient (SP) Programme at Alfaisal University

The continuous development of health care services and clinical practices with progress of medical education content and techniques makes the medical practices more safe and effective. Medical simulation is the most important aspect that guides clinical training to the stage of skill set mastery, which will insure provision of safe practice on patients and students. Utilization of Standardized Patients in medical schools started many years ago and it was recognized as a valid program in the early nineties [21].

Many educational health care organizations and associations around the world are using both SPs in clinical training and the OSCE exam, in conjunction with evaluations. This methodology has proven to be an effective tool which produces measurable results.

One of our primary goals at Alfaisal University, College of Medicine is to become a leader in Simulation Centre based OSCE's with tailor designed Curricula, developed specifically for each clinical task. Alfaisal University will soon become known as the most advanced and organized medical school in the Kingdom of Saudi Arabia.

Standardized Patients (SPs)

A standardized patient (SP) also called simulated patient or patient actor, is a healthy person carefully trained to act and play the role of an actual patient including psychosocial, physical and emotional roles under structured standardized scenarios and controlled environments. Standardized patients (SPs), also known as patient actors, are people trained in interview, communication, physical examination, and feedback techniques [21].

They memorize the script of a patient, including symptoms and past medical history, family situation, and even physical examination findings. Then they act out the patient's story for a student. After the encounter they give feedback on how well the student communicated during the encounter, comment on the quality and breadth of data, and evaluate the student's physical examination skills. Standardized Patients in the medical school started many years ago and it was recognized as viable program in the early nineties. Many educational health care organizations and associations around the world are using SPs in clinical training and OSCE exams coupled with evaluation as an effective tool for the examiners.

BENEFITS OF USING STANDARDIZED PATIENT

A standardized patient (SP) also called simulated patient or patient actor, is a healthy person carefully trained to act and play the role of an actual patient including psychosocial, physical and emotional roles under structured standardized scenarios and controlled environments.

Values and Benefits

1. Clinical Training
√ Risk free: learners practice skills and learn techniques in a safe environment without risk of harm for both patients and students.
√ Available: can be used anytime, anywhere because of their flexible schedules.
√ Realistic and valid: they are comparable to real patients.
√ Adaptable: flexible in adapting the role to meet specific needs of the trainee as directed by the trainer.
√ Reliable: symptoms, signs, and psychosocial aspects remain stable and consistent with each standardized repetition.
√ Controllable: Situation, setting and level of difficulty and amount of information given to the learner can be controlled
√ Able: to give constructive feedback in a learning environment

2. Financial Benefits

The SP program is an ideal resource to generate revenue by serving the needs of other medical education institutions and related industry (e.g. SCFHS) by providing them with resources and curricula (e.g. SPs, clinicians, technicians, instruments, A.V, simulators... etc.) supported by OSCE exams and clinical training.

In addition, clinical workshops may be coupled with faculty created programs.

Disadvantages of SPs

1   Moderate cost
2   Time consuming
3   Need extensive training
4   Requires dedicated space and personnel
5   Not appropriate for Operation room
6   Intervention is not possible

SP Bank at Alfaisal

Standardized patients are the main needed resource for our programme. At present we have 30 SPs as follows:

Age: 18-35 (25 SPs) 15 Males and 10 Females
Age: 36-45 (5 SPs) 3 Males and 2 Females

All SPs are recruited after following the criteria set by the recruitment committee. Recruitment process was as follows:

1   Announcement
2   Registration forms
3   Choosing candidates
4   Interviewing candidates and role playing
5   Final choosing 40 SPs from all candidates
6   Health examination: All SPs should pass it to assure that they are healthy
7   Approval

All SPs are trained for communication, history taking and physical examination skills.

Alfaisal Curriculum

At Alfaisal University, College of Medicine (CoM), we have adopted a PBL-based hybrid curriculum which is taught in three successive phases over the period of five years.

Professional (Clinical) Skills courses are taught in an integrated fashion with ongoing blocks in two successive phases as follows:

Phase-I
1   Communication Skills (PRO 115) ----------------- Semester-I
2   Professional Skills-I (Introduction to Basic Clinical Skills-PRO 234) --Semester-III

Phase-II
Professional Skills II, III and IV (Integrated with Clinical Sessions)-Semester – IV, V and VI.

Considering the importance of early introduction of clinical skills teaching in the pre-clerkship phase, we have designed an innovative clinical skills curriculum for the better delivery of the clinical skills objectives.

THE ALFAISAL MODEL FOR BASIC CLINICAL SKILLS

History taking and general physical examination remains an integral part of the clinical practice. The science is mostly an art that enables the physician to reach provisional diagnosis, order appropriate investigations and judge the prognosis. The clinical skills remain important way of gaining patient confidence and establishing the physician's rapport.

This course is offered during semester-1, year-1. The aim of this course is to enable the medical students in first year of medical curriculum to gain basic skills to take medical history and perform general physical examination. Additionally it is also meant to develop sufficient basic skills for performing two very important emergency management skills, namely, cardiopulmonary resuscitation and phlebotomy.

The course covers the clinical manifestations and the patho-physiological basis of common clinical signs. The course also covers the measurement of vital signs. The course is conducted through interactive lectures, small group sessions, self-study assignments, and practical sessions.

Rationale

People visit doctors for many reasons. Sometimes it is because something unexpected and catastrophic has happened to them, but usually it is because something isn't right. The general practitioner (GP) or family doctor is usually the first point of contact.

The doctor needs to try to work out why patients are there and what they are most concerned about. The first and major part of that is talking with the patient (communication skills). If a doctor listens carefully the patient will probably tell him what is wrong with him, what is concerning him, and

The physical examination helps doctors to confirm this or not. General physical examination is integral to clinical examination and is the second most important at the beginning to make a provisional diagnosis.

After taking a history, idea about the diagnosis is developed and the expected physical signs are explored, because there is a saying "you only find what you look for".

By the end of this course, the students are expected to:

1 Record a medical history
2 Describe various presenting complaints
3 Perform general physical examination of a patient thoroughly.
4 Perform basic clinical procedures such as CPR and phlebotomy

Course Strategies

Peer-Assisted Teaching Methods

Peer-assisted learning (PAL) – the concept of teaching sessions organized by students for students is a well-established learning tool used in many institutions. Indeed, within the literature, it is sometimes regarded as the quintessential method of learning and reviewing new material effectively and efficiently [22-38].

Teaching Methodology

- A group of selected students is trained for the weekly task prior to the sessions
- An explanation of the task is given to the whole class for 20-25 minutes (in the lecture hall) by lectures, demonstrations, videos, and role plays for history taking skills
- Students are divided into groups and taken to the small class rooms.
- They are provided with a hand-out and a checklist
- They are then asked to take a history from a patient/SP or perform a physical examination individually on a standardized patient or a simulator or a volunteer
- A trained student supervisor observes their performance, then guides and evaluates their performance for feedback (peer-assisted teaching)
- Two attendances are taken; one before the session and the second at the end

Course Evaluation

The course would be evaluated through written assignments, performance during course and end of course objective structured clinical examination (OSCE). Final grades ARE calculated according to the following apportionment;

Assessment and Assessment Strategies

a. Continuous (40%)

i   Attendance and professional behaviour------- (10%)
ii   Written assignment (minimum) ------------ (10%)
iii Mid-block test / Mid-course test (MCQs) --- (20%)

b. *Final End of Course Exam (60%)*
iv   Theory paper; MCQs (one best type), (30%)
v   OSCE (Objective Structured Clinical Examination) (30%)

Evaluation of the Course is done at the end with the help of a questionnaire.

Because of the shortcomings in teaching and evaluation of clinical skills in addition to our own experience of teaching medical students, we have identified a need for a clinical skills teaching model that could be used in most medical schools which is both conserves time and is low cost. We call this delivery system the "Alfaisal Model" of Professional Skills.

THE ALFAISAL MODEL FOR INTEGRATED CLINICAL SKILLS

Professional Skill-II, III and IV (PRO 245, PRO 356 and PRO 365) are offered simultaneously to male and female medical students studying in semester-4, year-2, semester-5, year-3, and semester-6, year-3 respectively. The courses run for 16-18 weeks parallel to the system blocks of semester-4, 5 and 6 curriculums (Table-1).

Table 1. Showing Integration of Professional Skill courses with System Blocks

PRO-245						
	S.N.	Course Code	Year	Sem	Course Title	Credits
SEM-4	1	NEU 241	2	4	Neuroscience Block (10-wks)	5
	2	HNS 242	2	4	Head and Neck Block (4-wks)	2
	3	SKN 243	2	4	Skin Block (2 w-ks)	2
	4	PRO 245	2	4	Professional Skills-II Block Integrated with above system Blocks (16-wks)	2
PRO 356						
SEM-5	1	MSK 351	3	5	Musculoskeletal Block (3-wks)	2
	2	GIT 352	3	5	Gastrointestinal Block (6-wks)	3
	3	Endocrine Block 353	3	5	Endocrine Block (4-wks)	2
	4	REP 354	3	5	Reproductive Block (4-wks)	2
	5	PRO 356	3	5	Professional Skills-III Block Integrated with above system Blocks (17-wks)	2
PRO 365						
SEM-5	1	CVS 361	3	6	Cardiovascular Block (5-wks)	3
	2	RES 362	3	6	Respiratory Block (4-wks)	2
	3	URN 363	3	6	Renal Block (4-wks)	2
	4	HEM 364	3	6	Hem/Onc Block (3-wks)	2
	5	PRO 365	3	5	Professional Skills-IV Block Integrated with above system Blocks (16-wks)	

Each block contains target skill sets which have been selected as a key foundation for acquisition by medical student.

Objective

The courses assist medical students to integrate critical thinking with practical skills by means of developing connections between basic science knowledge and clinical presentation:

Training during the professional courses involves: History taking, symptomatology recognition, clinical examination, common diagnostic methods, and the acquisition and deployment of necessary procedural skills related to system blocks.

Group Apportionment

Male and Female medical students are divided into 2 large groups as A and B (45-50 students/group) which have a 2-hour session/week at their respective hospital or AU campus. Each group is further divided into 4-subgroups (10-12 students) supervised/facilitated by a clinician, faculty member or an intern (Table-2).

Course Delivery

1   Week-1 of each block: 2-hour session (A lecture followed by a demonstration) by a clinician on symptomatology, SOAP history taking and common diagnostic methods relevant to the system block at AU campus.

2   Week-2 of each block: Students visit the respective hospitals where they are divided into 4-groups. Each group is supervised by a clinician. Task for each group remains the same i.e. history taking and performance of physical examination on a real patient or standardized patient (SP). Students need to adhere to each hospital dress code policy and regulations. Students need to maintain respectful communication with patients, their families, peers, tutors and all members of medical care team. During hospital rotations students are exposed to patients for real patient interaction

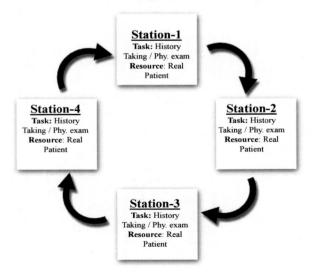

Alfaisal Model of Clinical Skill Sessions at the Hospital

Table 2. Showing Typical Weekly Schedule for Professional Skills Courses

Time	Sun Sem-1 Male	Fem	Sem-3 Male	Fem	Sem-5 Male	Fem	Mon Sem-1 Male	Fem	Sem-3 Male	Fem	Sem-5 Male	Fem	Tue Sem-1 Male	Fem	Sem-3 Male	Fem	Sem-5 Male	Fem	Wed Sem-1 Male	Fem	Sem-3 Male	Fem	Sem-5 Male	Fem	Thurs Sem-1 Male	Fem	Sem-3 Male	Fem	Sem-5 Male	Fem
8:00 to 8:50		PBL																			Lab F1-F4					Lab F5-F8				
9:00 to 9:50													PRO 115		Lab F5-F8															
10:00 to 10:50			PRO 356 GRA	PBL					Lab F1-F4		PRO 234 GRA		Lab M1-M4		PRO 115		LAB				PRO 356 GR B	PBL			Lab M5-M8		PBL		PRO 234 GRB	
11:00 to 11:50																														
12:00 to 1:00	There will be no classes scheduled from 12:00 – 13:00 officially or unofficially						There will be no classes scheduled from 12:00 – 13:00 officially or unofficially						There will be no classes scheduled from 12:00 – 13:00 officially or unofficially						There will be no classes scheduled from 12:00 – 13:00 officially or unofficially						There will be no classes scheduled from 12:00 – 13:00 officially or unofficially					
1:00 to 2:00 pm				PBL	PRO 356 GRA		Elective Course for Year I		PRO 234 GRA						Lab M5-M8				Lab M1-M4		Elective Course for Year 2		PBL	PRO 356 GRB	TBL		TBL		PRO 234 GRB	PBL
2:00 to 3:00 pm																	LAB													
3:00 to 3:30																														
3:30 to 5:00 pm	Elective Courses Year 1		PBL				Lab M5-M8		Elective Courses Year 2				Elective Courses Year 1		Lab F5-F8				Lab F1-F4		Elective Courses Year 2						Lab M1-M4			

3 Week-3 of each block: 4 -stations are set each with a simulator/instrument, SP, or a volunteer at the AU simulation lab. Two stations are supervised by clinicians, one by an Alfaisal University faculty member and one by an intern. Students rotate after 25-30 minutes. Each student gets an opportunity for hands-on experience

Alfaisal Model of Clinical Skill sessions at the Simulation Lab

Station-1
Task: History Taking
Resource: Standardized Patient (SP)

Station-2
Task: Phy. exam
Resource: (SP), simulator

Station-3
Task: Phy. exam
Resource: (SP), simulator

Station-4
Task: Procedural skill
Resource: simulator

4 Week-4 of each block: All students visit hospitals on their specified days and time
5 Week-5 of each block: 4 -stations are set each with a simulator/instrument, SP, or a volunteer at the AU simulation lab. Two stations are supervised by clinicians, one by an Alfaisal University faculty member and one by an intern. Students rotate after 25-30 minutes. Each student gets an opportunity for hands-on experience

Assessment

a. Continuous (30%)

1   Attendance (10%): This reflects overall attendance of all sessions at AU and respective hospitals. It also includes their professional behaviour and attitude

2   Observed performance evaluation (OPE) (10%): Observed performance evaluations are feasible, inexpensive and qualitatively effective methods of teaching clinical skills [14, 15]. Evaluation of performance is done during sessions at the respective hospitals. For each of the bedside teaching sessions at the hospitals, tutors are expected to observe the performance of students for a given task and then document evaluation of each student on the sheet provided to them by the course director. For this purpose, structured observed performance evaluation (OPE) sheets with guidelines for the tutors and observations for history taking, physical examination, and information given skills were created (Table-3).

Clinical MCQs (10%): Scenario based MCQs to test the psychomotor skills. Specially constructed Clinical MCQs were introduced to test the knowledge component of basic clinical skills.

b. End of Course

OSCE (70%): The OSCE is a valid tool to test the psychomotor skills which are the basis of all clinical skills. This would comprise of a series of clinical stations with tasks for the students to demonstrate their ability of a particular skill, such as history taking and physical examination.

Feedback: One of these course goals is to ensure that students of AlFaisal College of Medicine receive an excellent learning experience. This wouldn't be possible without continuous and ongoing feedback from faculty as well as equally important input from students.

Table 3. Showing Observed Performance Evaluation Sheet (OPE)

Wk	Date and Day	Gp. #	Session/ Activity	Student Name and ID	Performance Evaluation					Comments
					5	4	3	2	1	

Tutor's Name: --- Signature: ---.
5 = 100%, 4 = 80%, 3 = 60%, 2 = 40%, 1 = 20%.

Faculty evaluation: Students are highly encouraged to evaluate each tutor they were supervised by during this course by completing "tutor evaluation form".

Sessions Evaluation: for a comprehensive evaluation process, students are also encouraged to evaluate each session.

REFERENCES

[1]   *Teaching Clinical Skills-E-Learning Modules* www.faculty.londondeanery.ac.uk/e-learning/teaching-clinical-skills.

[2]   *Recommendations for Clinical Skills Curricula for Undergraduate Medical Education.* Association of American Medical Colleges (AAMC), 2005. Retrieved from https://www.aamc.org/download/130608/.../clinicalskills_oct09.

[3]   Corbett, E. C., Whitcomb, M. *The AAMC Project on the Clinical Education of Medical Students. Clinical Skills Education.* Association of American Medical Colleges, Washington, DC, 2004.

[4]   Okuda, Y., Bryson, E. O., DeMaria, S. Jr, Jacobson, L., Quinones, J., Shen, B., Levine, A. L. The utility of simulation in medical education: What is the evidence? *Mt. Sinai J. Med.* 2009; 76(4):330-40.

[5]   Nutter, D., Whitcomb, M. *The AAMC Project on the Clinical Education of Medical Students.* Association of American Medical Colleges, Washington, DC, 2001.

[6]   Hawkins, R. E., Swanson, D. B., Dillon, G. F., et al. The introduction of clinical skills assessment into the United States Medical Licensing Examination (USMLE): description of USMLE step 2 clinical skills (CS). *J. Med. Licensure Discipline* 2005; 91:21-25.

[7]   Jackson, M. B., Keen, M., Wenrich, M. D., Schaad, D. C., Robins, L., Goldstein, E. A. Impact of a pre-clinical clinical skills curriculum on student performance in third-year clerkships. *J. Gen. Intern. Med.* 2009; 24(8):929-33.

[8]   Lam, T. P., Irwin, M., Chow, L. W. C., Chan, P. Early introduction of clinical skills teaching in a medical curriculum-factors affecting students' learning. *Medical Education* 2002; 36(3):233-40.

[9]   Devi, K. T. A., Yasmin, K. S., Viswanathan, N. [Early introduction of clinical skills in the pre-clinical phase of an integrated medical curriculum]. *J. Contemp. Med. Edu.* (2013), [cited June 24, 2014]; 1(3): 142-144.

[10]   Kiguli, S., Kijjambu, S., Mwanika, A. Introducing clinical skills training to pre-clerkship medical students in a resource constrained medical school. *Medical Education* 2006; 40(5):473.

[11]   Furman, G. E., Smee, S., Wilson, C. Quality Assurance Best Practices for Simulation-Based Examinations. *Sim. Healthcare* 2010; 5:226-231.

[12]   Gimpel, J. R., Boulet, J. R., Errichetti, A. M. Evaluating the clinical skills of osteopathic medical students. *J. Am. Osteopath. Assoc.* 2003; 103:267-279.

[13]   Gimpel, J. R., Weidner, A. C., Boulet, J. R., Wilson, C., Errichetti, A. M. Standardized patients and mechanical simulators in teaching and assessment at colleges of osteopathic medicine. *J. Am. Osteopath. Assoc.* 2007; 107:557-561.

[14] Lane, J. L., Gottlieb, R. P. Structured Clinical Observations: A Method to Teach Clinical Skills With Limited Time and Financial Resources. *Pediatrics* 2000; 105 (4): 973-7. *Med. Teach.* 2002, 24(1):57-61.

[15] Kassebaum, D. G., Eaglen, R. H. Shortcomings in the evaluation of students' clinical skills and behaviors in medical school. *Acad. Med.* 1999; 74(7):842-849.

[16] George, J. H., Doto, F. X. A simple five-step Method for Teaching Clinical Skills. *Fam. Med.* 2001; 33(8):577-8.

[17] Virdi, M. S., Sood, M. Effectiveness of a five-step method for teaching clinical skills to students in a dental college in India. *J. Dent. Educ.* 2011 Nov.; 75(11):1502-6.

[18] Issenberg, S. B., McGaghie, W. C., Hart, I. R., Mayer, J. W., Felner, J. M., Petrusa, E. R., Waugh, R. A., Brown, D. D., Safford, R. R., Gessner, I. H., Gordon, D. L., Ewy, G. A. Simulation technology for health care professional skills training and assessment. *JAMA* 1999; 282(9):861-6.

[19] Scalese, R. J., Obeso, V. T., Issenberg, S. B. Simulation technology for skills training and competency assessment in medical education. *J. Gen. Intern. Med.* 2007; 23(suppl. 1):46-49.

[20] Rodgers, D. L. *High-fidelity patient simulation: A descriptive white paper report.* Retrieved from sim-strategies.com/downloads/Simulation%20White%20Paper2.

[21] Standardized Patient Practices: Initial Report on the Survey of US and Canadian Medical Schools. *Medical Education Online* 2009; 14:7.

[22] Blank, W. A., Blankenfeld, H., Vogelmann, R., Linde, K., Schneider, A. Can near-peer medical students effectively teach a new curriculum in physical examination? *BMC Medical Education* 2013, 13:165.

[23] Bruke, J., Fayaz, S., Graham, K., Matthew, R., Field, N. Peer-assisted learning in the acquisition of clinical skills: A supplementary approach to musculoskeletal system training. *Med. Teach.* 2007; 29:577-582.

[24] Bulte, C., Betts, A., Garner, K., Durning, S.: Student teaching: views of student near-peer teachers and learners. *Med. Teach.* 2007, 29(6):583-590.

[25] Burke, J., Fayaz, S., Graham, K., Matthew, R., Field, M.: Peer-assisted learning in the acquisition of clinical skills: a supplementary approach to musculoskeletal system training. *Med. Teach.* 2007, 29(6):577-582.

[26] Busari, J. O., Prince, K. J., Scherpbier, A. J., Van Der Vleuten, C. P., Essed, G. G.: *How residents perceive their teaching role in the clinical setting: a qualitative study.*

[27] Escovitz, E. S. Using senior students as clinical skills teaching assistants. *Acad. Med.* 1990; 65(12):733-734.

[28] Glynn, L. G., Mac Farlene, A., Kelly, M., Cantillon, P., Murphy, A. W. Helping each other to learn - a process evaluation of peer-assisted learning. *BMC Med. Educ.* 2006; 6:18.

[29] Henning, J. M., Weider, T. G., Marty, M. C. Peer-assisted learning in clinical education: Literature review. *J. Athl. Train.* 2008; 43(3):84-90.

[30] Nestel, D., Kidd, J. Peer-assisted learning in patient-centred interviewing: The impact on student tutors. *Med. Teach.* 2005; 27(5):439-444.

[31] Nikendei, C., Andreesen, S., Hoffmann, K., Junger, J.: Cross-year peer tutoring on internal medicine wards: effects on self-assessed clinical competencies-a group control design study. *Med. Teach.* 2009, 31(2):e32-e35.

[32] Peter, W., Markus, S., Bernd, K., et al. Undergraduate technical skills training guided by student tutors. Analysis of tutors` attitude, tutees acceptance and learning progress in an innovative teaching model. *BMC Med. Educ.* 2008; 8:18.

[33] Saleh, M., Sinha, Y., Weinberg, D. Using peer-assisted learning to teach basic surgical skills: medical student's experiences. *Med. Educ. Online.* 2013; 18:10.

[34] Stibert, B. I., Lake, F. R. Peer-assisted learning in teaching clinical examination to junior medical students. *Med. Teach.* 2012; 34:392-7.

[35] Ten Cate, O., Durning, S.: Peer teaching in medical education: twelve reasons to move from theory to practice. *Med. Teach.* 2007, 29(6):591-599.

[36] Tolsgaard, M. G., Gustafsson, A., Rasmussen, M. B., Hoiby, P., Muller, C. G., Ringsted, C.: Student teachers can be as good as associate professors in teaching clinical skills. *Med. Teach.* 2007, 29(6):553-557.

[37] Weyrech, P., Celebi, N., Schrauth, M., Maltner, A., Lammerding-Koppel, M., Nikendei, C. Peer-assisted versus faculty staff-led skills laboratory training: A randomised control trial. *Med. Educ.* 2009; 43(2):113-120.

[38] Yu, T. C., Wilson, N. C., Singh, P. P., Lemanu, D. P., Hawken, S. J., Hil, A. G. Medical students-as-teachers: A systematic review of peer-assisted teaching during medical school. *Adv. Med. Educ. Pract.* 2011; 2:157-172.

In: Health and Disease   ISBN: 978-1-63463-052-8
Editor: Paul Ganguly   © 2015 Nova Science Publishers, Inc.

Chapter 9

THE WHY, THE WHAT AND THE HOW OF SIMULATION BASED EDUCATION: PREPARING FOR THE FUTURE

N. Harrison, L. Owen, S. Somerville, K. Stirling and J. Ker[*]
University of Dundee, Dundee, United Kingdom

ABSTRACT

The use of simulation, throughout the continuum of professional development for health and social care is essential if we are to achieve the WHO millennium goals and consistently deliver high quality care to the peoples of the world. As an educational technique, simulation is not new and dates back to the 11th century. Since these early days, simulation has evolved alongside the advances made in our wider understanding of education. The adoption and development of simulation continues to intensify, driven by advances in technology, lessons learnt from other high reliability organisations and an increasing recognition of the importance of quality improvement and patient safety. It now plays a pivotal role in our undergraduate and postgraduate healthcare education.

This chapter considers 'The Why?', 'The What?' and 'The How?' of simulation, simple yet complex questions which will highlight both the opportunities and challenges of simulation based education and its role in the future of the education of health and social care practitioners for quality healthcare. It provides educators with a theoretical and practical basis from which to successfully utilise simulation as a powerful education tool, embedded into a curriculum to augment learning from clinical experience.

INTRODUCTION

The use of simulation, throughout the continuum of professional development for health and social care is essential if we are to achieve the WHO millennium goals and consistently deliver high quality care to the peoples of the world.

---

[*] J. Ker, e-mail address: j.s.ker@dundee.ac.uk, b.c.charnley@dundee.ac.uk.

The recognition of the importance of simulation in education originated from its impact in other high-reliability organisations, such as aviation, the military and the nuclear industry [1-3]. This benefit, combined with a number of high profile adverse events in health care has highlighted its potential to enhance the delivery of high quality health care and in turn improve patient outcomes.

Simulation also has a vital role in ensuring our healthcare systems continue to improve and meet constantly changing demands. It can enhance educators' exploration of innovative, efficient and effective ways to prepare healthcare professionals for the future workplace. Quality improvement, the science of implementation, patient safety and the development of human factors training in health care can all utilise simulation to prepare individuals and teams as well as enhance the design of delivery systems.

The use of simulation in medical education is not new. Life-sized statues where used in the teaching of acupuncture by the Chinese Imperial Physician Wang Wei-Yi in the 11th century [5]. However the development of Resusci Anne in 1958, initiated by Åsmund Laerdal saw the start of the use of simulation in modern health care training [6]. In line with technological advances, the last 50 years have seen the development of physiologically driven manikins and the incorporation of computer-assisted simulation into the learning journey. In 1989 a team from the NASA research team pioneered the use of virtual reality in simulation which has led to the development of the virtual reality operating environment [7, 8].

Today the use of simulation has broadened to incorporate the use of simulated health and social care environments, simulated patients, advanced part task trainers and information technology. This will provide exciting ways to educate all those involved in the organisational effectiveness of healthcare systems as well as develop the health and social care professionals of the future. Understanding of adverse events and the need for human factors training have led to the use of simulation for teaching both technical and non-technical skills [9-12].

One of the major challenges for educators in the 21st century will be the provision of faculty expertise in simulation based education to provide the standards and resilience in practitioners to ensure healthcare globally functions like high reliability organisations.

In response to the emerging demands for the use of simulation, a number of associations, societies and government groups have been formed to harness expertise and stimulate growth in best evidence around the use of simulation.

This chapter considers 'The Why?', 'The What?' and 'The How?' of simulation, simple yet complex questions which will highlight both the opportunities and challenges of simulation based education and its role in the future of education of health and social care practitioners for quality healthcare.

The theoretical underpinning and the current evidence is shared through examples to help educators identify how they can successfully and sustainably incorporate and adapt the use of simulation into their curricular programmes along the continuum of education.

Box 1.

Gaba describes simulation as a:
Technique—not a technology—to replace or amplify real experiences with guided experiences that evoke or replicate substantial aspects of the real world in a fully interactive manner [4].

THE 'WHY?'

Some of the drivers behind the utilisation of simulation in modern healthcare education were highlighted in the introduction. In this section we discuss these drivers in more depth, review the educational underpinning for the use of simulation and then analyse the current evidence base.

Drivers for the Utilisation of Simulation

The service, political and education drivers for the use of simulation are been summarised in Figure 1 below and subsequently explored in more depth.

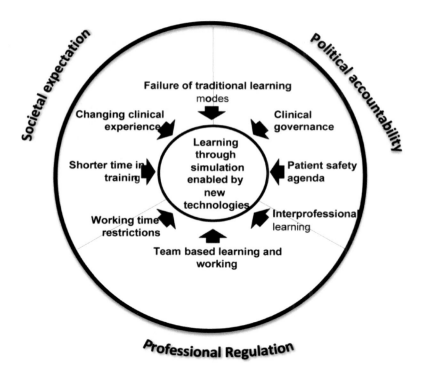

Adapted from Bradley P. The history of simulation in medical education and pos future directions. Med Educ. 2006 Mar;40(3):254-62.

Figure 1. Service, political and education drivers.

1. Technological Drivers

Although new whole body simulators such as that described by Abrahamson and Denson as early as 1960 had advanced physiological functionality, Bradley [13] asserts that simulation was not readily adopted at that time because the need for anything other than an apprenticeship model of learning had not been realized [13].

The change in educational delivery toward more integrated curricula and the enhanced availability of new technology such as mobile learning and e-learning has been at the centre of the dramatic increase in the use of simulation in medical education as part of a framework to deliver technology enhanced learning.

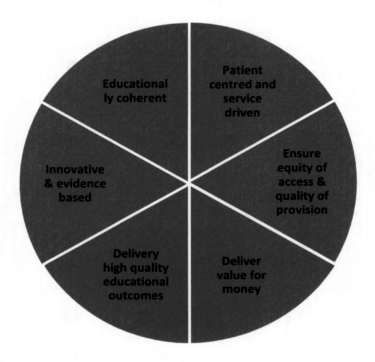

Adapted from Technology Enhanced Learning framework DOH 2013

Figure 2. Technology Enhanced Learning framework DOH 2013.

2. Curricular Drivers

Curricular reform has been influenced by enhanced knowledge of education, changes in healthcare delivery and knowledge of quality health care dimensions. Medical education has responded to these with an enhanced focus on communication skills development, team based and problem based learning approaches, and greater integration of doctors as members of the multi-professional skills team [14].

Increase in the use of simulation has also been driven by changes in doctors working practice and changes to the structure of training programmes. The consequence of these changes has often lead to a reduced time for speciality training as well as reducing the available time for expert faculty to dedicate to teaching and mentoring activities [14]. Trainees now see fewer patients, leaving them less prepared for practice [15]. Simulation based medical education offers alternative strategies which can be readily programmed into timetables, are reproducible, are deliverable on demand, provide greater efficiency and can address the limited availability of realistic learning opportunities [16].

3. Health Care Delivery Drivers

In-patient hospital stays have reduced and more patients are being treated in ambulatory settings [17]. Patients are no longer kept in hospital for prolonged periods of convalescence. Those patients who are in hospital are more unwell, and therefore less able to consent and participate in the teaching and training of students and junior doctors. Simulation based education can support the development of prepared practitioners.

4. Changes in Patient Expectations

Whilst experiential learning in real clinical encounters still remains the gold standard of medical teaching practice, the public agenda is that practitioners should already have competence before encountering patients in the context of full informed consent in the clinical care setting. Simulated health care environments and specialist simulators have a role to play in addressing patients' expectations. The issue of learning on non-consenting patients has also come to light in recent years [18], and has become a concern amongst professionals and the public [19].

5. The Patient Safety Agenda

A number of public scandals and enquiries highlighting failings in the system by individual practitioners, teams and regulatory bodies has focused the public's attention on safety and has had significant political impact on professional regulation [20]. The reports into Shipman [21], the Bristol heart inquiry [22], and Mid-Staffordshire [23] in the UK have had a profound influence on societal expectations and the national political agenda. The 1999 report by the United States Institute of Medicine, "To err is human" [24], revealed endemic failures in the healthcare system as well as the extent and cost of errors. "An organisation with a memory" [25] identified similar concerns in the UK setting. The concept of healthcare causing patient harm, an anathema to the Hippocratic imperative to "first does no harm" heralded the rise of the modern patient safety agenda. The National Patient Safety Foundation in the UKwas established in 1997 to drive forward the patient safety mission. Medical simulation has clearly become an important part of the solution by creating a safe environment to learn, rehearse and assess the complex skills needed for practitioners and teams to offer the safe medical care required, and in fact have been described as an ethical imperative [26].

All of these drivers have influenced and enhanced the use of simulation in healthcare education.

Educational Underpinning and Theory

To analyse any simulation based education event it is essential to have an understanding of the theoretical underpinning. Theory is a group of assumptions and ideas which help in the understanding and interpretation of a phenomenon. A theory should be comprehensive, coherent and internally consistent, and helpful in informing and guiding practice in medical education in general, and in understanding, planning, delivering and evaluating simulation based medical education [27]. Four of the commonly used educational theories of particular relevance to simulation are described here. Although they are described separately they can and do often link together.

Experiential Learning

Kolb's model [28] emphasises learning based on the individual's experience, and although it has been criticised as being over simplified it identifies the main trigger for learning as being a concrete experience which one can reflect upon and then, as a means of perceiving, form an abstract conceptualisation. This then as part of the cycle leads to critical reflection and active experimentation.

In the world of simulation, a scenario based learning event offers a concrete experience which then provides a structured opportunity for reflection and formulation of an abstract conceptualisation of what has been learnt. This can then be generalised, adapted and used in another context (active experimentation).

The simulated setting allows the concrete experience to occur in a setting which is safe, both from the point of view of patient safety as well as from the learner's perspective. The teacher role is that of facilitator who guides the learner through the process of reflection to enable connections and genralisations to be made.

Social Cognitive Theory

Social Cognitive theory encompasses both behaviourist and cognitivist approaches to understanding learning.

The behaviourist approach emphasises the external behaviour of people and their reactions to situations. It addresses the concept of a stimulus –response relationship where a given stimulus, if rewarded will be repeated whereas unrewarded responses will become reduced. Skinnerian behaviourism modifies this concept to include successive graduations towards the desired final behaviour. In behaviourist theories no account is taken of internal processes. In the context of simulation feedback serves to offer the reward for desirable behaviours.

The cognitivist approach emphasises the interaction of the learner with their environment as they assimilate new behaviours into their existing concepts and understanding in order to build or challenge existing knowledge or application of knowledge.

Skills and drills in acute care and resuscitation scenarios are typical examples of where social cognitive theory can be used.

Situated Learning

Situated learning is one of several theories where group participation in a sociocultural setting is regarded as key to learning. It is a theory which explains the power of the apprenticeship model of learning commonly used in health care learning, where a whole community contribute to the development of the apprentice, rather than a single expert.

The learning which occurs is through collaboration, social interaction and connectivity with the practice community. This theory suggests that when a new learner enters the community of practice they do so at the periphery or edge. Lave and Wegner called this legitimate peripheral participation [29]. The novice observes then performs less vital tasks and gradually with increasing skill and experience move towards the centre of the community of practice as they learn the knowledge, values and discourse of the whole group which will include experts, peers and more advanced apprentices. The participation in discourse (or talk) within the community is vital to the learning process. Situated learning theory encompasses cognitive apprenticeship theory and informal learning theories. It is also closely related to experiential learning model as it includes learning by doing and participating in he shared experience of the community.

A simulation based learning event that focuses on the team and the context of the scenario can by analysed using this theory.

Deliberate Practice

Deliberate practice is a term introduced by Ericsson where he identified the development of psychomotor skills in experts in terms of hours of deliberate practice, as a means of explaining variation in individual performances [30].

His theory described stages of development of skills competence from novice to autonomy and mastery together with the concept of continuous improvement.

Although his initial work was carried out in relation to speed typists and musicians the concepts have been applied in the context of medical education and simulation [31].

Much of the literature suggesting advantages of simulation focus on the opportunity that simulation offers for opportunity for repetition and practice of healthcare performance.

Application of Educational Theories

Kaufman and Mann discuss in detail a number of theoretical approaches to medical education [32]. They suggest an opportunistic and pragmatic approach to applying these to medical education contexts. They offer a very helpful summary of themes which connect many of them to inform practice.

These are shown in table 1 and can be applicable in simulation based education.

The Evidence Base for SBE

There has been a dramatic increase in the published literature on simulation in medical education over the past thirty years.

Table 1. Theoretical approaches to medical education

1. All theoretical frameworks view the learner as an active contributor in the learning process
2. The entire context of learning is more important that any one variable alone
3. Learning is integrally related to the solution and understanding of real life problems
4. Individual past experience and knowledge are critical in learning, actions and acquiring new knowledge
5. Learner's values, attitudes and beliefs influence their learning and actions, and building learner's self-awareness in his area is important for their development
6. Individuals as learners are capable of self-regulation that is, of setting goals, planning strategies and evaluating their progress
7. The ability to reflect on one's practice (performance) is critical to lifelong self-directed learning
8. Learning occurs not only individually, but in collaboration with others

The simulation research community have identified the key areas of simulation research which already offer robust evidence for the effectiveness of simulation as well as identifying the key gaps in our knowledge and understanding and areas where further research is needed [33].

Medical education is also known to cross boundaries between the traditions of natural science and the social sciences and although some have argued that randomised controlled trails are not the only way of generating sufficiently robust and persuasive evidence of educational effectiveness and workplace transfer [34, 35], the methodologies of systematic reviews and meta-analysis are the most relied upon for evidence of effectiveness of simulation. Systematic reviews have tended to be specialty specific, or with a focus on a particular skill or skill set. Seymour [36] demonstrated evidence that simulation was as effective in training surgeons for laparoscopic cholecystectomy as training on patients. Similarly Chaer [37] identified better patient outcomes for angioplasty following simulation based training. Draycott [38, 39] demonstrated the effectiveness of simulation based training programmes in obstetrics with better outcome measures quantified as improved APGAR scores and better patient outcomes in cases of peri-natal shoulder dystocia.

Another area where there appears to be measured improved patient outcomes is Central Venous Catheter (CVC) associated line infection and insertion complications as reported by Barsuk et al. [40, 41].

Systematic reviews of the use of simulation in surgical training practice have clearly demonstrated the benefit of simulation based training [42-44]. The wider medical education community however, need to seek to understand which specific specialist skills have evidence of improvement, and which aspects of simulation based training contribute to a positive educational impact with a positive transfer to patient outcomes [45].

A Best Evidence Medical Education Review in 2005 [46] identified that although there was a relative paucity of strong evidence for simulation skills transfer there were a number of features of high fidelity simulation that were associated with good evidence of positive impact on learning. These features are shown in box 1:

Box 1.

Provision of feedback
Allowing repetitive practice
Integration within a curriculum
Provision of range of difficulties
Adapting to multiple learning strategies
Range of clinical scenarios
Safe, educationally supportive learning environment
Active learning based in individual needs

Other more recent systematic reviews and meta-analyses have shown positive effects for outcomes of knowledge, skills and behaviours, and moderate effects for patient related outcomes [47]. Cook et al. [47] performed a meta-analysis of 609 studies of technology enhanced simulation to identify the outcomes of interventions and the impact of instructional design. They included published evidence across a wide range of skills and medical specialties, rather than focussing on a single skill or set of skills. Their wide inclusion criteria contained papers in the analysis using any technology enhanced simulation. They excluded the use of role-play and simulated or standardized patients where there was no technology enhancement. They found a moderate to large, statistically significant positive result for simulation training. They demonstrated educational gains for knowledge acquisition, time skills, process skills, product skills, behaviour. There was a moderate effect on outcomes of patient care. There was some inconsistency in the meta-analysis with two included studies demonstrating a negative effect on patient outcomes.

Research Opportunities

Simulation is commonly considered as a tool to enhance teaching and learning of technical and non-technical skills. There is limited literature describing the utility of simulation in testing systems or process, or as a research tool. Simulation has been used to identify behavioural markers in team performance. Shmutz [48] and Kim [49] describe the utility of simulation to evaluate team performance and also to develop an instrument to measure team performance. Fletcher [50] has also effectively used simulation as a research tool in the development of behavioural markers for evaluation and feedback for performance in anaesthetic practice. Research has also used simulation to both evaluate and improve patient outcomes by identifying performance features of management of septic shock and critical illness situations and usability studies [51]. In–situ simulation has been used to test a healthcare system protocol and develop a safe and timely stroke thrombolysis service [52]. In –situ simulation can effectively be used in learning from critical incidents and near-miss episodes.

The Future: What Next?

The simulation research community have indicated the priority areas for simulation based education research: the number 1 priority identified was to study the impact of medical school simulation learning on residents' performance [45]. Other research likely to influence simulation in the future includes research questions shown in Box 2 . There is significant opportunity for research using simulation for human factors orientated investigations such as the impact of fatigue on human performance and incident analysis.

Box 2. Research questions likely to influence simulation in the future

1. Learning acquisition, retentions of skills and cognitive load e.g., How do theories of learning and teaching inform the design of simulation interventions?
2. De-briefing e.g. what are the relevant characteristics of debriefing that lead to effective learning?
3. Learner characteristics e.g. how learner motivation affects the acquisition and retention of skills in simulation based activities
4. Impact on learning theory e.g. how do theoretical concepts and empirical findings about learning in non-medical domains apply in healthcare?
5. Role of the instructor e.g. what characteristics optimize trainee learning experience?
6. System challenges e.g. how can institutions address operational scale to ensure meeting educational outcomes?

Simulation also offers utility for systems, process and team testing before systemic changes, and following critical incidents and near misses. Simulation may also be used to explore and test the design of Technology Enhanced learning in health care practice.

THE 'WHAT?'

Understanding what can be taught effectively using simulation based education is fundamental to its integration into healthcare curricular programme. The potential for the use of simulation is principally defined by its design; the fidelity of the activity in relation to actual practice and the interactivity of the environment created.

What is learnt using simulation is defined by the learning outcomes which need to be constructively aligned with the learning activity and the debriefing and feedback. Often there are unexpected learning outcomes from participating in the learning experience and these also need to be explored to enhance practice [52].

What is taught and learnt using simulation is also dependent on the degree that the learner is willing and able to engage with the simulated environment. Educators need to design simulation activities that meet the requirements and level of expertise of the learner. Simulation can be used to learn both Technical skills and Non-Technical Skills as classified below.

Box 3.

Technical Skills	Non-technical Skills
History taking Physical examination Communication skills Procedural skills Manual handling	Communication and Teamwork Leadership Professionalism Situational Awareness Task management Decision making

Technical Skills Training

The utilisation of simulation for the development of technical skills has been shown to deliver sustained improvements in confidence, knowledge and an overall reduction in medical errors [53, 54]. In this section we outline what different technical skills can be learned using simulation.

Procedural Skills

Studies have shown that part task trainers can effectively be used to enhance procedural skills in relation to venepuncture, cannulation, preparing intravenous infusions and blood glucose measurement [55, 56]. Additionally, more sophisticated part task trainers and manikins have been shown to be effective in teaching central line insertion [57], lumbar puncture [58] and nasogastric tube insertion [59]. Haptic models and full sized manikins can be used within surgical specialities to improve trainee's capabilities in relation to endoscopic proficiency [60], laparoscopic surgery [61, 62] and surgical proficiency [63, 64] including suturing technique [65].

The examples provided above are a snapshot of the wider literature available. The construct of the learning activity using simulation should be designed to support learning, deliver effective feedback and enhance the transformation of practice and the transfer of learning into the clinical setting [54, 66, 67]. Deliberate practice as already identified is crucial for the acquisition and maintenance of procedural skills and aids the development of expert performance [30].

Examination Skills

Examination skills were one of the earliest documented applications of simulation. There is evidence that the Mayan and early Egyptian cultures had anatomical models which were used for educational purposes [5]. Simulation is used widely to teach examination techniques pertinent to the systems of the human body [58, 68]. This often involves the use of simulated patients and, for more intimate examinations, part task trainers. Since the 1970s, the use of simulated patients in simulation based learning events has widened and some institutions are enrolling them in learning intimate examinations   such as teaching associates [69-72]. Simulation has been associated with a significant improvement in performance of intimate examinations such as breast and pelvic examination techniques [73, 74]. Wanggren et al. [72] identified that trainees exhibited less stress and anxiety following a mentored gynaecology simulation teaching session with professional patients. However Chen et al. [68] identified that although students were willing to participate in a programme of peer examination there were cultural issues relating to intimate examination and they reported that a proportion of students still lacked confidence to transfer this learning into their clinical practice.

Consultations Skills

Consultations skills are essential for medical practice and the regulatory bodies with responsibility for education have prioritised consultation skills in alignment with government policy; for example in the GMC Tomorrow's Doctors 2009. Simulation can effectively be used to create a safe environment where these skills can be developed [75] with evidence from studies which examined the preparedness of medical students from three medical schools across the United Kingdom for clinical practice as newly qualified doctors [76]. One of the key findings of this report identified that many medical curricula did not prepare students sufficiently for performing complex communication tasks, for example breaking bad news.

Simulated practice can however provide an opportunity for videoing of sessions for self-review and effective debrief and feedback, essential for the development of more complex consultation skills [77-79]. The development of simulation activities with complex consultation scenarios has also allowed a greater understanding of the effect that stress can have on a trainee's consultation skills [80-83] and there is evidence of how it can prepare practitioners for challenging communication situations in clinical practice.

Resuscitation

Even though Resusci-Anne revolutionised education in life support, it took over ten years for this product to become an established part of resuscitation training programmes. The Resusci-Anne and other products are currently being used to deliver a wide range of resuscitation training programmes.

In the United Kingdom, the Resuscitation Council delivers fourteen separate courses to train individuals in skills relating to Adult, Paediatric and Newborn life support (all Immediate to Advanced) [84]. Publications evaluating the effectiveness of resuscitation training across healthcare disciplines have shown demonstrable improvements in practice [85-88]. In their comprehensive review of 114 resuscitation publications Mundell et al. concluded that simulation-based resuscitation training is highly effective when compared with no-intervention [89]. Mosley et al. reviewed a similar level of publications and identified that although there was an identifiable improvement in the knowledge and skills of those who attend resuscitation training programmes, there was evidence of skill decay in as little as three months [90]. This emphasises the importance for simulation to be adopted as part of an integrated programme rather than an isolated event.

Acute Care Skills

In 2012, the National Confidential Enquiry into Patient Outcome and Death published its report 'Time to Intervene?' [91]. This report identified that one third of in-hospital cardiac arrests and subsequent attempts to resuscitate could have been prevented. The authors called for better assessment of patients on hospital admission, more effective systems to recognise and respond when acutely ill patients deteriorate and improvements in the decision-making process around what care is likely to benefit acutely unwell patients.

Simulation has an essential role to play both in developing confidence and competence of practitioners. Applications such as in-situ simulation are being championed by acute care teams who are using simulation as a technique to recreate critical aspects of their working practice [92]. Acute care teams are publishing evidence regarding the power of simulation in improving patient safety [93, 94], emergency airway management [94, 95] and using tools such as team STEPPS to improve aspects of team working including the recognition and management of patients with life-threatening conditions such as severe sepsis and septic shock [58, 96, 97].

Disaster Management Training

Real and virtual environments have been developed to train physicians in managing traumatically injured patients [98], casualty resuscitation [96], disaster management training [99, 100] and reacting to a pandemic outbreak [101].

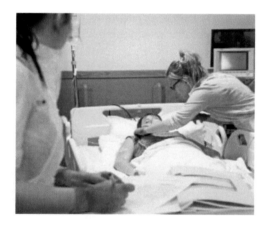

As the complexity of technical skills simulation activities has increased it has been complemented by a growing body of non-technical skills simulation based training most notably in the arena of Human factors such as crisis resource management training [102].

Non-Technical Skills Training

The publication of 'To Err is Human' was the catalyst for an international drive towards a culture of patient safety within healthcare institutions. It recommended that healthcare organisations make patient safety a declared and serious aim by establishing team training programmes that incorporated proven methods of team training, such as simulation. Since the time of this report the utilisation of simulation for non-technical skills training has become a priority to address some of the deficiencies identified in this report.

Communication Skills and Team Working

The power of simulation to recreate substantial aspects of the real world has been shown to improve patient safety [104], interprofessional practice [105, 106], communication skills [107] and team working [108]. The utilisation of handover tools such as SBAR have been shown to improve team communication [76, 103].

Simulation has proven value in championing the advancement of inter-professional team working and developing effective leaders. Calhoun et al. [109] developed a simulation activity to challenge the notion of hierarchy correlating with expertise. As part of this scenario the lead physician made an intentional drug error that proved fatal for the manikin in the scenario. This article critiqued the necessity of team work and effective communication in 'speaking up' to ensure patient safety regardless of the physician's status. Roberts et al. [110] addressed two key issues that limit healthcare staff engaging with simulation; the belief that simulation takes a lot of time and that you must be part of an established team.

Roberts et al. created a simulation programme that exposed ad-hoc members of a trauma team to a combination of simulation activities and behaviour training that resulted in improved leadership, team working and communication skills in their practice.

Human Factors Training

The popularity of Human Factors training has accelerated over the last decade. Human factors can be defined as 'the scientific discipline that takes a systems approach to understanding and optimizing the interactions among humans and their work system' [111].

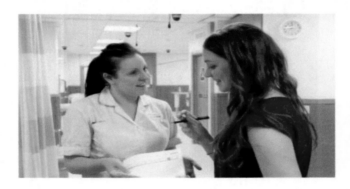

Human factors training has a pivotal role to play in enhancing patient safety [112], reducing medical error [113] and improving team dynamics [114]. In 2005 Martin Bromiley [115], an airline pilot, lost his wife when she underwent a 'routine operation'. The resultant investigation highlighted significant lack of human factors that resulted in sub-optimal care levels. In 2007, Martin Bromiley founded the clinical human factors group to champion the embedding of human factors training in healthcare. Simulation and human factors training share common linkages. Applying the principles of human factors within a simulation activity allows a systematic deconstruction of intrinsic and extrinsic factors that have a direct correlation on the performance capacity of the individual and the healthcare team. The ability to pause and unpick critical incidences in a safe and controlled environment has been crucial in informing systems design and organisational change.

Clinical Assessment Using Simulation

The reduction in the time that medical students spend in clinical environments at undergraduate level has raised concerns about their preparedness for clinical practice [116, 117]. The current evidence suggests that it is difficult to standardise workplace based assessments due to the experience and availability of assessors, the opportunistic nature of workplace based assessments and the limitations of the assessment tools to provide reliable and objective assessments [118, 119]. These circumstances have created the opportunity for simulation to demonstrate the added value it can bring to assessment.

The Objective Structural Clinical Examination (OSCE) has been the benchmark for assessing clinical competency since its inception in 1979 [120]. Since this time assessment of both technical [121] and non-technical skills [50] have been adopted into educational curricula and clinical practice. The Publication of the Bristol Royal Infirmary Inquiry Report [122], the Shipman Inquiry [123] and the Francis Report [23] again highlighted the ethical and moral responsibility of medical schools to only graduate those who have reached a required level of competency [124]. At the University of Dundee the ward simulation exercise has been developed to assess a medical student's preparedness for clinical practice within a realistic simulated ward environment. Final year medical students are assessed on their ability to manage the simulated ward for thirty minutes, prioritise competing demands including timed interruptions, make safe decisions and manage the care of three simulated patients. Each simulated patient is trained to play a new admission, a patient with a communication issue or an acutely unwell patient. This exercise has also been adapted for assessment purposes at postgraduate level to assess trainees who have been identified as having performance concerns within their clinical practice [125, 126].

The Future: What Next?

Fincher et al. [137] have suggested that the most important research question currently in medical education is 'what is the impact of medical school simulation learning on resident's performance?' This question has been also been identified at the Utstein meeting in 2011 and the issue will remain important for all new developments [45]. As educators we must be cognizant of the need for education and educational research to keep pace with changes in the clinical environment. The importance of close links with clinical practice will become increasingly important as the speed of development gathers.

A recent example of this would be the use of ultrasound bedside scanning and the training required to implement this. We must ensure that we continue to deliver educational programs and develop simulation technology in line with future clinical advances.

THE 'HOW?'

We discussed earlier in this chapter the 'Why?' of simulation including the evidence and educational underpinning for its use in education. We then explored the "What" in terms of technical and non-technical skills learning and the use of simulation in assessment. This leads us to "How" we best achieve learning using simulation within an educational programme.

There is a danger that the advances in technology will become more important than the way in which simulation can be used within a structured curriculum to be most effective [32]. As Clarke states "Method not medium affects Learning" [128], and the use of simulation in isolation is not necessarily a productive learning experience. Consideration therefore must be made as to 'how' it can be best utilised.

Glavin asserts that in order to achieve the aim of learning as a permanent change in behaviour, delivery of this kind of session needs to be "grounded in other curricular activities" [129]. The purpose of using simulation for participants as recipients of a learning event is to support and enhance learning of new skills and build on existing knowledge in relation to a subject, to prepare learners for practice [32]. It provides opportunities for those with established skills and clinical roles for; Rehearsal, Reinforcement, Renewal, Re-design, Risk reduction, Regulation and Research [32].

Designing the Learning Activity

"Education is an agent of change" [130] and theoretically the foundations of simulation based education advocate this approach. It is not simply about knowledge transfer from teacher to learner, but also about transfer to clinical practice, and improvement in patient care and safety. In order to achieve this aim, we must carefully position an activity within a curriculum, ensure it is planned and focused and is driven by identified learning outcomes [131].

Table 2. Simulation Building Template

Simulation Building Template
1. Identify the learning need to be addressed
2. Describe the logistics for the activity – Participants needed, Equipment required
3. Define the Learning Outcomes and underpinning educational theory for your proposed teaching session.
4. Setting and Background Information
5. Brief for Narrator, Participants and Simulated Patient
6. Immersion in the Simulation Event – consider engagement, level of control, safety
7. Expected activity/Response/Intervention to Observe – i.e. - What do we expect to happen?
8. Conclusion of session using Simulation
9. Approach to Debrief and Feedback

The use of tools for simulation can enhance a learning event if they feature as part of the learners' educational schedule and performance evaluation [132]. Planning a simulation learning activity is key to its success and structured tools can be helpful in doing this . Gagne states the use of training technology must begin with clearly defined educational objectives [133].

Intended Learning Outcomes and Constructive Alignment

Intended learning outcomes (ILOs) are the intended result of a learning process and serve a number of purposes (see box 4).

Box 4.

The Purpose of Intended Learning Outcomes is to:
• Ensure curriculum coverage
• Inform learners of what they should achieve
• Inform teachers of what they should help learners to achieve
• Reflect the nature and characteristics of the profession into which the learner is being inducted
• Direct the delivery of feedback
• Align teaching with assessment and clarify what will be assessed

They should answer the question – what new knowledge, skills and attitudes would you like learners to demonstrate by the end of the educational session? ILOs are learner focused and therefore differ from the aims of a session (example in box 5). Considering this example, we can see how the construct of the ILO will affect the planned learning activity. The ILO promotes engagement with the learning activity and clearly describes what the learner should expect to achieve following the simulation session.

Box 5.

Aim
To teach students about the Calgary-Cambridge Model for structuring a clinical consultation.

Intended Learning Outcome
Students will be able to apply the Calgary-Cambridge Model to conduct a structured patient consultation in a simulated general practice setting.

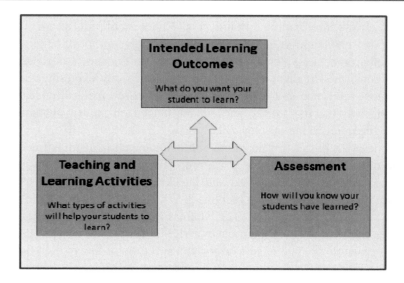

Constructive Alignment

When developing any simulation based teaching session, by writing clearly defined ILOs the educator can appropriately design the learning activity to reflect these. In doing so the educator can select when simulation is the most appropriate means of achieving the intended outcome [32]. Assessment of skills must align with both the intended learning outcomes and the learning activity and must be considered when designed the assessment [133]. Swanwick suggests that the process of immersion is probably more important than assessment, but that "assessment by its nature reinforces the intended outcomes of learning" [134]. Constructive alignment describes the relationship between 3 concepts the ILO, the teaching method and the Assessment as illustrated in the diagram below (Box 6).

Constructing Intended Learning Outcomes

Bloom's Taxonomy is commonly used in the design of intended learning outcomes and is a helpful way of conceptualising what you intend to achieve through your simulation activity [134]. "When there is alignment between what we want students to learn, what we teach, and what we assess, teaching is likely to be much more effective than when it is not" [133]. In order to write clear and helpful learning outcomes, to underpin our simulation activity, we should consider the following:

- Define the intended result of learning
- Consider the learners level of professional competence
- Consider constructive alignment with the curriculum
- Ensure they are specific, achievable and assessable

Fidelity and Realism

Realism is a term which is probably universally understood, and is used in simulation based education to lend support to the case for development of facilities, technology, techniques and environments which replicate the look, feel, smell, atmosphere of clinical practice. Artino considered realism as a phenomenon in a study exploring the relationship between motivation, relevance and realism in simulation based medical education [135]. A significant finding was the importance participants placed on realism in their motivation, closely related to their perception of relevance.

Participants describe physical, semantical and phenomenal realism as important in their intention to participate in simulation based learning [136]. The terms fidelity is also widely used in relation to simulation. Ostergaard and Dieckmann define fidelity as the similarity between the learning experience and the real one [137], Ker and Bradley describe it as "How well a learning event replicates reality" [32], whereas Maran and Glavin suggest the term is used to "describes aspects of the reality of the experience" [138].

The term is frequently applied to simulators on a spectrum of low to high fidelity, usually meaning simple to advanced. . A common misconception relating to fidelity is the role of technology in the generation of fidelity or authenticity in simulation based education. Alinier describes 'common misconceptions about simulation' and uses the example of trainees passively standing around an integrated patient simulator for the purpose of ECG interpretation [139]. This in itself is not higher fidelity simulation merely because it employs technology. In other words, fidelity is not generated solely by the technology but the experience of the users. The environment plays a significant role in the generation of contextual fidelity and is crucial in supporting transfer to the real world and in creating a suspension of disbelief to enhance learning [129]. There are multiple facets of a simulation experience which generate fidelity not simply the advanced technology. Maran and Glavin explain this in the context of "a continuum of medical education" [138].

The creating of fidelity is the responsibility of the facilitator during the Brief (preparation) and Immersion (activity) phases of the simulated event. The techniques and technologies of simulation have been developed with the aim of further suspending disbelief. It is interesting to note that the selection of a specific medium at times affects learning but not always as we might expect. Collins and Harden suggest the learner's actions are similar regardless of whether the patient is a colleague, an actual or simulated patient [140]. However Somerville identified that UG medical students experience was different when a manikin was replaced by an SP in acute care scenario [141]. Clearly fidelity has a role in the simulated learning activity and must be carefully considered within the context of the intended learning outcomes.

Simulators

There are now many different simulators available and selection of an appropriate simulator is one of the keys to the engagement and motivation of the participants [133].

The spectrum of simulation extends from basic skills acquisition to performing complex tasks and interpersonal communication in a multi-dimensional simulated environment. The simulators selected to support this learning should be influenced by factors which are relevant to the intended learning outcome [32]. When planning a simulation activity the selection of a simulator affects learning in respect to fidelity and feedback, therefore the following points should be considered:

a) Simulator Classification
Simulators are classified according to their function.

- Part task trainers, often replicating a body part, allow practice of a certain technical skill, for example an anatomical arm for venepuncture practice.
- Computer based systems and virtual reality simulation programs have been developed for e-learning. These programmes range from models of physiology and anatomy to online virtual learning environments using avatars for online learning. Haptic systems including models linked with virtual reality can provide kinaesthetic and tactile sensation for rehearse technical procedures.
- Integrated simulators combine a body part or whole body manikin with a computer which controls physiological parameters. The capability of these systems is advancing. More traditionally the manikins were controlled by the facilitator but using pre-determined algorithms they can now react automatically to interventions. The manikins may also incorporate realistic body parts for procedures.
- The use of actors, simulated and standardised patients is increasing within the simulation community. Simulated patients have been defined as 'a well person trained to simulate a patient's illness in a standardised way' [142]. These patients are

often utilised to teach communication skills and examination skills as well as being used in more complex scenarios to teach non-technical skills.

The choice of simulator will be driven by the clinical features that it can reproduce linked with the ILOs for the activity.

b) Simulated Environments

Simulated environments can be set up within educational institutions to replicate clinical areas and create a safe learning environment [143-145].

These aim to enhance learner engagement through increasing fidelity and supporting transfer of learning to the clinical environment.

The Teaching and Learning Activity: Brief – Immersion – Debrief

Gaba categorises 11 dimensions of simulation as a guide to promoting innovation by users of this "technique" [4].

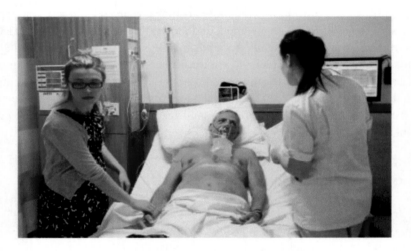

In this chapter we use the terms Brief, Immersion and Debrief to reinterpret and illustrate the elements of facilitating a simulation event:

- Brief – preparation for simulation,
- Immersion – the simulation activity
- Debrief – focused discussion following the activity

Brief

The Brief is often underestimated in the preparation for any simulated event. When not properly briefed a simulated event may result in harmful consequences, including learner humiliation and failure to achieve the ILOs. Aspects to be considered to ensure clear briefing include; preparation of a safe learning environment, assuring learners of confidentiality, orientation to the simulators and environment, introductions and clarification of role of staff, learners and patients. As simulation aims to recreate components of a clinical scenario from practice, we should always consider;

- o   who is participating, (e.g. professional background, individuals or teams)
- o   what is their level of experience (junior/senior/peers)
- o   what is the time limit you have for the session and debrief

As the facilitator you present the clinical situation and engage the participant(s) in the simulation to ensure they have a shared mental model of the learning activity. Using SBAR is a useful way to present a scenario, as the information is intended to be accurate and concise, and this is also the way we may expect a learner to conclude the session [148].

Brief
Prepare self, assistants and environment appropriately for the relevant session (plan)
Welcome participants and introduces the context of the intended activity (SAFE)
Define the learning outcomes – the purpose and importance of the session (i.e. constructive alignment)
Link relevance of the simulated activity to the practitioner or practice (i.e. curriculum integration)
Consider significance of process in relation to educational theory (e.g. Kolb's experiential cycle)

Immersion
"The scenario is the curriculum" [149]

In the short time that a simulated activity occurs an enormous amount of content can be covered. Whether the proposed session is focussed on a specific procedure, a communication exchange, or the assessment and management of a patient, levels of anxiety can be high. To minimise this affect and optimise learning, consider the following elements:

- Manufacture the reality of the setting and the facilities – having knowledge of simulator/specialist context/simulated patient.
- Maintain control of safety and simulation equipment. Correct miscues, if the learner has misinterpreted a situation and is progressing towards an unexpected pathway then it would be best to interrupt, pause or stop the activity [150].
- Consider the level of interaction by the facilitator with the individual or group [40]. It can be easy to dominate and overwhelm a simulated activity by your physical presence or vocal interruption. The degree to which this is appropriate depends on the purpose and ILO of the session.
- The complexity required – the degree of difficulty of a scenario depends on the intended learning outcomes and participants. Making the session too difficult or easy will deter junior and experienced participants respectively. It may also be appropriate to acknowledge the input and experiences in the group.

Different teaching methods can be used to structure the immersion phase of the simulation based education (SBE) activity. For procedural activities 4 and 2 stage approaches are common [152].

Facilitate effectively the relevant structured learning event, consider levels of facilitation
Allow participants to immerse in practice
Nurture engagement between 'expert' and learners (beware 'intrusion' of expert)
Relate 'new' activity to relevant clinical standards
Respond to and guide practice to seek change/improvement
Lend support throughout task and checks understanding of participants

Feedback and Debrief

Feedback and debrief are widely accepted as fundamental to the process of SBE [153], and it is beyond the scope of this chapter to explore all the literature relating to feedback and debrief. However, defining these terms is a helpful starting point for further differentiation and debate as at times these terms are used interchangeably and give rise to confusion. Salvodelli et al. [154] define feedback (FB) and debrief (DB) as follows:

- Feedback is 'corrective information in order to improve future performance'
- Debrief is 'a whole process of reflective practice, including feedback'

The aim of feedback and debrief is to close the loop between the elements of constructive alignment; intended learning outcomes, the SBE activity and the reflection/assessment. The process should focus on the ILOs, to enquire, encourage and embed learning from the simulated activity. The reflection involved in feedback and debrief presents individuals with an insight from experts and peers into their own abilities and behaviours, an insight into the known and unknown self [155]. Commonly used approaches to feedback and debrief include; Pendleton's' Rules [156], ALOBA – agenda-led outcome-based analysis [157] and advocacy with enquiry [158]. Inherent in these models is that the feedback conversation should be learner focussed and constructive.

Kneebone and Nestel advocate an approach to feedback where the learner sets the agenda for observation and discussion, focussing on the learners needs [159]. It is recognised however that recipients of feedback often do far less talking than the deliverer [160], and the process of debriefing can be disappointing and at worst evoke defensiveness in the learner depending on the perceived expertise and skill of the facilitator [161]. Video assisted debrief can be used to select episodes of effective and challenging performance, and is advocated as a means to enhance the learners ability to reflect 'on action'.

Video is particularly useful for more complex scenario and team based simulated activities [162]. It is important that the debrief and feedback process concludes with some form of action plan for future application and learning.

Applications to Practice

Chiniara et al. argue that the concept of Instructional Design is overlooked in the use of SBE [146]. They propose a framework and taxonomy "to assist educators in creating appropriate simulation learning experiences". Chiniara's framework includes the medium (mode of delivery), the simulation modality (e.g. part task or computer based), instructional method (techniques used for learning) and presentation (the intervention). De Freitas and Oliver have questioned how exploratory learning with simulation can be evaluated within the curriculum and advocate a checklist considering the 'context, learner specification, pedagogic considerations, and mode of representation (tools for use) [147].

This checklist is aimed specifically at the use of online simulated learning, but could be adapted as an analytical tool for researchers and as a pragmatic tool for practitioners to aid 'product selection' and utility.

The Future – What Next ?

Evaluation and development of local programs, resources and facilitators, need to ensure the efficacy and quality of the product being delivered. Much of the evaluation of simulation is undertaken by facilitators, looking at the learners experiences and there is commonly a feel-good factor amongst deliverers and recipients. However, there are still pockets of cynicism amongst individuals who see limited value in simulation based education. Some fail to engage or struggle to overcome the challenge of participating in SBE. This may be due to poor experiences or cultural differences [163]. There is evidence that simulation-based education improves the clinical skills and practices of healthcare professionals and translates into improved patient care [164]. However in spite of this, and the increasingly common use of simulation in healthcare education, there are gaps in the literature identifying how the use of simulation can influence learning and performance in the workplace [45]. There are developing trends in education research adopting video based methodologies within an interpretive paradigms, which pushes the research question to address how does it work or how does it not work? Bradley and Postlethwaite also urge that increased theoretical clarity with respect to learning theory may lead to different kinds of enquiry regarding interventions in SBE [165].

CONCLUSION

The "why what and how" of simulation based education has captured what is the current state of play and evidence for its use in modern curricula, in both undergraduate and postgraduate medical education. Simulation provides a structure for deliberate practice of technical and non-technical and is most useful when fully integrated into a curriculum [46]. Importantly, the use of simulation is not limited to the acquisition of core technical skills but can also successfully develop complex professional behaviours such as clinical reasoning and situational awareness.

Ultimately the aim of introducing simulation into any medical curriculum is to positively impact on reliability and resilience of performance in the workplace for enhanced patient outcomes. Predictability of transfer of learning from simulation to practice requires further evidence particularly around the discrepancies between environments and the impact this has on performance [166].

Additionally, simulation is currently used to learn skills and concepts rather than learning to transfer into the clinical environment. The use of in-situ simulation is increasing with research demonstrating improved quality and safety of healthcare delivery [167, 168]. It has the added advantage of identifying the effectiveness of a workplace which impacts on an individual's ability to transfer skills [169]. To further promote this important transfer of learning, it is may be that learning about transfer with increasing authenticity is required [170].

The costs associated with simulation based education are significant but the growing evidence for its impact on patient safety and the production of a better prepared workforce have the potential to offset these [171, 172]. There is also a potential to reduce long term costs by using simulation to trial and rehearse equipment, techniques and systems prior to their employment [173-177]. Currently simulation is being adopted globally as a technique to address the increasingly high profile issues of patient safety and quality improvement within clinical practice. Although there are areas of research still to be addressed, the growing body of evidence and greater public accountability of medical practice look set to intensify its use over the coming years. Simulation has the potential to be of immense value in health care learning if well supported and integrated [178]. The challenge is to ensure that's its potential is realised through appropriate and skilful research application to best prepare the healthcare team for tomorrow.

REFERENCES

[1]   Reason, J. (2000) Human error: models and management. *BMJ*. 320: 768-70.
[2]   Burke, C. S., Salas, E., Wilson-Donnelly, K., and Priest, H. (2004) How to turn a team of experts into an expert medical team: guidance from the aviation and military communities. *Quality and Safety in Health Care*. 13: i96-104.
[3]   Anon (2007) 'Out of this nettle, danger, we pluck this flower, safety': healthcare vs. aviation and other high-hazard industries. *Simulation in Healthcare*. 2: 213-7.
[4]   Gaba, D. The future vision of simulation in health care. *Quality and Safety in Health Care*. 2004. 13. i2-i10.
[5]   Owen, H. (2012) Early use of Simulation in Medical Education. *Simulation in Healthcare*. Apr.;7(2):102-16.
[6]   Tjomsland, N. and Baskett, P. (2002) Resuscitation greats: Armund S Laerdal. *Resuscitation*. 53: 115-9.
[7]   Delp, S. L., Loan, J. P., Hoy, M. G., et al. (1990). An interactive graphics based model of the lower extremity to study orthopaedic surgical procedures. *IEEE Transactions on Biomedical Engineering*. 37: 757-767.
[8]   Savata, R. (1993). Virtual Reality Surgical simulator: the first steps. *Surgical Endoscopy*. 15: 232-241.
[9]   Howard, S. K., Gaba, D. M., Fish, K. J., Yang, G., and Sarnquist, F. H. (1992) Anesthesia crisis resource management training: teaching anesthesiologists to handle critical incidents. *Aviation, Space, and Environmental Medicine*. 63: 763-70.
[10]   Gaba, D. M., Fish, K. J. and Howard, S. K. (1994) *Crisis Management in Anesthesiology*. Churchill Livingstone, New York.
[11]   Flin, R. and Maran, N. J. (2004) Identifying and training non-technical skills for teams in acute medicine. *Quality and Safety in Health Care*. 13 (1): 80-4.
[12]   Glavin, R. J. and Maran, N. J. (2003) Integrating human factors into the medical curriculum. *Medical Education*. 37: 59-64.

[13]   Bradley, P. The history of simulation in medical education and possible future directions. *Med. Educ.* 2006 Mar.;40(3):254-62.

[14]   Spencer, J. The clinical teaching context: a cause for concern. *Medical Education.* 2003;37(3):182-3.

[15]   Illing, J., Davies, C., Bauldauf, B. *How prepared are medical graduates to begin practice? A comparison of three diverse UK medical schools.* London: General Medical Council; 2008.

[16]   McLachlan, J. C., Patten, D. Anatomy teaching: ghosts of the past, present and future. *Medical Education.* 2006;40(3):243-53.

[17]   Health Do. Day surgery: operational guide Waiting, booking and choice. *Crown Copyright. Crown Copyright*; 2002. p. 40.

[18]   Rees, C. E., Monrouxe, L. V. Medical students learning intimate examinations without valid consent: a multicentre study. *Med. Educ.* 2011 Mar.;45(3):261-72.

[19]   Feldman, D. S., Novack, D. H., Farber, N. J., Fleetwood, J. The Ethical Dilemma of Students Learning to Perform Procedures on Nonconsenting Patients. *Academic Medicine.* 1999;74(1):79.

[20]   McIndoe, A. The future face of medical training--ship-shape and Bristol fashion. *The British Journal Of Theatre Nursing: Natnews: The Official Journal Of The National Association Of Theatre Nurses.* 1998;8(8):5.

[21]   Smith, J. *Shipman Fifth report. Safeguarding patients: lessons from the the past-proposals fo the future;* 2005.

[22]   Enquiry, B. R. I. *Learning from Bristol: The report of the public enquiry into childrenns heart surgery at The Bristol Royal Infirmnary* 1984-1995; 2001.

[23]   Francis, R. *Report of the Mid Staffordshire NHS Foundation Trust Public Inquiry.* [cited April 2014]; Available from: http://www.midstaffspublicinquiry.com/sites/default/files/report/Executive%20summary.pdf.

[24]   Linda, T., Kohn, J. M. C. and Molla, S., Donaldson, E. *To err is human: Building a safer health system.* Washington DC: Committee on Quality of Health Care in America, Institute of Medicine; 2000.

[25]   Donaldson, L. An organisation with a memory. *Clinical Medicine.* 2002 September 1, 2002;2(5):452-7.

[26]   Ziv, A., Wolpe, P. R., Small, S. D., Glick, S. Simulation-based medical education: an ethical imperative. *Simulation in healthcare: journal of the Society for Simulation in Healthcare.* 2006 Winter;1(4):252-6.

[27]   Rees, C. E., Monrouxe, L. V. Theory in medical education research: how do we get there? *Medical Education.* 2010;44(4):334-9.

[28]   Kolb, D. *Experiential Learning.* Englewood Cliffs, NJ: Prentice Hall Inc.; 1984.

[29]   Lave, J., Wegner, E. *Situated Learning: Legitimate peripheral partcipation.* Cambridge, UK: Cambridge University Press; 1991.

[30]   Ericsson, K. Deliberate practice and the acquisition and maintenance of expert performance in medicine and related domains. A. *Academic Medicine: Journal Of The Association Of American Medical Colleges.* 2004;79(10 Suppl.):S70-81.

[31]   McGaghie, W. C., Issenberg, S. B., Cohen, E. R., Barsuk, J. H., Wayne, D. B. Medical education featuring mastery learning with deliberate practice can lead to better health for individuals and populations. *Academic Medicine: Journal Of The Association Of American Medical Colleges.* 2011;86(11):e8-e9.

[32] Swanwick, T., editor. *Understanding Medical education: Evidence, Theory and Practice*. Ker J., Brdaley P., Simulation in medical education Second ed. Oxford: Association for the study of medical education; 2014.

[33] Dieckmann, P., Phero, J. C., Issenberg, S. B., Kardong-Edgren, S., Ostergaard, D., Ringsted, C. The first Research Consensus Summit of the Society for Simulation in Healthcare: conduction and a synthesis of the results. *Simulation In Healthcare: Journal Of The Society For Simulation In Healthcare*. 2011;6 Suppl.:S1-S9.

[34] Dieckmann, P., Gaba, D., Rall, M. Deepening the Theoretical Foundations of Patient Simulation as Social Practice. *Simul. Healthc*. 2007;2(3):183-93 10.1097/SIH.0b013e 3180f637f5.

[35] Monrouxe, L. V., Rees, C. E. Picking up the gauntlet: constructing medical education as a social science. *Med. Educ*. 2009;43(3):196-8.

[36] Seymour, N. E. M. D., Gallagher, A. G. P., Roman, S. A. M. D., O'Brien, M. K. M. D., Bansal, V. K. M. D., Andersen, D. K. M. D., et al. Virtual Reality Training Improves Operating Room Performance: Results of a Randomized, Double-Blinded Study. *Annals of Surgery*. 2002;236(4):458-64.

[37] Chaer, R. A., Derubertis, B. G., Lin, S. C., Bush, H. L., Karwowski, J. K., Birk, D., et al. Simulation improves resident performance in catheter-based intervention: results of a randomized, controlled study. *Ann. Surg*. 2006 Sep.;244(3):343-52.

[38] Draycott, T., Sibanda, T., Owen, L., Akande, V., Winter, C., Reading, S., et al. Does training in obstetric emergencies improve neonatal outcome? *BJOG: an international journal of obstetrics and gynaecology*. 2006;113(2):177-82.

[39] Draycott, T. J., Crofts, J. F., Ash, J. P., Wilson, L. V., Yard, E., Sibanda, T., et al. Improving neonatal outcome through practical shoulder dystocia training. *Obstet. Gynecol*. 2008;112(1):14-20.

[40] Barsuk, J. H., McGaghie, W. C., Cohen, E. R., Balachandran, J. S., Wayne, D. B. Use of simulation-based mastery learning to improve the quality of central venous catheter placement in a medical intensive care unit. *Journal Of Hospital Medicine: An Official Publication Of The Society Of Hospital Medicine*. 2009;4(7):397-403.

[41] Barsuk, J., Cohen, E., McGaghie, W., Wayne, D. Long-term retention of central venous catheter insertion skills after simulation-based mastery learning. *Acad. Med*. 2010; 85 (10 Suppl.):S9-12.

[42] Gurusamy, K., Aggarwal, R., Palanivelu, L., Davidson, B. R. Systematic review of randomized controlled trials on the effectiveness of virtual reality training for laparoscopic surgery. *British Journal of Surgery*. 2008;95(9):1088-97.

[43] Sturm, L. P., Windsor, J. A., Cosman, P. H., Cregan, P., Hewett, P. J., Maddern, G. J. A Systematic Review of Skills Transfer After Surgical Simulation Training. *Annals of Surgery*. 2008;248(2):166-79 10.1097/SLA.0b013e318176bf24.

[44] Sutherland, L. M., Middleton, P. F., Anthony, A., Hamdorf, J., Cregan, P., Scott, D., et al. Surgical simulation: a systematic review. *Ann. Surg*. 2006 Mar.;243(3):291-300.

[45] Issenberg, S., Ringsted, C., Ostergaard, D., Dieckmann, P. Setting a research agenda for simulation-based healthcare education. A synthesis of the outcome from an Utstein style meeting. *Simul. Healthc*. 2011;6:155-67.

[46] Issenberg, S. B., McGaghie, W. C., Petrusa, E. R., Lee Gordon, D., Scalese, R. J. Features and uses of high-fidelity medical simulations that lead to effective learning: a BEME systematic review. *Medical Teacher*. 2005;27(1):10-28.

[47] Cook, D. A., Hatala, R., Brydges, R., et al. Technology-enhanced simulation for health professions education: A systematic review and meta-analysis. *JAMA*. 2011;306 (9): 978-88.

[48] Schmutz, J., Manser, T. Do team processes really have an effect on clinical performance? A systematic literature review. *British Journal of Anaesthesia*. 2013 April 1, 2013;110(4):529-44.

[49] Bond, W. F., Deitrick, L. M., Arnold, D. C., Kostenbader, M., Barr, G. C., Kimmel, S. R., et al. Using simulation to instruct emergency medicine residents in cognitive forcing strategies. *Academic Medicine: Journal Of The Association Of American Medical Colleges*. 2004;79(5):438-46.

[50] Fletcher, G., Flin, R., McGeorge, P., Glavin, R., Maran, N., Patey, R. Anaesthetists' Non-Technical Skills (ANTS): evaluation of a behavioural marker system. *Br. J. Anaesth*. 2003 May 1, 2003;90(5):580-8.

[51] Ottestad, E., Boulet, J. R., Lighthall, G. K. Evaluating the management of septic shock using patient simulation. *Crit. Care Med*. 2007;35(3):769-75 10.1097/01.CCM.000025 6849.75799.20.

[52] Mardon, J. Use of Workplace Simulation to Enable Development of a Safe Stroke Thrombolysis Service Dr Julie Mardon University Hospital Crosshouse. *4th International conference Clinical Skills*. Prao, Italy; 2013.

[53] Siassakos, D., Crofts, J., Winter, C., Weiner, C., Draycott, T. The active components of effective training in obstetric emergencies. *BJOG*. 2009.116. 1028-1032.

[54] Kneebone, R., Kidd, J., Nestel, D., Asvall, S., Paraskeva, P., and Darzi, A. An innovative model for teaching and learning clinical procedures. *Medical Education*. 2002. 36. 628-634.

[55] Wright, J. A quantitative pilot study evaluating the effectiveness of a venepuncture and cannulation study day. *Nurse Education Today*. 2009. 29. 555-560.

[56] Morton, J., Anderson, L., Frame, F., Moyes, J., and Cmeron, H. Back to the future: teaching medical students clinical procedures. *Medical Teacher*. 2006. 28 (8). 723-728.

[57] Scholtz, A., Monachino, A., Nishisaki, A., Nadkarni, V., and Lengetti, E. Central Venous Catheter Rehearsals. *Journal of Simulation in Healthcare*. 2013. 8(5). 341-349.

[58] Wayne, D., Cohen, E., Singer, B., Moazed, F., Barsuk, J., Lyons, E., Butter, J., and Mcgaghie, W. Progress Toward Improving Medical School Graduates' Skills via a "Boot Camp" Curriculum. *Journal of Simulation in Healthcare*. 2014. 9(1). 33-39.

[59] Summer, L., Gonzalez, L., Jimeno, M., and Christensen, K. Development of a nasogastric tube insertion simulator: a collaborative interdisciplinary effort. *Computers, Informatics, Nursing*. 27(2). 105-113.

[60] Victor Wilcox, V., Trus, T., Salas, N., Martinez, J., and Dunkin, B. A Proficiency-Based Skills Training Curriculum for the SAGES Surgical Training For Endoscopic Proficiency (STEP) Program. *Journal of Surgical Education*. 2014. 71 (3).

[61] Andreatta, B., Hillard, M. and Krain, L. The Impact of stress factors in simulation-based laparoscopic training. *Surgery*. 2010. 631-638.

[62] Gauger, P., Hauge, L., Andreatta, P., Hamstra, S., Hillard, M., Arble, E., Kasten, S., Mullan, P., Cederna, P., and Minter, R. Laparoscopic simulation training with proficiency targets improves practice and performance of novice surgeons. *The American Journal of Surgery*. 2010. 199. 72-80.

[63] Aggarwal, R., Black, S., Hance, J., Darzi, A., and Cheshire, N. Virtual Reality Simulation Training can Improve Inexperienced Surgeons' Endovascular Skills. *Eur. J. Vasc. Endovasc. Surg.* 2006. 31. 588-593. (2006).

[64] Marshall, B., Wilson, B. and Carter, Y. Thoracic Surgery Skill Proficiency with Chest Wall Tumor Simulator. *Journal of Surgical Research.* 2012. 174. 250-256.

[65] Goova, M., Hollett, L., Tesfay, S., Gala, R., Puzziferri, N., Kehdy, F., and Scott, D. Implementation, Construct Validity, and Benefit of a Proficiency-Based Knot-Tying and Suturing Curriculum. *Journal of Surgical Education.* 2008. (65) 4. 309-315.

[66] Veloski, J., Boex, J., Grasberger, M., Evans, A., and Wolfson, D. Systematic review of the literature on assessment,feedback and physicians' clinical performance: BEME Guide No. 7. *Medical Teacher.* 2006. 28 (2). 117-128.

[67] Mezirow, J. (2000) *Learning as Transformation: Critical Perspectives on a Theory in Progress.* Joey Bass Publishing. San Fransico.

[68] Chen, J., Yip, A., Lam, C., and Patil, N. Does medical student willingness to practise peer physical examination translate into action? *Medical Teacher.* 2011. 33. e528-e540.

[69] Hendrickx, Kristin, et al. "Intimate examination teaching with volunteers: implementation and assessment at the University of Antwerp." *Patient education and counseling* 63.1 (2006): 47-54.

[70] Pickard, S., Baraitser, P., Rymer, J., and Piper, J. (2003) Can gynaecology teaching associates provide high quality effective training for medical students in the United Kingdom? Comparative study. *BMJ.* 327: 1389-92.

[71] Rochelson, B., Baker, D., Mann, W., Monheit, A., and Stone, M. (1985) Use of male and female professional patient teams in teaching physical examination of the genitalia. *Journal of Reproductive Medicine.* 30: 864-6.

[72] Wånggren, K., Pettersson, G., Csemiczky, G., and Gemzell-Danielsson, K. (2005) Teaching medical students gynaecological examination using professional patients - evaluation of students' skills and feelings. *Medical Teacher.* 27: 130-5.

[73] Naylor, R., Hollett, L., Valentine, J., Mitchell, I., Bowling, M., Ma, A., Dineen, S., Bruns, B., and Scott, D. Can medical students achieve skills proficiency through simulation training? *The American Journal of Surgery.* 2009. 198. 277-282.

[74] Dilaveri, C., Szostek, J., Wang, A., and Cook, D. Simulation training for breast and pelvic physical examination: a systematic review and meta-analysis. *BJOG.* 2013. 120. 1171-1182.

[75] Maguire, P. and Carolyn, P. "Key communication skills and how to acquire them." *BMJ: British Medical Journal* 325.7366 (2002): 697.

[76] Cornell, P., Townsend-Gervis, M., Vardaman, J., and Yates, L. Improving Situation Awareness and Patient Outcomes Through Interdisciplinary Rounding and Structured Communication. *JONA.* 2014. 44(3). 164-169.

[77] Kurtz, S., Silverman, J., Draper, J. *Teaching and learning communication skills in medicine.* Oxford: Radcliffe Medical Press; 1998.

[78] Maguire, P., Roe, T., Goldberg, D., Jones, S., Hyde, C., O'Dowd, T. The Value of feedback in teaching interviewing skills to medical students. *Psychol. Med.* 1978; 8: 695-704.

[79] Maguire, P., Fairbairn, S., Fletcher, C. Consultation skills of young doctors: benefits of feedback training in interviewing as students persist. *BMJ.* 1986; 292: 1573-1578.

[80] Pottier, P., Dejoie, T., Hardoiun, J., Loupp, A., Planchon, B., Bonnaud, A., and Lebalnc, V. Effect of stress on clinical reasoning during simulated ambulatory consultations. *Medical Teacher*. 2013. 35. 472-480.

[81] Tobler, K., Grant, E. and Marczinski, C. Evaluation of the Impact of a Simulation-Enhanced Breaking Bad News Workshop in Pediatrics. *Journal of Simulation in Healthcare*. 2014. 00:00-000. 1-7. DOI: 10.1097/SIH.0000000000000031.

[82] Merckaert, I., Liénard, A., Libert, Y., Bragard, I., Delvaux, N., Etienne, A.-M., Marchal, S., Meunier, J., Reynaert, C., Slachmuylder, J.-L., and Razavi, D. Is it possible to improve the breaking bad news skills of residents when a relative is present? A randomised study. *British Journal of Cancer*. 2013. 109. 2507-2514.

[83] Vyas, D., Lackey, G. and McCulloh, R. Acute Overdose. *Journal of Simulation in Healthcare*. 2013. 8(4). 272-8.

[84] *The Resuscitation Council*. http://www.resus.org.uk/pages/courses.htm [Accessed 26.5. 14].

[85] Schillemana, K., Siewb, M., Lopriorea, E., Morleya, C., Walthera, F., and te Pasa, A. Auditing resuscitation of preterm infants at birth by recording video and physiological parameters. *Resuscitation*. 2012. 83. 1135-1139.

[86] Passali, C., Pantazopoulos, I., Dontas, I., Patsaki, A., Barouxis, D., Troupis, G., and Xanthos, T. Evaluation of nurses' and doctors' knowledge of basic and advanced life support resuscitation guidelines. *Nurse Education in Practice*. 2011. 11. 365-369.

[87] Lyon, R., Clarke, S., Milligan, D., and Clegg, G. Resuscitation feedback and targeted education improves quality of pre-hospital resuscitation in Scotland. *Resuscitation*. 2012. 83. 70-75.

[88] Kazaurea, H., Romanb, S. and Sosab, J. Epidemiology and outcomes of in-hospital cardiopulmonary resuscitation in the United States, 2000-2009. *Resuscitation*. 2013. 84. 1255-1260.

[89] Mundell, W., Kennedy, C., Szosteka, J., and Cook, D. Simulation technology for resuscitation training: A systematic review and meta-analysis. *Resuscitation*. 2013. 84. 1174-1183.

[90] Mosley, C., Dewhurst, C., Molloy, S., and Shaw, B. What is the impact of structured resuscitation training on healthcare practitioners, their clients and the wider service? A BEME systematic review: BEME Guide No. 20. *Medical Teacher*. 2012. 34: e349-e385.

[91] National Confidential Enquiry into Patient Outcome and Death. Time to Intervene? *A review of patients who underwent cardiopulmonary resuscitation as a result of an in-hospital cardiorespiratory arrest*. 2012.

[92] Kobayashi, L., Patterson, M., Overly, F., Shapiro, M., Williams, K., and Jay, G. Educational and Research Implications of Portable Human Patient Simulation in Acute Care Medicine. *Academic Emergency Medicine*. 2008. 15.1166-1174.

[93] Miller, K., Riley, W., Davis, S., and Hansen, H. In Situ Simulation: A Method of Experiential Learning to Promote Safety and Team Behavior. *J. Perinat. Neonat. Nurs*. 2008. 22(2). 105-113.

[94] Zirkle, M., Blum, R., Raemer, D., Healy, G., and Roberson, D. Teaching Emergency Airway Management Using Medical Simulation: A Pilot Program. *Laryngoscope*. 2005. 115. 495-500.

[95] Hubert, V., Duwat, A., Deransy, R., Mahjoub, Y., and Dupont, H. Effect of Simulation Training on Compliance with Difficult Airway Management Algorithms, Technical Ability, and Skills Retention for Emergency Cricothyrotomy. *Anesthesiology*. 2014. 120. 999-1008.

[96] Capella, J. Smith, S. Philp, A. Putnam, T. Gilbert, C. Fry, W. Harvey, E. Wright, A. Henderson, K. Baker, D. Ranson, and ReMine, S. Teamwork Training Improves the Clinical Care of Trauma Patients. *Journal of Surgical Education*. 2010. 67 (6). 440-443.

[97] Nguyen, B., Underwood, L., Van Ginkel, C., Wong, M., Lee, D., Lucas, A., Palaganas, J., Banta, D., Denmark, T., and Clem, K. An educational course including medical simulation for early goal-directed therapy and the severe sepsis resuscitation bundle: An evaluation for medical student training. *Resuscitation*. 2009. 80. 674-679.

[98] Sohn, V., Runser, L., Puntel, R., Sebesta, J., Beekley, A., Theis, J., Merrill, N., Roth, B., and Rush, R. Training Physicians for Combat Casualty Care on the Modern Battlefield. *Journal of Surgical Education*. 2007. 64(4). 199-203.

[99] Scott, L., Carson, D. and Greenwell, B. Disaster 101: A novel approach to disaster medicine training for health professionals. *The Journal of Emergency Medicine*. 2010. 39 (2). 220-226.

[100] Rega, P. and Fink, B. Immersive Simulation Education: A Novel Approach to Pandemic Preparedness and Response. *Public Health Nursing*. 2013. 31(2). 167-174.

[101] Gomes, J., Borges, M., Huber, G., and Carvalho, P. Analysis of the resilience of team performance during a nuclear emergency response exercise. *Applied Ergonomics*. 2014. 45 780-788.

[102] Howard, S., Gaba, D. and Fish, K. Anesthesia crisis resource management training: teaching anesthesiologists to handle critical incidents. *Aviat. Space Environ. Med.* 1992. 63. 763-770.

[103] Randmaa, M., Mårtensson, G., Swenne, C., and Engström, M. SBAR improves communication and safety climate and decreases incident reports due to communication errors in an anaesthetic clinic: a prospective intervention study. *BMJ Open*. 2014.4.1-9.

[104] Ironside, P., Jeffries, P., Martin, A. Fostering Patient safety competencies using multiple – patient simulation experiences. *Nursing Outlook*. 2009. 57. 332-337.

[105] Van Soeren, M., MacMillan, K., Cop, S., Kenaszchuk, C., and Reeves, S. Development and evaluation of interprofessional care practices through clinical simulation. *Journal of interprofessional care*. 2009. 23(3). 304-306.

[106] Dadiz, R., Weinsvhnreider, J., Schriefer, J., Arnold, C., Greves, C., Crosby, E., Wang, H., Pressman, E., and Guilet, R. Interdisciplinary Simualtion-Based Training to Improve Delivery Room Communication. *Journal of Simulation in Healthcare*. 2013. 8 (5). 279-29.

[107] Kameg, K., Mitchell, A., Clochesy, J., Howard, V., Suresky, J. Communication and Human Simulation in Psychiatric Nursing. *Issues in Mental Health Nursing*. 2009. 30. 503-508.

[108] Miller, K., Riley, W. and Davis, S. Identifying key nursing and team behaviours to achieve high reliability. *Journal of Nursing Management*. 2009. 17. 247-255.

[109] Calhoun, A., Boone, M., Miller, K., and Pian-Smith, M. Case and Commentary: Using Simulation to Address Hierarchy Issues During Medical Crises. *Journal of Simulation in Healthcare*. 2013. 8(1). 13-19.

[110] Roberts, N., Williams, R., Schwind, C., Sutyak, J., McDowell, C., Griffen, D., Wall, J., Sanfey, H., Chestnut, A., Meier, A., Wohltmann, C., Clark, T., and Wetter, N. The impact of brief team communication, leadership and team behavior training on ad hoc team performance in trauma care settings. *The American Journal of Surgery*. 2014. 207. 170-178.

[111] Clack, L., Kuster, S., Giger, H., Giuliani, F., and Sax, H. Low-hanging fruit for human factors design in infection prevention still too high to reach? *American Journal of Infection Control* 42 (2014) 679-81.

[112] Youngson, G. and Flin, R. Patient safety in surgery: non-technical aspects of safe surgical performance. *Patient Safety in Surgery*. 2010. 4:4.

[113] Endsley, M. Toward a theory of situation awareness in dynamic systems. *Human Factors* 1995b. 37(1). 32-64.

[114] Norris, E. and Lockey, A. Human factors in resuscitation teaching. *Resuscitation* 83 (2012) 423-427.

[115] Bromiley, M. *Clinical Human Factors Group*. http://chfg.org/.

[116] Calman, S., Mcregor, R. and Spector, N. How Can We Assure Procedural Competence in Pediatric Residents in an Era of Diminishing Opportunities? The Answer is Simulation-Based Training. *The Journal of Pediatrics*. 2010. 156(6). 865-866.866.e1.

[117] Perkins, G. Simulation in resuscitation training. *Resuscitation*. 2007. 73. 202-211.

[118] Aaron, S. Moving up the Pyramid: Assessing Performance in the Clinic. *Journal of Rheumatology*. 2009. 36.1101-1103.

[119] General Medical Council. *Workplace Based Assessment: a guide for implementation*. 2010.

[120] Harden, R. and Gleeson, F. Assessment of medical competence using an objective structural clinical examination (OSCE). *Association for the Study of Medical Education*. 1979.

[121] Macleod, R., Mires, G. and Ker, J. Direct observed procedural skills assessment in the undergraduate setting. *The Clinical Teacher*. 9(4). 228-232.

[122] *Bristol Royal Infirmary Inquiry Report*. The Inquiry into the management of care of children receiving complex heart surgery at the Bristol Royal Infirmary. 2001.

[123] *The Shipman Inquiry. Independent Public Inquiry into the issues arising from the case of Frederick Harold Shipman*. 2005.

[124] Roberts, C., Newble, D., Jolly, B., Reed, M., and Hampton, K. Assuring the quality of high-stakes undergraduate assessments of clinical competence. *Medical Teacher*. 2006. 28(6). 535-543.

[125] Ker, J., Hesketh, A., Anderson, F., Johnston, D. (2006) Can a ward simulation exercise provide the realism required to provide evidence for full registration decisions for borderline PRHOs? – the results of a feasibility study. *Medical Teacher*. 2006. 28(4). 330-334.

[126] Stirling, K., Anderson, F., Hogg, G., Hanslip, J., Byrne, D., and Ker, J. Using Simulation to Support Doctors in Difficulty. *The Clinical Teacher*. 2012. 9; 285-289.

[127] Fincher, R., White, C., Huang, G., and Schwartzstein, R. 'Toward Hypothesis-Driven Medical Education Research: Task Force Report From the Millennium Conference 2007 on Educational Research'. *Academic Medicine*. 2010. 85(5): 821-828.

[128] Clark, R. E. (1994). "Media will never influence learning." *Educational technology research and development* 42(2): 21-29.

[129] Glavin, R. J. (2011). "Skills, training, and education." *Simulation in Healthcare* 6(1): 4-7.

[130] Cooper, S., et al. (2010). "Rating medical emergency teamwork performance: development of the Team Emergency Assessment Measure (TEAM)." *Resuscitation* 81 (4): 446-452.

[131] Somerville, S. *2013 SCSN/ASPiH Scottish Symposium,* Edinburgh, April 2013, Short papers-oral presentation of the following: "What are medical students' perceptions of the use of simulation in developing Human Factors skills, (for improving patient safety) in the context of an acutely unwell patient?"

[132] Motola, I., et al. (2013). "Simulation in healthcare education: A best evidence practical guide. AMEE Guide No. 82." *Med. Teach.* 35(10): e1511-e1530.

[133] Gagne, R. M., Wager, W. W., Golas, R. C., Keller, J. H., Russell, J., (2005) *Principles of instructional design* 5th edition p. 231.

[134] Biggs, J. and C. Tang (2011). *Teaching for quality learning at university*, McGraw-Hill International.

[135] Artino, A. R. and Durning, S. J. (2012) Media will never influence learning: but will simulation. *Medical Education*, 46, 630-635.

[136] Dieckmann, P., et al. (2007). "Deepening the theoretical foundations of patient simulation as social practice." *Simulation in Healthcare* 2(3): 183-193.

[137] Dieckmann, P. and Ringstead, C. Chp. 4 p. 52, cited in Forrest, K., et al. (2013). *Essential Simulation in Clinical Education,* John Wiley and Sons.

[138] Maran, N. J. and R. J. Glavin (2003). "Low-to high-fidelity simulation-a continuum of medical education?" *Med. Educ.* 37(s1): 22-28.

[139] Alinier, G. 2007. A typology of educationally focused medical simulation tools. *Medical Teacher* 2007; 29: e243-250.

[140] Collins, J. P. and Harden, R. M., 1998 AMEE medical education guide no 13, Pear patients, simulated patients and simulators in clinical examinations. *Med. Teacher* 20; 508-521.

[141] Somerville, S. 'Are the performances of students in a formative OSCE affected, when a medium fidelity simulator is substituted for a simulated patient?' *Research conducted for the Education and Research Module and presented as a poster at the Scottish Clinical Skills Conference Sept.* 2012.

[142] Barrows, H. S. (1993). "An overview of the uses of standardized patients for teaching and evaluating clinical skills. AAMC." *Academic Medicine* 68(6): 443-451.

[143] Dacre, J., Nicol, M., Holroyd, D., and Ingram, D. (1996) The development of a clinical skills centre. *Journal of the Royal College of Physicians of London.* 30: 318-24.

[144] Boulay, C. D. and C. Medway (1999). "The clinical skills resource: a review of current practice." *Med. Educ.* 33(3): 185-191.

[145] Bradley, P. and J. Bligh (1999). "One year's experience with a clinical skills resource centre." *Med. Educ.* 33(2): 114-120.

[146] Chiniara, G., et al. (2013). "Simulation in healthcare: A taxonomy and a conceptual framework for instructional design and media selection." *Med. Teach.* 35(8): e1380-e1395.

[147] De Freitas, S., Oliver, M. 2006. *Computers and Education* 46; (2006) 249-264.

[148] Haig, K. M., et al. (2006). "SBAR: a shared mental model for improving communication between clinicians." *Joint Commission Journal on Quality and Patient Safety* 32(3): 167-175.

[149] Salas, E., et al. (2005). "Using simulation-based training to improve patient safety: what does it take?" *Joint Commission Journal on Quality and Patient Safety* 31(7): 363-371.

[150] Weller, J. M. (2004). "Simulation in undergraduate medical education: bridging the gap between theory and practice." *Med. Educ.* 38(1): 32-38.

[151] Joyce, B. R. and Showers, B. Improving in service training: the messages of research. In: *Educational Leadership* 1980.

[152] Bullock, I. (2000). "Skill acquisition in resuscitation." *Resuscitation* 45(2): 139-143.

[153] Issenberg, S. B. (2006). "The scope of simulation-based healthcare education." *Simulation in Healthcare* 1(4): 203-208.

[154] Savoldelli, G. L., et al. (2006). "Value of debriefing during simulated crisis management: oral versus video-assisted oral feedback." *Anesthesiology* 105(2): 279-285.

[155] Luft, J., Ingham, H. (1955). "The Johari window, a graphic model of interpersonal awareness". *Proceedings of the western training laboratory in group development* (Los Angeles: UCLA).

[156] Pendleton, D., Schofield, T., Tate, P., Havelock, P. *The consultation: an approach to learning and teaching:* Oxford University Press, Oxford; 1984.

[157] Silverman, J. as cited in Chowdhury, R. R., Kalu, G. Learning to give feedback in medical education. *The Obstetrician and Gynaecologist.* 2004;6(4):243-7.

[158] Rudolf et al. *Anesthesiology Clin.* 25 (2007) 361-376. Debriefing with good judgement: combining rigourous feedback with genuine enquiry.

[159] Kneebone and Nestel Learning Clinical skills – the place of simulation and feedback. *Clin. teacher* 2005 vol. 2 no. 2.

[160] Molloy, E. (2009). "Time to pause: giving and receiving feedback in clinical education." *Clinical education in the health professions*: 128-146.

[161] Carless, D. (2006). Differing perceptions in the feedback process. *Studies in Higher Education,* 31(2), 219-233.

[162] Ostergaard, D. and Rosenberg Jas cited in Forrest, K., et al. (2013). *Essential Simulation in Clinical Education,* John Wiley and Sons.

[163] Chung, H. S., et al. (2013). "It is time to consider cultural differences in debriefing." *Simulation in Healthcare* 8(3): 166-170.

[164] McGaghie, W. C., et al. (2010). "A critical review of simulation-based medical education research: 2003-2009." *Med. Educ.* 44(1): 50-63.

[165] Bradley, P. and K. Postlethwaite (2003). "Simulation in clinical learning." *Med. Educ.* 37(s1): 1-5.

[166] Silverman, J. and Wood, D. F. (2004) New approaches to learning clinical skills. *Medical Education.* 38: 1021-3.

[167] Wheeler, D., Geis, G., Mack, E., LeMaster, T., and Patterson, M. (2013) High-reliability emergency response teams in the hospital: improving quality and safety using in situ simulation training. *BMJ Qual. Saf.* 2013;22:507-514.

[168] Theilen, U., et al. "Regular in situ simulation training of paediatric medical emergency team improves hospital response to deteriorating patients." *Resuscitation* 84.2 (2013): 218-222.

[169] Gardner, Aimee King, et al. "In Situ Simulation to Assess Workplace Attitudes and Effectiveness in a New Facility." *Simulation in Healthcare* 8.6 (2013): 351-358.

[170] Gott, S. P., Kane, R. S. and Lesgold, A. (1995) *Tutoring Transfer of Technical Competence.* Armstrong Lab., Brooks Air force base, TX.

[171] Kneebone, R. L., Nestel, D., Moorthy, K., et al. (2003) Learning the skills of flexible sigmoidoscopy – the wider perspective. *Medical Education.* 37: 50-8.

[172] Grantcharov, T. P., Kristiansen, V. B., Bendix, J., Bardram, L., Rosenberg, J., and Funch-Jensen, P. (2004) Randomized clinical trial of virtual reality simulation for laparoscopic skills training. *British Journal of Surgery.* 91: 146-50.

[173] Kobayashi, L., Shapiro, M. J., Sucov, A., et al. (2006) Portable advanced medical simulation for new emergency department testing and orientation. *Academic Emergency Medicine.* 13: 691-5.

[174] Vadodaria, B. S., Gandhi, S. D. and McIndoe, A. K. (2004) Comparison of four different emergency airway access equipment sets on a human patient simulator. *Anaesthesia.* 59: 73-9.

[175] Sanders, J., Haas, R. E., Geisler, M., and Lupien, A. E. (1998) Using the human patient simulator to test the efficacy of an experimental emergency percutaneous transtracheal airway. *Military Medicine.* 163: 544-51.

[176] Lim, T. J., Lim, Y. and Liu, E. H. C. (2005) Evaluation of ease of intubation with the Glide-Scope or Macintosh laryngoscope by anaesthetists in simulated easy and difficult laryngoscopy. *Anaesthesia.* 60: 180-3.

[177] Anderson, K., Gambhir, S., Glavin, R., and Kinsella, J. (2006) The use of an anaesthetic simulator to assess single-use laryngoscopy equipment. *International Journal for Quality in Health Care.* 18: 17-22.

[178] Aggarwal, R., Mytton, O., Debrew, M., et al. (2010). Training and Simulation for patient safety. *Quality and Safety in Health Care.* 19: i34-i43.

In: Health and Disease
Editor: Paul Ganguly

ISBN: 978-1-63463-052-8
© 2015 Nova Science Publishers, Inc.

Chapter 10

ENHANCING LABORATORY MEDICINE TEACHING THROUGH CONSTRUCTIVE ALIGNMENT OF THE MEDICAL CURRICULUM

Ahlam Alshedoukhy[1,], Abiola Senok[2] and Khurshid Anwar[1]*

[1]Department of Pathology and Pharmacology, College of Medicine, Alfaisal University, Riyadh, Saudi Arabia
[2]Department of Microbiology and Immunology, College of Medicine, Alfaisal University, Riyadh, Saudi Arabia

ABSTRACT

Pathology and the laboratory sciences represent a fundamental link between the basic sciences and clinical medicine. This branch of medical science encompasses anatomical pathology, haematology, microbiology, immunology, clinical chemistry and molecular pathology. In recent years, medical curriculum reform has changed the ways in which students engage with and are taught the laboratory medicine disciplines. In this chapter, we will discuss the concept of constructive alignment which has as a core principle the alignment of teaching and assessment modalities with pre-defined outcomes in a way that encourages deep learning approaches. How the utilization of this concept can provide a framework for advancement of the teaching of laboratory medicine disciplines in the training of twenty-first century doctors will be discussed.

Keywords: Anatomic Pathology, Microbiology, Laboratory Medicine, Constructive alignment, Problem based learning

---

[*] Corresponding author: Dr. Ahlam Alshedoukhy. Department of Pathology and Pharmacology, College of Medicine, Alfaisal University, P. O. Box 50927, Riyadh, Saudi Arabia. Tel: +966-11-2157696, fax: +966-11-2157651, e-mail: aalshedoukhy@alfaisal.edu.

INTRODUCTION

Pathology is the precise study and diagnosis of disease. The word pathology is from Ancient Greek "πάθος (pathos)" which may be translated into English as either "experience" or "suffering", and "λογία, (logia)", "an account of" or "the study of" [1].

Pathology represents a fundamental link between the basic sciences and clinical medicine, and between the normal and the abnormal [2, 3]. It is also referred to as laboratory medicine discipline and we will be using these two terminologies interchangeably in this chapter. This branch of medical science encompasses several disciplines namely anatomical pathology, haematology, microbiology, immunology, clinical chemistry and molecular pathology (Table 1). The Royal College of Pathologists in the United Kingdom (UK) has described pathology as the science at the heart of modern medicine and these laboratory medicine disciplines remain vital to the diagnosis and management of patients [4].

In this chapter we will discuss how medical curriculum reform has changed the ways in which students are taught and how they engage with the laboratory medicine disciplines. The concerns about the adequacy of current training of undergraduate medical students in the discipline of laboratory medicine will be addressed. We will explore some of the teaching modalities that can be used to convey the knowledge of pathology within an integrated curriculum with special reference to constructive alignment of content and assessment.

HISTORICAL PERSPECTIVES

In the past few decades, there has been a shift in the delivery of the medical education curriculum. This curriculum reform has been driven in part by the steady increase in advances in medical knowledge which requires that the new generation of physicians should have the skills of self-directed lifelong learners with critical thinking and problem solving abilities [5].

Table 1. Definitions of the disciplines and sub-disciplines encompassing pathology

Discipline	Sub-discipline	Definition
Anatomical pathology	Histopathology	General and organ-specific disease processes at the gross and microscopic levels
	Cytopathology	The pathology of dispersed cells (e.g. cervical smears, needle aspirates)
	Autopsy	The study of disease in the dead
Haematology		The cells of the blood, coagulation mechanisms, blood transfusion
Clinical chemistry		The chemicals of the blood, body fluids and tissues
Microbiology	Bacteriology Parasitology Mycology Virology	Infectious diseases, their causes, control and treatment
Immunology		The immune system and diseases caused by abnormal activity or underactivity
Molecular pathology		Analysis of diseases at the level of genes and their chromosomes

The need for curricular reform from the factually overloaded traditional medical curriculum was identified in the UK, by the General Medical Council's standards as set out in Tomorrow's Doctors in 1993 and 2002 [6, 7]. In the US, accreditation bodies such as the Liaison Committee on Medical Education [8, 9], The American Medical Association [8] and the General Professional Education of the Physician report echoed the need for curricular reforms [3, 5, 8, 9]. These recommendations aimed at a reduction in the amount of factual learning in medicine, promoting integrative teaching and learning across specialties and limiting the curriculum to what undergraduates need to know at qualification as general physicians. This has led to the development of pedagogies and learning techniques such as problem based learning (PBL) which has moved medical education from the traditional discipline-based curricula towards an integrated curricula. The ethos of the PBL curriculum is to enable students see the clinical relevance of the basic sciences, to make links with other subjects and to learn the complex process of clinical decision-making.

In the pre-PBL traditional curriculum, laboratory medicine was usually a component of the clinical years of the medical curriculum with department-led didactic courses in pathology, microbiology, immunology and clinical chemistry [8-12]. With these dramatic curricular reforms in undergraduate medical education, faculty in laboratory based disciplines now find themselves involved in courses that are significantly different from those which they encountered as medical students. The discipline based courses of microbiology, immunology, pathology, haematology and clinical chemistry have now been replaced by centrally managed, problem based integrated curricula, with emphasis on self-directed learning and problem solving skills. The downside of this is that many medical schools now include these disciplines within the PBL cases in the pre-clinical years, and sometimes the pathology content remains poorly defined and opportunities to be engaged in the laboratory practical aspects of these disciplines are becoming significantly reduced [13].

For clinicians in virtually every specialty, the care of patients depends upon the request for the right laboratory investigations, appropriate collection of specimens and accurate interpretation of laboratory investigations. As such, the medical school curricula must ensure that students become well-rounded physicians with knowledge of and appreciation for the role of laboratory medicine in patient care. Unfortunately, there are only few examples of the successful integration of pathology teaching, both anatomic pathology and other disciplines of laboratory medicine, in the clinical years of medical school [14, 15]. This imbalance in the approach to the content and teaching of the laboratory medicine disciplines has raised a lot of concerns. A recent report from the Centres for Disease Control and Prevention in the US concluded that "current medical student training in laboratory medicine is "inadequate" and "despite the integral role of laboratory testing in the practice of medicine, formal teaching of laboratory medicine is a relatively neglected component of the medical school curriculum" [16].

TEACHING PATHOLOGY / LABORATORY MEDICINE

Progressive curricular reforms during the past two decades have had a profound effect on the way in which pathology is taught to medical undergraduates.

The main concepts regarding educational approaches in the teaching of laboratory medicine disciplines have been addressed in the literature under the following categories:

i   The syllabus and curriculum
ii   Timing and duration
iii Methods of teaching and learning
iv   Assessment
v   Teacher training

These categories arose either from the weight given to them in the literature or from their importance in current educational thinking (curricular issues, problem based learning and assessment). In terms of the syllabus, there is no shortage of recommendations regarding what to teach. Detailed syllabi are available for most of the disciplines and sub-disciplines shown in Table 1. These are developed by national and international interest groups comprising of experts in medical education and content experts for these disciplines [17-21]. However, there are few attempts to define the approaches for teaching and outcomes for learners.

Objectives of Pathology Syllabus

The main goals of undergraduate pathology teaching have always been to provide:

- A language or framework for the description of disease, aetiological agents, transmission processes as well as the knowledge of the host-microbe interactions
- To provide a basis for the understanding of functional and structural changes in disease so that clinical signs and symptoms can be understood and interpreted.

The pathology teaching objectives described in the literature largely focus on two main themes [22-28]. These are:

- Teaching students the mechanisms of disease from the molecular basis, and the understanding of aetiological agents and factors, microscopic and gross appearance of lesions.
- Teaching students how to use a medical laboratory including appropriate specimen selection, collection, transportation, processing and interpretation of result.

As pathology bridges the gap between basic sciences and clinical medicine, a proper understanding of pathological processes is crucial for medical practice. It is of essence that the scope of the pathology curriculum should address core disease entities that a new medical graduate should know about. It has been suggested that as most of the new graduates will have their careers starting in primary care, more consideration and emphasis should be given to the pathological basis of the common diseases that will be seen in such setting [29]. However, within this premise and in an era of curricular reforms, the timing and duration for the teaching of the laboratory sciences within an integrated curriculum has become a critical question. Surveys calculating the number of hours allocated for the teaching of disciplines in pathology have appeared in literature. Unfortunately, some of these surveys appear to have generated data with the sole purpose of fighting pathology's corner [18, 30, 31].

It is indeed striking how much time is dedicated to time calculations when the more fundamental question should be whether the hours and methods of teaching correlate with what is learned and the degree of alignment with outcomes. We believe that the alignment of the pathology syllabus with assessment and outcomes in a way that promotes integration without any loss of the core elements of the laboratory medicine syllabus is the critical goal which should be actively pursued.

In addition, such alignment will provide a framework within which to address the various ongoing debates regarding how best to teach laboratory medicine such as the discussions on the use of hands-on laboratory sessions versus web-based microscopy; issues relating to the relevance of autopsy sessions as well as how best to integrate laboratory medicine with the clinical disciplines during the clerkship years [14, 15, 17, 32-34].

It is now universally agreed by medical educators that it is crucial to define what qualifying medical students need to know, what skills they are expected to acquire as well as the values and attitudes they should develop. However, the challenge remains how best to design and align pathology curriculum with expected outcomes. The role of assessment tools and modalities in this alignment is also important. This alignment is particularly important for those considering how to teach laboratory medicine to medical undergraduates as they now have to do so in the context of: increasing integration [3, 35], centralized curriculum management [9, 36, 37], reduced contact time [3, 6, 7, 17, 38, 39], a decline in duration and availability of laboratory facilities, understaffing and rising class sizes [40].

It should be added that pathology faculty need to be active participants and play a pivotal role in this process of curriculum design as the discipline of pathology remains central to medical science [41]. In the coming section, we will address how the application of the concept of constructive alignment can be a powerful tool in achieving this goal.

THE CONCEPT OF CONSTRUCTIVE ALIGNMENT

Constructive Alignment, a term coined by John Biggs is one of the most influential ideas in higher education [42, 43]. The essence of this concept is to guide teaching, direct learning and assess the outcomes. A core principle in constructive alignment is that we start by defining the outcomes we intend students to learn, the teaching and assessment modalities are then aligned to those outcomes. This makes constructive alignment a very good example of an outcomes-based education. Indeed constructive alignment forms the underpinning concept behind the current requirements for programme specification, declarations of Intended Learning Outcomes and assessment criteria, as well as the use of criterion based assessment.

Biggs [42, 43] has identified three different approaches to studying namely:

i   Deep learning approaches: characterised by a preference to work conceptually and are driven by intrinsic curiosity

ii   Strategic learning approaches: characterised by a focus on obtaining high marks and organised studying

iii   Surface learning approaches: characterised by an intention to achieve a pass, avoid too high workload, misunderstanding requirements, and/or thinking that factual recall is all that is required.

In a study assessing assessment results and approaches to learning among second year medical students, Reid et al. have demonstrated that marks correlated positively with deep and strategic approaches and negatively with surface approaches across a range of assessment methods [44]. In 2008 Yong Loo Lin School of Medicine, National University of Singapore successfully implemented the five year revised undergraduate medical curriculum in which assessment and teaching learning activities had been constructively aligned to the expected graduate outcomes for each phase of training [45].

Therefore, we can surmise that in the undergraduate learning environment particularly in the medical training, the desired goal is deep learning and this is achievable via incorporation of the concept of constructive alignment in curricula design.

There are four main steps in implementing constructive alignment in curriculum design:

i   Defining the desired learning outcome
ii   Choosing teaching and learning activities that can enable the students to attain the desired learning outcomes
iii Assessing students actual learning outcomes to see how well they match what was intended
iv   Grading the student learning

Figure 1 below, show how the components are linked in the implementation of constructive alignment.

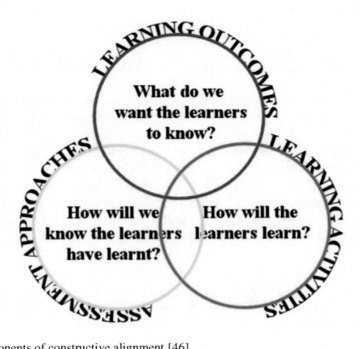

Figure 1. Components of constructive alignment [46].

DESIGNING THE LABORATORY MEDICINE CURRICULUM USING THE PRINCIPLE OF CONSTRUCTIVE ALIGNMENT

With regards to the laboratory medicine curriculum, we propose a schema wherein the goals and objectives which have formed the bedrock of pathology teaching are incorporated with integrated self-directed learning pedagogies but developed in the curriculum using the concept of constructive alignment.

Such an approach will of course start with a clear definition (by faculty from laboratory medicine disciplines) of the expected outcomes for competent new medical graduates. A key outcome is that these new doctors can make independent decisions and are capable of making proper diagnosis based on the application of acquired knowledge. In defining learning outcomes, different levels of learning can and should be defined for different aspects of the discipline content. This is important so that we avoid the traditional error of factual overload whilst we stimulate a high degree of intellectual curiosity which is integral for deep learning experience. This will provide us with the basis of the learning outcomes for designing our curriculum. We can mix the levels of learning required in such a way that we have some lower level outcomes that deal with the basic facts, as well as having higher level outcomes that require the students to apply acquired knowledge to deal with new situations of varying complexities. As an example for a particular disease entity, low level outcomes would be to have a grasp of basic mechanism of the disease processes whilst the higher level outcome will be to make a correlation with the patient's clinical presentation and appropriate choice of investigations. The ultimate goal is to enable the student to formulate appropriate diagnosis and management strategy. This approach will enhance critical thinking and deep learning.

At the same time, we need to introduce and utilize activities that will cause the students to be actively engaged with the learning process at a deeper level. In many institutions, course description documents usually define the amount of study hours in terms of contact time in lectures and tutorials. However, our personal experience and recent studies have shown that these are not the most effective way for the majority of students to learn as they quickly adopt passive learning approaches. Therefore strategies that require active participation and encourage high-level learning should be carefully designed to stimulate problem solving skills. This should also be integrally linked with the assessment modality that will be adopted and thus be in keeping with the saying "assessment drives learning". If we want students to consider that we expect them to synthesize concepts and link them together then we should consider teaching and assessment activities that encourage and emphasise such behaviour. During the teaching process, the students should be continually stimulated to consider the application of the knowledge being garnered.

In our experience at Alfaisal University, we have found that small group exercises are an excellent modality to promote such integrative alignment of outcome with teaching and assessment. This can take various formats such as case studies, PBL, clinico-pathological correlation sessions (CPC) and laboratory practical sessions.

In Alfaisal University, we are in the process of adopting this ethos in the teaching of the pathology disciplines. In addition, within our hybrid PBL curriculum we are extending the teaching of pathology across the pre-clinical and clinical years. For anatomical pathology, we are adopting the utilization of CPC and team based learning (TBL) sessions in which small groups are encouraged to actively take part in the learning process.

Looking into the future we envisage the possibility that traditional lectures will give way to flip class rooms and pathology will mostly be taught using scenario based TBL sessions which will be a stimulus for the students to acquire knowledge with more reasoning and to evaluate the topics more critically.

Moreover, scenario based TBL sessions can be easily merged with PowerPoint® slides showing gross and histological images, aetiological agents, transmission cycles and preventive measures. Subsequently, the theory and practical sessions can be beautifully amalgamated for better understandings of the difficult topics. In clerkship years, the same methodology can be used where clinical subjects can be supplemented by sessions of pathology mostly in the form of CPC which is now regarded as one of the cornerstones of the spirally integrated curriculum.

Currently, for microbiology, during the pre-clinical years, hands-on laboratory sessions are being conducted utilizing case scenarios which students have to work through to reach a diagnosis. These sessions are designed bearing in mind the varying levels of learning outcomes which we want our students to attain. The basic knowledge of infectious disease agents is integrated with the knowledge of the pathological processes which are manifested in the patient's clinical presentation.

Based on these, a determination of appropriate specimen choice and tests (including the identification of important pre-analytical variables) and the interpretation of tests to reach a diagnosis can be made. In these practical sessions, the opportunities to practice obtaining certain specimen types and carry out some of the tests give added real life experience which the students enjoy immensely.

During the clerkship years, the clinical microbiology sessions are tailored for the specific rotation the students are undergoing. This helps the students learn to how to apply the principles of clinical microbiology contextually in the day to day management of patients.

In relation to assessment, our guiding principle is to ensure that our assessment tools are crafted to assess the ability of the students to apply the knowledge gained in learning activities and test critical thinking process.

Furthermore, the multiple choice questions and short answer questions which make up the written paper in our exams are designed to test analytical thinking and application of knowledge.

These objectives are attained by increasing the number of questions which reflect critical thinking (C2 and C3 types) rather than simple recall (C1 type). Our approach discourages students from playing the assessment game in which they go for a mark 'trawl' in exams.

CONCLUSION

The disciplines encompassed in pathology / laboratory medicine remain central and crucial to medical science. Faculty in the field of laboratory medicine need be actively engaged in the ongoing curricular reforms. We need to adapt our teaching in such a way that minimizes factual overload, fosters integration and stimulates deep learning in students. The constructive alignment of teaching modality and assessment with pre-defined outcomes achieves that and provides a framework for the advancement of the teaching of these disciplines in the training of the new generation of twenty-first century doctors.

REFERENCES

[1]   http://en.wikipedia.org/wiki/Pathology Last accessed 28th May 2014.

[2]   Godfrey, R.: Medical education. All change? *Lancet* 1991, 338: 297-299.

[3]   Kumar, K., Daniel, J., Doig, K., Agamanolis, D.: Teaching of pathology in United States medical schools, 1996/1997 survey. *Hum. Pathol.* 1998, 29: 750-755.

[4]   www.rcpath.org. Last accessed 28th May 2014.

[5]   Bloom, S. W.: Structure and ideology in medical education: an analysis of resistance to change. *J. Health Soc. Behav.* 1988, 29: 294-306.

[6]   Keik, Reid: General Medical Council. *Tomorrow's doctors.* 1993.

[7]   Keik, Reid: General Medical Council. *Tomorrow's doctors.* 2002.

[8]   Enarson, C., Burg, F. D.: An overview of reform initiatives in medical education. 1906 through 1992. *JAMA* 1992, 268: 1141-1143.

[9]   Kassebaum, D. G., Cutler, E. R., Eaglen, R. H.: The influence of accreditation on educational change in US medical schools. *Acad. Med.* 1997, 72: 1127-1133.

[10]   Benbow, E. W., Rutishauser, S., Stoddart, R. W., Andrew, S. M., Freemont, A. J.: Pathologists and problem-based learning. *J. Pathol.* 1996, 180: 340-342.

[11]   Davis, W. K., White, C. B. M.: *Managing the curriculum and managing change.* Dordrecht Kluwer Academic Publishers; 2002.

[12]   Prichard, R. W., Davis, J. S., Matsen, J. M.: Teaching pathology to medical students in the 1990s: a 1989 symposium of the Association of Pathology Chairmen. *Hum. Pathol.* 1992, 23: 98-103.

[13]   Burton, J. L.: Teaching pathology to medical undergraduates. *Current Diagnostic Pathology* 2005, 11: 308-316.

[14]   Haspel, R. L., Bhargava, P., Gilmore, H., Kane, S., Powers, A., Sepehr, A., Weinstein, A. R., Schwartzstein, R. M., Roberts, D. H.: Successful implementation of a longitudinal, integrated pathology curriculum during the third year of medical school. *Arch. Pathol. Lab. Med.* 2012, 136: 1430-1436.

[15]   Magid, M. S., Cambor, C. L.: The integration of pathology into the clinical years of undergraduate medical education: a survey and review of the literature. *Hum. Pathol.* 2012, 43: 567-576.

[16]   Smith, B. R., Aguero-Rosenfeld, M., Anastasi, J., Baron, B., Berg, A., Bock, J. L., Campbell, S., Crookston, K. P., Fitzgerald, R., Fung, M., Haspel, R., Howe, J. G., Jhang, J., Kamoun, M., Koethe, S., Krasowski, M. D., Landry, M. L., Marques, M. B., Rinder, H. M., Roberts, W., Schreiber, W. E., Spitalnik, S. L., Tormey, C. A., Wolf, P., Wu, Y. Y.: Educating medical students in laboratory medicine: a proposed curriculum. *Am. J. Clin. Pathol.* 2010, 133: 533-542.

[17]   Dick, F., Leaven, T., Dillman, D., Torner, R., Finken, L.: Core morphological concepts of disease for second-year medical students. *Hum. Pathol.* 1998, 29: 1017-1020.

[18]   Iversen, O. H.: The teaching of general pathology in European undergraduate education programs in medicine. *Pathol. Res. Pract.* 1986, 181: 365-369.

[19]   Kirkpatrick, C. J.: How do we teach pathology? Bridging the gap between theory and practice. *J. Pathol.* 1989, 157: 157-159.

[20] Southwick, F., Katona, P., Kauffman, C., Monroe, S., Pirofski, L., del Rio, C., Gallis, H., Dismukes, W.: *IDSA Guidelines for Preclinical Microbiology and Infectious Diseases*. 2010.

[21] Southwick, F., Katona, P., Kauffman, C., Monroe, S., Pirofski, L. A., del Rio, C., Gallis, H., Dismukes, W.: Commentary: IDSA guidelines for improving the teaching of preclinical medical microbiology and infectious diseases. *Acad. Med.* 2010, 85: 19-22.

[22] Athanasou, N. A., McGee, J. O.: How do we teach pathology? The Oxford Clinical Pathology Course. *J. Pathol.* 1988, 156: 267-269.

[23] Harvey, J. M.: The undergraduate pathology course in the medical faculty of the University of Western Australia. *Pathology* 1993, 25: 426-429.

[24] Young, B.: Teaching anatomical pathology in an integrated self-directed learning programme: the Newcastle experience. *Pathology* 1993, 25: 423-425.

[25] Crotty, K., Pamphlett, R.: Present and future pathology teaching at the University of Sydney. *Pathology* 1993, 25: 81-86.

[26] Valdes-Dapena, M., Valdes-Dapena, A. M.: A senior elective program in anatomic pathology. *Arch. Pathol. Lab. Med.* 1989, 113: 330-332.

[27] Pawlowski, Z. S., Goullier-Fleuret, A., Bruschi, F.: Undergraduate teaching of medical parasitology. *Parasitol. Today* 1998, 14: 127-128.

[28] Singh, S., Singh, P.: An innovative approach to teaching microbiology to undergraduates. *Med. Educ.* 2009, 43: 1091-1092.

[29] Stevens, A., Lowe, J.: *Pathology*, 2nd edn. Edinburgh: Mosby; 2000.

[30] Davis, J. S., Mistry, F. D.: The pathology curriculum in US medical schools. 1986 survey by the Association of Pathology Chairmen. *Arch. Pathol. Lab. Med.* 1987, 111: 1088-1092.

[31] Kumar, K., Indurkhya, A., Nguyen, H.: Curricular trends in instruction of pathology: a nationwide longitudinal study from 1993 to present. *Hum. Pathol.* 2001, 32: 1147-1153.

[32] Benbow, E. W.: Autopsy demonstrations to medical students: audit by questionnaire. *J. Pathol.* 1990, 162: 177-179.

[33] Linder, E., Lundin, M., Thors, C., Lebbad, M., Winiecka-Krusnell, J., Helin, H., Leiva, B., Isola, J., Lundin, J.: Web-based virtual microscopy for parasitology: a novel tool for education and quality assurance. *PLoS Negl. Trop. Dis.* 2008, 2: e315.

[34] Lundin, M., Lundin, J., Helin, H., Isola, J.: A digital atlas of breast histopathology: an application of web based virtual microscopy. *J. Clin. Pathol.* 2004, 57: 1288-1291.

[35] Marshall, R., Cartwright, N., Mattick, K.: Teaching and learning pathology: a critical review of the English literature. *Med. Educ.* 2004, 38: 302-313.

[36] Reid, W. A.: Pathology in the undergraduate medical curriculum. *J. Pathol.* 1992, 167: 173-174.

[37] Reynolds, C. F., 3rd, Adler, S., Kanter, S. L., Horn, J. P., Harvey, J., Bernier, G. M., Jr.: The undergraduate medical curriculum: centralized versus departmentalized. *Acad. Med.* 1995, 70: 671-675.

[38] Anderson, J. R.: Pathology and the undergraduate curriculum. *J. Pathol.* 1988, 155: 6-8.

[39] Nash, J. R., West, K. P., Foster, C. S.: The teaching of anatomic pathology in England and Wales: a transatlantic view. *Hum. Pathol.* 2001, 32: 1154-1156.

[40] Lepoff, R. B.: Academic medical centers and managed care. *Arch. Pathol. Lab. Med.* 1995, 119: 598-599.

[41] Weedon, D.: Whither pathology in medical education? *Med. J. Aust.* 2003, 178: 200-202.

[42] Biggs, J.: What the Student Does: teaching for enhanced learning. *Higher Education Research and Development* 1999, 18.

[43] Biggs, J.: *Teaching for Quality Learning at University* 2nd edn. Buckingham: Society for Research into Higher Education/Open University Press.; 2003.

[44] Reid, W. A., Duvall, E., Evans, P.: Relationship between assessment results and approaches to learning and studying in Year Two medical students. *Med. Educ.* 2007, 41: 754-762.

[45] Barrow, M., McKimm, J., Samarasekera, D.: Strategies for planning and designing medical curricula and clinical teaching. *Medical Education in Practice* 2010, 4: 2-8.

[46] http://arc.caut.hku.hk/ConsAlign.html. Last accessed 28th May 2014.

In: Health and Disease
Editor: Paul Ganguly

ISBN: 978-1-63463-052-8
© 2015 Nova Science Publishers, Inc.

Chapter 11

EVALUATION AND ASSESSMENT OF A CURRICULUM: HOW DO WE DO THAT?

*Akef Obeidat**

College of medicine, Alfaisal University, Kingdom of Saudi Arabia

ABSTRACT

Evaluation of undergraduate medical education programs is necessary to meet accreditation standards; however, implementation and maintenance of an adequate evaluation process is challenging. The increasing globalization of medicine necessitates the need for definition of standards and for introduction of effective and transparent accreditation systems. In addition to global variability in content and delivery of medical education programs, systems of quality assurance oversight are not universal. This chapter presents a summary of developments in curriculum evaluation in medical education in recent decades and discusses key aspects of curriculum evaluation based on recent practical experiences.

INTRODUCTION

Medical education is continually evolving, necessitating an ongoing programmatic evaluations to determine the worth of programmatic components and whether overall goals and objectives are being attained [1]. Reviewing the literature provided relatively little practical guidance in conducting methodologically rigorous research or evaluation studies in education [2]; especially about establishing systems to define and maintain the quality of undergraduate medical education programs that encompass multiple aspects of quality. Structured evaluation of the curriculum is needed to monitor its implementation to enable continual improvement and evaluate the effectiveness of the change.

* Corresponding author: Akef Obeidat. College of medicine, Alfaisal University, Kingdom of Saudi Arabia. E-mail address: aobeidat@alfaisal.edu, akefobeidat@hotmail.com.

Although there is no doubt that systematic evaluations are powerful tools for formulating optimal structures of curricula; most evaluation studies in the field of medical education focus only on the new curricula or even on renewed components of a curriculum; they rarely investigate concrete educational objectives and their recognition in a systematic manner.

The major reason for assessing the effectiveness of a curriculum is to ensure that the goals of the program have been achieved and that graduates are well prepared to face the challenges of medical practice and well equipped to address the changing healthcare needs of the community. There is an increased public and professional demand for accountability in education.

Evaluation of teaching is traditionally realized in terms of student ratings. There is a large body of knowledge available regarding the psychometric properties of student ratings; curriculum evaluation is rarely done in a systematic manner. Acquired expertise and the actual performance of the graduates are the central indicators for the quality of a curriculum. However, grades warded for final exams definitely do not suffice as indicators for skills transferred into practice [3].

Evaluations of curricula have to go beyond students' ratings of courses. There is a need to investigate proximal goals, conditions, and long-term effects of university education. The evaluation of a curriculum investigating its effectiveness has to analyze concrete educational goals and their realization [4]. Therefore, neither student ratings of courses nor student ratings of the curriculum can provide sufficient information.

There is a need for 360° evaluations involving all stakeholders. Australian Medical Council lists eight relevant standards to address the requirements for delivery of high quality medical education and include the need for "ongoing monitoring of curriculum content, quality of teaching, assessment and student progress," the need for "teacher and student feedback," and "using the results of evaluation for course development."

Schools are required to analyze "the performance of student cohorts in relation to the curriculum and the outcomes of the medical course" and "evaluate the outcomes of the course in terms of postgraduate performance, career choice and career satisfaction." Finally, schools are required to report "outcome evaluation to academic staff, students and the full range of groups with an interest in graduate outcomes (Australian Medical Council: Assessment and Accreditation of Medical Schools: Standards and Procedures) [5]. Those are Similar to those specified by the Liaison Committee for Medical Education for North American medical schools: Functions and Structure of a Medical School [6].

In this chapter; the author provides (a) a brief overview of the literature concerning program evaluation as applied to medical education (b) discusses key aspects of undergraduate medical curriculum evaluation based on recent practical experiences under the following headings:

1   Development, benchmarking, and assessment of competence; from course design to competency based outcomes
2   A curriculum has to be dynamic and responsive to changes in the rapidly progressing, volatile world of medical education
3   The power of self-evaluation: Creating a culture of reflection and action involving all stakeholders
4   Development of a comprehensive whole-program evaluation with a focus on outcomes, processes, and environments

5   Qualitative and quantitative measures to be used in evaluating a curriculum
6   Evaluation across the whole spectrum of medical education; Evaluating a course, clerkship, or components of a residency based on accreditation requirements
7   Accreditation and international quality assurance of medical education
8   Alternative Quality Assurance Methods:
   A   Quality assurance of medical education through national accreditation
   B   Other mechanisms for recognition of medical education programs:
      a   International collaboration and partnerships
      b   International conventions
      c   The publication of global databases
      d   Governmental evaluation
      e   Self-evaluation
      f   Program Evaluators
      g   Benchmarking: Progress testing as an example
      h   Curriculum mapping

I. DEVELOPMENT, BENCHMARKING, AND ASSESSMENT OF COMPETENCE; FROM COURSE DESIGN TO COMPETENCY BASED OUTCOMES

The traditional way of designing modules and programs was to start from the content of the course. Teachers decided on the content that they intended to teach, planned how to teach this content and then assessed the content. This type of approach focused on the teacher's input and on assessment in terms of how well the students absorbed the material taught. Course descriptions referred mainly to the content of the course that would be covered in lectures. This approach to teaching has been referred to as a teacher-centered approach.

Among the criticisms of this type of approach in the literature is that it can be difficult to identify precisely what the student has to be able to do in order to pass the module or program.

International trends in education show a shift from the traditional "teacher centered" approach to a "student centered" approach. This alternative model focuses on what the students are expected to be able to do at the end of the module or program. Hence, this approach is commonly referred to as an outcome-based approach. Statements called intended learning outcomes, commonly shortened to learning outcomes, are used to express what it is expected that students should be able to do at the end of the learning period [7].

Assessment is an intrinsic component of outcome-based education. Outcome-based education and performance assessment are closely related paradigms. Outcome-based education involves an educational approach in which the decisions about the curriculum and evaluation are driven by the learning outcomes that students should achieve. In this approach, the product (student learning outcomes) defines the process (instructional methods and learning opportunities).

It is assessment and evaluation that often drives the curricula of medical schools and students measure their progress through the curriculum by the examinations they have passed.

Patient and other stakeholder have the right to know that physicians who graduate from medical school and subsequent residency training programs are competent and can practice their profession in a compassionate and skilful manner. It is the responsibility of the medical school to demonstrate that such competence has been achieved, and the responsibility of accreditation agencies to certify that the educational programs in medical schools can do what they promise [8].

In order to assist medical schools in their efforts to respond to these concerns and to develop a consensus within the medical education community on the attributes that medical students should possess at the time of graduation, and to set forth learning objectives for the medical school curriculum; different regulatory and accreditation bodies that are concerned with accrediting medical school or involved with the physicians licensure processes developed a set of objectives to assist medical schools in changing their curricula and to develop strategies for improving the general professional education of the physician.

In 1981, the Association of American Medical Colleges (AAMC) created a panel on the General Professional Education of the Physician and College Preparation for Medicine (GPEP Panel) to develop strategies for improving the general professional education of the physician. The Association hoped that the GPEP Panel would lead not only to agreement on the knowledge and skills that all physicians should possess to practice medicine in the 21st century, but also would promote debate on the personal qualities, values, and attitudes that those pursuing careers in medicine should possess. In its final report in 1984, the panel asserted that all physicians regardless of specialty should possess a common foundation of knowledge, skills, attitudes, and values, and recommended that each medical school faculty specify the attributes appropriate for students graduating from its school and adopt learning objectives for the curriculum consistent with those attributes. In keeping with this recommendation, in 1985 the Liaison Committee on Medical Education (LCME, [9]) added to the accreditation standards for the medical student education program a requirement that "a medical school must define its objectives and make them known to faculty and students."

The Association of American Medical Colleges (AAMC) formed an advisory group to recommend guidelines to US medical schools on the objectives of medical education (Report I Learning Objectives for Medical Student Education-Guidelines for Medical Schools, AAMC, 1998) [10]. This report contains detailed goals and objectives that could guide individual schools in establishing objectives for their own programs. The Medical Schools Objectives Project (MSOP) identified attributes based on society's expectations of a good physician. They were grouped into four categories: (a) physicians must be altruistic; (b) physicians must be knowledgeable; (c) physicians must be skilful; and (d) physicians must be dutiful (AAMC, 1998). In the United States, the Liaison Committee for Medical Education (LCME) is the accreditation agency for North American medical schools (US and Canada). North American medical education institutions are now required to document educational outcomes in light of their institutional purposes and missions. Some individual medical schools in the US have developed their own competences.

The Accreditation Council for Graduate Medical Education (ACGME) in the US also specified learning outcomes for the training of the doctor (ACGME, 2003) [11]. The International Institute of Medical Education has produced an international consensus on the learning outcomes or minimum essential requirements expected of a student on graduation from medical school (IIME, 2002) [12].

Likewise, in Canada, physician groups developed the essential competences and roles of their profession. The CanMEDS 2000 Project Societal Needs Working Group [13] reported seven roles of specialist physicians: (a) medical expert, (b) communicator, (c) collaborator, (d) manager, (e) health advocate, (f) scholar, and (g) professional (CanMEDS, 2000) [13]. Within each of these categories, a number of specific attributes or objectives were identified.

The General Medical Council (GMC) has the responsibility to ensure that graduates of a UK medical school have met the requirements for their next posts.

They have also published a detailed document called "Tomorrow's Doctors, Outcomes and standards for undergraduate medical education, 2009" [14]. It places greater emphasis on learning outcomes and on the assessment of the outcomes.

The outcomes specified by these different bodies have similarities and embrace a similar set of competences or abilities. Other bodies have also contributed to this field and published their reports. They include; Accreditation Council for Graduate Medical Education (ACGME) Outcomes Project and American Board of Medical Specialties (ABMS), (2000) "Toolbox of Assessment Methods" [15], Scottish Deans' Medical Curriculum Group, 2002 [16]; The Tuning Project for Medicine-learning outcomes for undergraduate medical education in Europe, 2007 [17]; Federation of Royal Colleges of Physicians UK, Generic Curriculum for the Medical Specialties, 2006 [18]; Implementing Bologna in your institution, 2014 [7].

Benchmarking course/program objectives is the first step in designing quality medical education program. Courses/ clinical rotations directors; need to refer to the aforementioned documents, for the intended objectives of their particular course/rotation. For detailed description on how to build and assess a competency (outcome-based) curriculum, I refer the reader to Shumway and Harden [8]; and Mukhopadhyay and Smith [19].

For more test oriented objectives that might be useful in designing individual blocks; I refer the reader to the following document:

1   USMLE Step 1; Content Description and General information [20].
2   The Medical Council of Canada. 2005, Objectives for the Qualifying Examination [13].
3   NBME subject Exam's content outline [21], presents the percentage of each discipline's contents in each of the 10 systems the exam tests. These exams are constructed to be appropriate for a broad range of curricular approaches. This distribution of the contents of each discipline to different body systems can be utilized as a guide while constructing the courses/modules or clinical rotations.

How to Evaluate Curriculum Outcomes

When writing learning outcomes, it is important to write them in such a way that they are capable of being assessed.

Clearly, it is necessary to have some form of assessment tool or technique in order to determine the extent to which learning outcomes have been achieved. Examples of direct assessment techniques are the use of written examinations, project work, portfolios, grading system with rubrics, theses, reflective journals, performance assessment, etc. Examples of indirect assessment methods are surveys of employers, comparison with peer institutions, surveys of past graduates, retention rates, analysis of curriculum, etc.

The challenge for teachers is to ensure that there is alignment between teaching methods, assessment techniques, assessment criteria and learning outcomes. This connection between teaching, assessment and learning outcomes helps to make the overall learning experience more transparent. In terms of teaching and learning, there is a dynamic equilibrium between teaching strategies on one side and learning outcomes and assessment on the other side [7].

It is important that the assessment tasks mirror the learning outcomes since, as far as the students are concerned, the assessment is the curriculum: "From our students' point of view, assessment always defines the actual curriculum" [22]. They will learn what they think will be assessed, not what may be on the curriculum or even what has been covered in lectures.

To the teacher, assessment is at the end of the teaching-learning sequence of events, but to the student it is at the beginning.

If the curriculum is reflected in the assessment, the teaching activities of the teacher and the learner activities of the learner are both directed towards the same goal.

In preparing for the assessment, students will be learning the curriculum [23]. The curriculum should be designed so that the teaching activities, learning activities and assessment tasks are coordinated with the learning outcomes. Learning outcomes can: [7]

o   Help to ensure consistency of delivery across modules and programs.
o   Aid curriculum design by clarifying areas of overlap between modules and programs.
o   Help course designers to determine precisely the key purposes of a course and to see how components of the syllabus fit and how learning progression is incorporated.
o   Highlight the relationship between teaching, learning and assessment and help improve course design and the student experience.
o   Promote reflection on assessment and the development of assessment criteria and more effective and varied assessment.

In a study by Spiel et al. [3], they conducted 25 preliminary interviews with representatives of the four key stakeholder groups of Austrian medical education: (a) advanced students in medical education at university, (b) graduates who completed the obligatory full-time internship in various hospitals, (c) university teachers of the students, and (d) clinical supervisors. They have excluded patients from the interview. For the assessment of physicians' expertise beyond individual skills, which can be experienced by the patients (e.g., if the application of an injection hurts or not), the extensive questioning of patients seems to be suitable only to a limited extent; they argue.

Based on these interviews, they have defined seven different general areas of expertise (outcomes). To measure these outcomes, they have developed questionnaires to obtain comprehensive information about the effectiveness of curricula. They considered two bases of reference: the learners' and the teachers' views. Both groups, learners and teachers, were asked to evaluate the seven areas of expertise (outcomes). Whereas the teachers were asked to assess to what degree the learners actually possess the skills (external ratings), learners were asked to assess to what extent they believe to possess them (self-ratings); on the assumption that learners' self-ratings provide information about the subjective assessments of acquired skills, while external ratings by teachers provide information on how learners use and apply these skills and how they are reflected in their behavior.

The results of the study were very interesting. I refer the reader to the article [3] to see the results.

In general, they have found that there is a significant discrepancy between educational objectives and their realization. The acquired skills of students and graduates were assessed as very low and concluded that it is empirical to reform medical education.

II. A CURRICULUM HAS TO BE DYNAMIC AND RESPONSIVE TO CHANGES IN THE RAPIDLY PROGRESSING, VOLATILE WORLD OF MEDICAL EDUCATION; THE COLLEGE OF MEDICINE AT THE UNIVERSITY OF DUNDEE AS AN EXAMPLE

The medical school at the University of Dundee introduced a new curriculum in 1995. The curriculum combined six aspects: the spiral curriculum with three interlocking phases; a systems-based approach with themes running through the curriculum that provided a focus for the students' learning; a core curriculum with options; educational strategies with elements of problem-based learning (PBL); community-based learning; and student-centered approaches to teaching and learning that encouraged students to take more responsibility for their own learning; the student assessment approach that emphasized the overall objectives of the course; and an organizational and management structure with the allocation of resources designed to support the educational philosophy.

In 1997, an outcome-based approach was adopted for all five years of the curriculum, task-based learning was introduced as the framework for student learning in phase 3 and the portfolio assessment process was introduced as the medical students' final examination.

In 2003, Davis and Harden [24] looked at how the curriculum responded to changes with time; which aspects of the curriculum were still in place; and what new approaches have been added. They used evidence from a number of sources, which included internal reviews, external reviews, and student examination data.

A   The internal review data included:
  1   Results of the academic standards processes of the medical school that include both staff and student evaluations; analysis of student progress; student performance in degree examinations; peer review of teaching; review of some of the more novel elements, such as portfolio assessment and student diaries; and regular program review
  2   The University of Dundee quality assurance processes and quality awards
B   External reviews included formal review by various accreditation authorities (the Scottish Higher Education; General Medical Council; the Quality; Assurance Agency for Higher Education in the UK) and external examiner reports. Informal evaluative reviews wre also collected from visitors to the medical school.
C   Student examination data: They have used data from the progress test introduced in 2000 that provided evidence relating to the efficacy of the spiral design as well as Portfolio assessment data

There systematic program evaluation resulted in number of suggested corrective/ improvement measure at 6 levels: (a) The curriculum, (b) Teaching and learning: student support, (c) Teaching and learning: educational facilities, (d) Assessment, (e) Organization and management: committee structures, (f) Organization and management: administrative support.

III. THE POWER OF SELF-EVALUATION: CREATING A CULTURE OF REFLECTION AND ACTION INVOLVING ALL STAKEHOLDERS

Fetterman et al. [25] described their approach in evaluating the Stanford University School of Medicine's newly revised undergraduate medical education curriculum, through what they called as "empowerment evaluation"; an evaluation method that involves all stakeholders in an open process of review, critique, and improvement. They based their approach to curriculum evaluations on the following approaches:

A   Developing a culture of evidence: disseminating formative feedback and data about the curriculum to help inform decision making. Reporting processes are established to improve stakeholder access to evidence (evaluation data and findings) and to provide regular opportunities for reviewing and discussing the evidence.

B   Using a critical friend (office of quality assurance).

C   Encouraging a cycle of reflection and action: Structured opportunities allow stakeholders to reflect on evaluation data, set priorities, and develop action plans for revising the courses and curriculum.

D   Cultivating a community of learners: Under the empowerment evaluation model, the assumption is that each stakeholder, regardless of his or her status within the institution, has a unique and important perspective on curricular issues that should be shared and valued. As stakeholders engage in dialogue and discussion, they learn from one another and, in the process, are able to broaden and deepen their understanding of issues affecting individual courses and, more broadly, the curriculum.

E   Developing reflective practitioners. Faculty, students, and administrators develop the habit of continually reflecting on their practices and programs, both individually and as part of a larger group or community. By establishing a habit of regular self-assessment, stakeholders become reflective practitioners.

In applying those approaches to evaluation they have implemented a systematic cycle of reflection and actions across the curriculum.

As a result, course and clerkship directors, deans, and administrators frequently make requests for reports, data, and consulting assistance from the Division of Evaluation to help inform their strategic planning.

They applied several familiar evaluation tools including focus groups and surveys. The process is follows:

1   They conducted focus groups midway through each quarter of the program, in order to measure student responses to the new curriculum while courses were still in progress. Key findings were immediately disseminated to course directors and administrators. This process allowed numerous directors to make midcourse corrections based on the preliminary feedback.

2   They developed tailored, end-of-quarter online course evaluation forms to collect evidence about individual courses, the curriculum, and student life. Faculty received results four to six weeks after course completion.

3   They analyzed qualitative and quantitative data, using both standard questions across the curriculum and questions rooted in specific concerns of course directors.

4   Student ratings and comments were summarized into brief, written reports that provided a "dashboard view" of each course's key strengths and weaknesses

5   They instituted an ongoing practice of holding course director meetings within six weeks of the conclusion of each quarter to review and discuss evaluation findings. Meetings were facilitated by the evaluation director, who served as a critical friend, coaching faculty through the process of reviewing results and setting priorities for revisions. During these meetings, faculty directors could discuss the students' evaluations of individual courses and their educational experience during the quarter as a whole. Faculty members then shared their perspectives, bringing their knowledge and insights about the course to bear on the discussion, including additional data regarding student performance on exams (pass/fail rates) and reflections on gaps and redundancies in course content, either within individual courses or in the curriculum as a whole.

6   A variety of data sources (e.g., faculty and student surveys and comments, focus-group findings, and exam scores) were highlighted in quarterly and annual reports to the curriculum committee, with emphasis placed on highlighting crosscutting curricular issues.

7   Once revisions to courses and the curriculum were implemented, the cycle came full circle as the stakeholders reviewed evaluation data the following year to assess the impact that the planned changes had had on the curriculum.

To measure the effectiveness of this approach of curriculum evaluation, they have used number of internal and external metrics. For internal metrics, they have compared evaluation results before and after stakeholders began using this approach. They have found improvements in student ratings for course and clerkship courses. As for external metrics; they have used the following:

1   The median United States Medical Licensing Examination (USMLE) Step 1 score and failure rates for three years before and after the introduction of empowerment evaluation

2   Student performance during the first postgraduate year of training (graduating students matching at competitive academic residencies).

3   Graduates' performance in first year of residency as reported by residency program directors.

IV. DEVELOPMENT OF A COMPREHENSIVE WHOLE-PROGRAM EVALUATION WITH A FOCUS ON OUTCOMES, PROCESSES, AND ENVIRONMENTS

Gibson et al. [26] described the development of a comprehensive whole-program evaluation and improvement strategy for their new undergraduate medical education program at University of New South Wales (UNSW) in Sydney, Australia. They described the process of developing a multicomponent model that defines the quality of the educational program and outlined how they were addressing evaluation of each quality component.

Their Program Evaluation and Improvement Group formulated six strategic principles to guide development of a program evaluation and improvement strategy. They adopted a holistic view of evaluation, based on the principles that, both student and staff experiences are important and provide valuable information, there is a need to measure student and graduate outcomes, and an emphasis on action after evaluation is critical. The need for a multiple-aspects view of the academic quality was also considered important. Finally, they agreed that the evaluation process should also seek to develop explicit and systematic means for fostering and recognizing the commitment of faculty and professional staff to the continuing improvement of the program.

The adopted 4 program quality aspects (PQA);

a   Curriculum and resources
b   Staff and teaching
c   Student experience, and
d   Student and graduate outcomes

They considered that articulation of these program quality aspects (PQAs) was a necessary condition for the development of a model for continuing comprehensive evaluation and improvement of the program. For each PQA, they formulated three to four components to describe the principal building blocks of the PQA; and for each PQA they formulated a key quality indicator or indicators (Table 1): Note that only components and key quality indicators pertinent to this chapter were included in the table.

This was followed by the creation of working parties to establish the practical processes required to enable evaluation of, improvement of, and reporting on the quality of the medicine program. These working parties were aligned with the PQAs. The creation of these working parties enabled additional staff and students to participate in the program evaluation and improvement processes.

Before establishing specific projects, each working party reviewed their respective indicators to identify relevant available data, areas where instrument development needed to occur, and the reporting, communication, and implementation implications for indicator development.

Various tools have been used for collecting evaluative data, including using the university's data bases on issues pertaining to teaching loads, resources, and evaluations; faculty and student surveys; as well as semi structured focus groups and interviews. The data generated have been analyzed and findings communicated to faculty leaders, academics, and students.

Table 1. Program Quality Aspects (PQAs) and Key Quality Indicators of the Undergraduate Medical Curriculum of the Faculty of Medicine of the University of New South Wales, Sydney, Australia [26]

Program quality aspects	Components	Key quality indicators
Student Experience (SE)	Learning and teaching	1. Satisfaction with learning and teaching (includes activities) 2. Student perception of quality of learning and teaching materials 3. Student perception of quality of physical environment 4. Student perception of quality of learning culture
Student and Graduate Outcomes	Student capabilities	Assessment results profile Attitude to medicine/career Progression patterns of students
	Graduate capabilities	External capability assessments Perceived self-efficacy (referenced to capabilities)
	Career outcomes	Paths, diversity, changes, and achievements of graduates
Staff and Teaching	Quality of teaching	Student satisfaction with learning and teaching Alignment of teaching, learning and assessment External assessments of quality of teaching
Curriculum and Resources	Quality of curriculum design	Stakeholder judgments of quality of curriculum design Evaluation and improvement processes informing change

Modified (to be in line with the purpose of this chapter) from; Kathryn A. Gibson, Patrick Boyle, Deborah A. Black, Margaret Cunningham, Michael C. Grimm, and H. Patrick McNeil, 2088. Enhancing Evaluation in an Undergraduate Medical Education Program; Academic Medicine; 83: 787-793.

V. QUALITATIVE AND QUANTITATIVE MEASURES TO BE USED IN EVALUATING A CURRICULUM

Durning et al. [27]; argue that variety of measurements can, and should, be used. Both qualitative (descriptive) as well as quantitative (numerical scores) assessments can, and in many cases, should be used for program evaluation as the quantitative measurements alone may overlook important findings that are revealed through qualitative analysis.

They advocate that particularly for new innovations (a new educational program and/or a new component of an existing educational program) and/or formative program evaluation, at least one qualitative measurement in addition to quantitative measurements should be implemented; because qualitative measurements complement the quantitative data and can be particularly useful for detecting unexpected outcomes.

Qualitative data can also serve as a rich database for hypothesis generation that can subsequently be confirmed with further qualitative and/or quantitative data.

In a paper by Dagenais and colleagues [28]; they review measures that have been used in medicine for evaluating academic programs and curriculum assessment methods.

They propose the following curriculum assessment methods; which I will list in the way they were described in the article with the authors' comments.

A   Qualitative Tools
   1   Curriculum Guidelines (curriculum contents): They believe that traditional guidelines address curriculum content rather than knowledge transfer and are neither linked to student learning nor linked to competence after completion of the program. They encourage, linking the content of courses in a curriculum to national guidelines as this may be a useful exercise and it provides some comparative information about the program

   2   Competency Documents: Competency statements or lists of competencies for students can be the basis for an internal assessment of the curriculum.

   3   Discussions and Focus Groups:
     a   Discussions: Revolve around the courses and cover organization, content, teaching methods, clinical experience, student assessment, and evaluation methods. Participants traditionally include the course director, members of the curriculum committee, student representatives, and the associate dean for academic affairs. Such face-to-face interactions between students and faculty are based on the information gathered through the evaluation questionnaires and have the advantage of clarifying the problems identified and enabling the faculty to respond to criticism. To limit confrontational situations, the evaluations of individual faculty members by students are not part of the discussion.

     b   Focus groups: Refer to structured discussions of limited duration with a randomly selected group of people. The moderator of the focus group is generally not a faculty member and has experience in facilitating interactions. The participants are stimulated by the ideas of one another, which are thought to be an advantage. Focus groups can explore thoughts and feelings of participants better than questionnaires. Focus groups are particularly useful to identify problems and find solutions, but have the major disadvantages of being time-consuming and requiring considerable faculty participation.

B   Quantitative Tools
   1   Competency Examinations: Performance based competency tests are valuable means of demonstrating to the public the standards of care to which the profession is committed. They may be the best way to measure the effectiveness of a clinical curriculum, and they have been used as curriculum assessment tools in medical education; they argue. They noted that some questions need to be

answered before they can be adopted as outcome measures. For example: Are the current school's competency documents comprehensive enough or too detailed? Are all necessary competencies being evaluated? And are the skills being tested a reflection of skills needed in practice?

2   Board Examinations: Performance of students on the examinations developed by board examining bodies for example, "the Medical Council of Canada Qualifying Examination (MCC), National Board of Medical Examiners (NBME), and United States Medical Licensing Examinations (USMLE) are a frequently reported curriculum assessment tool". The primary role of board examinations is to assure society that graduating students are competent, which of course is also a major goal of each medical school. May be useful measures of training programs, providing that examination questions fairly cover the content of the curriculum and are consistent with the educational goals of the institution.

Drawbacks of board examinations: The values of standardized licensure examinations to determine the success of innovative programs have been questioned for medicine. Dagenais et al. [28] question its sensitivity as a tool. They feel that a restructuring of these examinations is required to ensure that the entire curriculum is properly covered. They believe that, variations in the results between schools can be due to the fact that not all schools give study time prior to the examinations and that some candidates enroll in private preparatory courses. Also, may be due to the fact that, the students of some schools had built up banks of old examination questions, while student at other schools had not. It has also been pointed out that the evaluation of the effectiveness of a medical curriculum should not rely solely on standardized tests using multiple-choice questions. Results on board examinations should be reviewed with caution for the following reasons: First, the content of the medical board examination may better reflect a traditional than an unconventional program. Secondly, the multiple-choice format of board examinations is very familiar to students in conventional programs, but varied testing methods are more likely to be used in modified programs. In fact, studies of board examination questions suggest that the format of the questions can influence student performance. (For references, see Marie E. Dagenais et al. [28])

3   Oral Comprehensive Examination: Structured oral examination has been reported to result in higher overall and inter rater reliabilities than multiple choice questions to assess knowledge acquisition and problem-solving skills of surgical residents

4   Surveys: They believe that questionnaires are widely used curriculum assessment tools because they provide a lot of information rapidly, at a small cost, and with minimal staff involvement.

a   Student Surveys: These surveys provide information on the quality of university and faculty services, practice and postgraduate education plans, and the adequacy of time allotted to various areas of undergraduate instruction. Educators ask students to rate their level of competence or level of preparation for the program competencies. This provides immediate feedback from graduating students on the entire curriculum.

Pabst et al. [29] argue that at early stages of the curriculum it will be the atmosphere created by the teacher that matters. They;

i   Recommend repeated questionnaires during undergraduate and postgraduate phases as well as later while physicians are practicing.

ii   Recommend that the evaluations should be performed by discipline experts themselves in cooperation with statisticians and experts in didactics.

iii   Believe that it is important to secure high response rates as otherwise during the discussions of academic committees in particular it will often be argued that the data are not representative.

iv   Believe that the type of survey also affects the results: It seems to be important to include open questions, which have often given evaluators important clues for further improvements

v   Believe that anonymous evaluations can be very useful to obtain opinions not mentioned in front of fellow students.

b   Alumni Surveys: Alumni can give significant information on the strengths and weaknesses of the curriculum and on the importance of its various components. Surveys of alumni can also reveal practice patterns, learning behaviors, and levels of satisfaction with the profession, three areas that may provide information about the effectiveness of the curriculum. However, these surveys have inherent limitations. If the length of time between the end of university training and data gathering is long, it becomes difficult to separate the effects of a curriculum from those of experience. The level of interest or lack of interest of alumni for certain aspects of practice can introduce biases in their responses to questions about university programs. For these reasons, it has been recommended that surveys be limited to individuals who have graduated in the past ten years. (For references, see Dagenais et al. [28])

c   Evaluation by Instructors: Some authors have used questionnaires filled out by instructors to rate the competency of graduating students

d   Patient Satisfaction Survey: Student-patient interactions are important but difficult to evaluate. Patients are able to evaluate communication skills and empathy, so it is logical that a patient-centered curriculum be evaluated by the patients receiving the care. However, there is a tendency for patients to become attached to students, which may lead to artificially high ratings on patient satisfaction questionnaires. To counteract this, standardized patients have been used to rate humanistic skills, history-taking, and examination skills of medical students. [30, 31, 32], Patients can comment on their comfort and perhaps their perception of resident comfort and skill with the procedure (i.e., checklist and/or interview). They might also comment on the resident's explanation of risks/benefits and their satisfaction with the procedure performed (i.e., interview).

5   Clinical Productivity: Educators tend to be reluctant to use clinical output or income as an assessment tool. However, there are two justifications for using these variables. First, students need to learn to be efficient, and second, students who are more positive and enthusiastic about their training might be more productive.

In summary; a range of evaluation tools were used, focusing on clinical productivity, instructor effectiveness surveys, graduating student surveys, patient feedback surveys, and board examinations.

VI. EVALUATION ACROSS THE WHOLE SPECTRUM OF MEDICAL EDUCATION; EVALUATING A COURSE, CLERKSHIP, OR COMPONENTS OF A RESIDENCY BASED ON ACCREDITATION REQUIREMENTS

Durning et al. [27]; purposed a framework for program evaluation based on accreditation requirements and is intended for course, clerkship, and residency or fellowship directors as well as those who oversee them, such as chairs of departments, deans, and perhaps chief operating officers of hospitals.

They proposed a basic three-phase structure for program evaluation readily applies to existing programs and new programs, curricula, or interventions. The proposed framework emphasizes the role of baseline, process, and product (outcome) information for undergraduate medical education and for postgraduate medical education (residency), both quantitative and qualitative, for describing program "success."

Process measurements are those collected about the trainees, the faculty, and the program that are made during the curriculum.

Outcome measurements occur after (or at least at the very end of) the course, clerkship, or residency training program.

They believe that the advantages of such an approach include:

1 With this approach, goal is to understand how the program is working rather than simple classification of graduates (e.g., competent or not competent).

2 This three-phase framework of program evaluation could foster collaboration across the medical education continuum, as the baseline measurements for a 3rd-year clerkship director may comprise the outcome measurements of a 2nd-year course director and the outcome measurements of a clerkship director can serve as baseline measurements for a residency training program director.

Many of the measurements used in this article are derived from expectations of the LCME or Residency Review Committees of the ACGME.

They believe that: (a) All those responsible for the program's performance should have input into defining the questions to be asked and data to be gathered about the program.

(b) Stakeholders include anyone with an interest in the course, clerkship, or residency training program such as medical school deans, department chairs, university presidents, hospital chief executive officers, and the public.

Pertinent to this chapter, I will only present their proposed measures that apply to undergraduate medical education.

The three phases are:

a Baseline measurements (before): are necessary to determine "how learners change," and they are especially important to determine the effect of curriculum as opposed to selection of trainees and they allow academic managers to put program outcomes into context (they argue)

b   Process measurements (during): are those that monitor the activities of learners during the training program. These measurements are often collected prospectively, that is, in real time.

c   Product measurements (after): are outcome measurements.

For the baseline measurements; they propose the following;

1   Student self-assessment
2   Exams (United States Medical Licensing Examination (USMLE), pretest)
3   Clinical performance evaluation (Objective Structured Clinical Examination (OSCE))
4   Compliance with requirements (e.g., immunizations)
5   GPA prior to clinical years
6   Introduction to Clinical Medicine Grades
7   MCAT scores
8   Critical Incident Reports

For the process measurements; they propose the following;

1   Patient logs
2   Procedure logs
3   Hours
4   End-of-clerkship critiques
5   Student exit interviews
6   Clinical performance evaluation
7   Portfolios
8   Reflective exercises
9   Attendance rates

For the product measurements; they propose the following;

1   Surveys (4th year, graduates, program director)
2   Placing graduates (i.e., location, choice)
3   Future exams (United States Medical Licensing Examination (USMLE), in-training, Examination (ITE)
4   Clinical performance evaluations
5   Narratives of trainee performance (e.g., 360 degree evaluation, peer assessment)
6   Review of write-ups
7   Attitudinal
8   Student portfolios
9   Professional development plans
10   End of clerkship exams (National Board of Medical Examiners (NBME), analytic, pattern)
11   Critical incident reports

12   Peer Evaluations
13   360 degree evaluations

VII. Accreditation and International Quality Assurance of Medical Education

There is significant variation in the structure and quality of undergraduate medical education around the world. Accreditation processes can encourage institutional improvement and help promote high-quality education experiences. Globalization in medicine and medical education is leading towards common trends in curricular management and medical education that should facilitate defining common standards. This necessitates the need for measures to protect the practice of medicine. There are increasing pressures for international quality assurance of medical education; therefore, international recognition of basic medical education programs is needed; this will be beneficial to medical colleges and all stakeholders. However, there are no mechanisms in place at present for the international recognition of medical educational institutions and programs.

Physicians are educated in countries with diverse educational systems, including variations in teaching traditions, curricular models, instructional methods, clinical opportunities, assessment principles, and available resources. In addition, approximately one-third of countries with medical schools do not have a system of accreditation or other quality assurance oversight of medical education programs that is conducted by an independent or governmental body [33] Experiences from well-established accreditation systems, which combine counseling and guidance with review and control, have proved accreditation to be an effective quality assurance tool [34].

Policies of the Liaison Committee on Medical Education (LCME), ensure a level of uniformity in the education offered by US institutions, however, assessing the quality of medical education has also been recognized as an important need outside North America. Numerous organizations promote accreditation efforts and quality assurance methodology around the world. The World Federation for Medical Education (WFME) is a global association dedicated to enhancing the quality of education and training of medical doctors around the world. The WFME is not an accrediting body, but, through its creation of a document of global standards (the Trilogy of WFME Standards for Quality Improvement in Medical Education), covering standards for basic medical education, postgraduate medical education, and continuing professional development for medical doctors, it promotes the establishment of accreditation systems (www.wfme.org).

The 3 documents should be seen as an entity, underlining the need for coordination of the three phases of medical education. The 3 sets of standards are built on the same principles, using 9 areas and 33-38 sub-areas corresponding to performance indicators. The standards use 2 levels of attainment: basic standards ("musts") for accreditation purposes and standards for quality development ("shoulds") for reform processes.

The standards cover all aspects of medical education, i.e. organization, structure, process, content, environment and outcome. The standards have already influenced medical education significantly worldwide [34].

In the United States, the US Department of Education's National Committee on Foreign Medical Education and Accreditation (NCFMEA) determines whether the educational programme in a foreign medical school and the standards and processes used to accredit it are comparable to those in the United States or not [35]. NCFMEA voluntarily reviews the accreditation systems used by accrediting bodies around the world to determine whether those systems are comparable to LCME standards. While WFME and other, regional organizations are involved with accreditation efforts around the world, no unified process or quality assurance standards have been universally adopted [33].

A program for promotion of accreditation was formulated within the WHO/WFME strategic partnership. Essential to this development was the definition of a WFME advisor function and the development of a manual for WFME advisors. The WFME, the Copenhagen-Lund University Centre for International Medical Education (CLUCIME) and the Open University Centre for Education in Medicine (OUCEM) in the UK are now working together on training programs for advisors and assessors [36].

International Databases of Medical Schools

Three major databases with global coverage list a different number of medical schools. These are: the WHO World Directory of Medical Schools; the Foundation for the Advancement of International Medical Education and Research (FAIMER) International Medical Education Directory (IMED), and the Institute for International Medical Education (IIME).

None of these databases contain reliable information about the quality of the medical programs listed. The information is often out of date and in some cases can be misleading (For references, please see Hans Karle 2008 [2]) [36].

AVICENNA Directories

In response to requests from member states, the World Health Organization (WHO) has decided to develop new Global Directories of Health Professions Education Institutions (AVICENNA Directories [37]). The World Health Organization has published a World Directory of Medical Schools since 1953. The last printed edition (7th ed., 2000) lists institutions of basic medical education in 157 countries. After the year 2000, updating has been done electronically, the latest covering information received before the end of 2007. In August 2007, the WHO and the University of Copenhagen signed an agreement, which gave the University responsibility for the development and administration of the new directory with the assistance of the World Federation for Medical Education (WFME) which has a long-standing collaboration with WHO. In 2011, all rights to the database were transferred from the University to WFME. From August 2008, the data of the World Directory of Medical Schools has been available on AVICENNA Directories website. Information concerning individual schools and countries is continuously updated in response to requests from medical schools and national authorities. The mission of the AVICENNA Directories will be to facilitate transparency in understanding of the human resources for health, and of the educational background of health professionals. Fundamental information will support improvement of the quality of education, especially by providing information on the quality of education and training and by guiding users to other sources containing more specific and detailed information. The information about medical schools and their programs is of general worldwide interest. AVICENNA Directories have the following advantages:

A   It is an important tool in quality assurance.
B   It is a valuable tool for the registration agencies, which are responsible for licensing to practice in medicine.
C   It is an instrument to promote international collaborations.
D   It provides information for potential students or staff wishing to learn about an individual school or faculty or about all schools in a particular country.
E   Finally, as a reliable and comprehensive database, it becomes a powerful research tool and an instrument for networking between schools.

It intends to cover educational institutions for all academic health professions, and to increase the amount of information provided about institutions and programs, including number of admissions and graduates, attrition rates, ownership, management and funding sources. More importantly, quality-related information will be added, such as accreditation status (operating agency, the criteria used, type of procedure, etc.).

This plan will provide a process of meta-recognition of medical schools programs. Such an approach of "accrediting the accreditors" will stimulate establishment of national accreditation systems and respect the work already being carried out by existing reliable accreditation agencies, and avoid unnecessary bureaucracy. The result will be the creation of a global network of recognized accrediting agencies within medical education [36].

In summary; the establishment of new accreditation systems in countries without quality assurance instruments and the modification of existing accreditation systems to meet the WHO/WFME Guidelines is a high priority. A method of "accrediting the accrediting agencies" based on WHOM/WFME Guidelines will stimulate the establishment of national accreditation systems. The WFME will, therefore, together with FAIMER and other partners, develop a database of accrediting and/or recognizing agencies.

VIII. ALTERNATIVE QUALITY ASSURANCE METHODS

A. Quality Assurance of Medical Education through National Accreditation

The Task Force that defined the World Health Organization (WHO) / WFME Guidelines for Accreditation in Basic Medical Education considered that organizations such as the WHO or the WFME should not assume an accrediting agency role. It was therefore recommended that accreditation should be a national responsibility. The Foundation for Advancement of International Medical Education and Research (FAIMER) has developed and continues to update a Directory of Organizations that Recognize/Accredit Medical Schools (DORA).

This database is freely available on the FAIMER website (http://www.faimer.org/orgs. html). DORA contains a list of countries with identified accreditation authorities, the names of the organizations, and website links if available. Information on whether the process is mandatory or voluntary and on whether the accrediting body is an independent entity or a government authority is provided, if known. The inclusion of an accreditation body in DORA does not indicate that FAIMER has endorsed the authority or verified the level of quality of overseeing provided. FAIMER is not an accrediting agency and has no relationship with the organizations listed.

Zanten et al. [33]; Provide an overview of medical school accreditation processes in 91 countries around the world, highlighting variations by region. Their study revealed that medical school accreditation is not universal. They concluded that a robust accreditation system, functioning either as an autonomous entity or as part of a government's ministry of health or education, can be useful in encouraging institutions to conduct self-review and improvement. It can also ensure that medical students receive high-quality education experiences based on established standards. Their baseline data for current worldwide accreditation practices are a necessary preface to future studies investigating relationships between accreditation processes and medical outcomes.

B. Other Mechanisms for Recognition of Medical Education Programs

Other mechanisms for recognition of medical education programs are needed Initiatives to address this issue include [34]:

a   International collaboration and partnerships: The International Database for Enhanced Assessments and Learning (IDEAL) consortium, set up in Hong Kong in 2001 invites medical schools internationally to share materials and to enhance assessment of medical students'. The Universities Medical Assessment Partnership (UMAP) is a UK-based collaborative project, aimed at "raising standards in written assessment in undergraduate medicine", which now has 15 partners after starting with 5 medical schools in 2003 [38]. "Despite the pitfalls of inter-institutional collaboration, the expected benefits of joining forces seem to have an attractive appeal, as is shown by various recent initiatives. The main advantage of cooperative assessment is that it creates opportunities for comparing curricular effectiveness and identifying problem areas in schools" [38]

b   International conventions

c   The publication of global databases allowing meta-recognition of accredited institutions and programs.

d   Governmental evaluation based on comparison of programs with general regulations without use of institutional self-evaluation or site visits

e   Self-evaluation including the use of external examiners without formal accreditation and by national examinations before licensure. The introduction of institutional self-evaluation at regular intervals is of utmost importance. Furthermore, review of self-evaluation reports and site visits by teams of trained and experienced experts ensures that program development follows nationally adopted criteria and is consistent with international standards. Using international standards as a template for national criteria guarantees a foundation for international recognition, while allowing for institutional self-determination. Internal quality management systems should be considered as an acceptable alternative to external review and accreditation [36]

f   Program Evaluators: Internal evaluators are intra- or interdepartmental experts who evaluate educational program. This could include an education committee, a medical education office, or other members of the medical school faculty and/or administration. External evaluators are often academic managers from different institutions who evaluate an educational program. As external evaluators are not involved with the local curriculum or program politics, external evaluators can potentially provide greater objectivity and a clearer perspective of programmatic strengths and needs. The program being evaluated benefits from ideas for improvement and high visibility and the external evaluators' programs might benefit from new ideas for conducting program evaluation at their own institutions [27].

Noteworthy at this stage is to describe the recent experience by the college of medicine at Alfaisal University/ Kingdom of Saudi Arabia, in establishing an internal evaluation process. In order to facilitate the process; a curriculum review office (CRO) was established immediately after graduating the first batch of students. The mandate of this office was to review courses/blocks in terms of the following attributes and provide recommendations to the Director of Academic affairs:

A   Placement in the overall curriculum structure
B   Credits assigned
C   Learning objectives/ outcomes
D   Structure of the curriculum (Sequential instructional order)
E   Resource material provided to the students
F   Resource faculty
G   Assessment
H   Review of students' feedback

The following will be the steps of the review process:
I.   Each block is assigned to two members who will review the blocks independently. They have an access to following items:

1   Curriculum outline
2   Block document (syllabus)
3   Course specification document: as mandated by the National Commission for Assessment and Academic Accreditation (NCAAA)
4   Power-point presentations of lecturers
5   PBL/TBL cases/questions
6   Examination papers
7   Course reports: as mandated by the National Commission for Assessment and Academic Accreditation (NCAAA)
8   Students' evaluation

II.   Evaluating objectives and contents of undergraduate medical curriculum courses

Benchmarking course/program objectives is the first step in designing quality medical education program. Courses/ clinical rotations directors; need to benchmark the intended objectives of their particular course/rotation. The CRO members evaluating course goals and objectives check these parameters against college goals and objectives for alignment. Each educational session (e.g., lecture, laboratory, and small-group session) is expected to have specific learning objectives addressing varying cognitive levels that are written in behavioral terms which describe knowledge, skills, and attitudes students should demonstrate as a result of the educational session.

These should be clearly stated in the course syllabus as well as the course specification document, mandated by National Commission for Assessment and Academic Accreditation (NCAAA) [39]; the local accrediting agency; which is responsible for academic accreditation in higher education institutions beyond the secondary education.

The NCAAA has identified broad categories or types of learning outcomes in five groups or domains, knowledge, cognitive skills, interpersonal skills and responsibility, communication, IT and numerical skills, and psychomotor skills, and has described in general terms the level of knowledge and skill expected for different qualifications.

There are differences in how these learning outcomes are developed by students and an important aspect of program and course planning is to plan for teaching processes and forms of assessment that will be appropriate for these different types of intended learning outcomes.

In the process; course content is compared to course goals and the stated learning objectives, and curricular content published by NCAAA. Organization and integration of content, pedagogy, quality of lecture slides, and ease of navigation of electronic course management tools are assessed (on Moodle). CRO members look for horizontal and vertical integration of curricular content. They also look into evaluations of clinical clerkships to assess parameters such as inpatient and outpatient experiences, opportunity to perform procedures, and comparability of student experiences across clerkship.

III.   Assessment

The concept of exam blueprints was introduced. These allow course directors to assure and evaluate, fair representation of course content and testing at the desired range of cognitive levels. This insures that each examination question is mapped to (a) a specific learning objective and (b) the cognitive domain that is being tested.

Assessment office provides the CRO with detailed analysis of multiple choice question-based examinations in terms of: test reliability, alignment between test questions and objectives and content, level of cognitive domain being tested, item difficulty, item discrimination value, grade distribution, and format and quality of questions.

IV.   Students' Feedback

End-of-course evaluations by students are semi-quantitative (Likert scale) with opportunity for anonymous comments. CRO members that review student evaluations look for themes pertaining to: quality of lectures; course organization; clarity of learning objectives; quality of problem-based learning sessions, team-based learning sessions, small group sessions; clarity and content of examination questions; and level of knowledge necessary for examination in light of course and lecture objectives.

V.   Different tools (Performas) were used as templates for developing an in-house tool for the review process. The purpose of this Performa is to provide documentary evidence from which the reviewers have formulated their recommendations.

VI.   Once the independent review is completed (in most situations it should be completed within two weeks), the reports are presented to curriculum review office and a final report is generated after the review of all members. This final report with an executive summary of recommendations is sent to Head of Academic affairs, Curriculum Committee and will be copied to the members of College Board.

G   Benchmarking: Progress testing as an example

Sound benchmarking can yield information to support curriculum evaluation to raise educational standards across schools. Recently, the use of data obtained from progress testing in different medical schools around the globe has been used as a benchmarking tool.

Progress testing is defined by Freeman et al. [40] as" a form of assessment where groups of learners of different seniority (i.e. different classes in a curriculum) are given the same written test. The test is comprehensive by sampling all relevant disciplines in a curriculum usually determined by a fixed blueprint. The test is repeated regularly in time".

Progress testing has been established in many medical schools internationally as the primary method for assessing applied medical knowledge. The tests require students to apply their learning in a clinical context, to integrate clinical science with clinical practice and to extend their knowledge of clinical science into later years of the program. Progress tests are aimed at assessing the functional knowledge of medical students. As students' progress through their program, test scores increase, this indicates that knowledge is advancing towards that expected of them. Progress tests are therefore useful for assessing the extent to which curricular objectives are met [41, 42, and 43].

Progress testing, as an alternative form of multiple choice tests, was introduced in the University of Missouri in 1991 and the University of Maastricht, in the Netherlands, in 1996. It is now administered in five out of eight medical schools in the Netherlands; 13 medical schools in Germany, where it began as a student initiative; a number of medical schools working together in the UK and the United States; and in other individual medical schools globally. Most of these medical schools use progress testing for summative assessment, with the notable exception of Germany, where it is used formatively in all medical schools.

The University of Otago, in New Zealand, has been using progress testing formatively since a successful trial in 2003. (For references, please see [44]).

In an article by Yielder et al., they are promoting the idea of introducing progress testing as potential for collaboration and benchmarking across Australian and New Zealand medical schools for the following reasons:

1   There could be considerable strategic benefits in collaborating with other medical schools in the development of question banks and the evaluation and validation of test items. This would enable broad curriculum coverage to be achieved spreading

the load of producing assessment material, sharing of resources, and a degree of standardization and benchmarking across programs.

2   There is good potential for collaboration, since progress testing is curriculum independent, meaning that the questions aim to assess the program outcomes rather than specific content at set points within the program.

3   The cross-sectional and longitudinal implementation of progress testing also provides an additional research opportunity within the medical program. The data obtained would allow for comparison in the growth of different knowledge areas within a program and provide cross-sectional data about student cohorts and test items

4   It would also facilitate the potential for cross-institutional comparisons and raise the possibility of collaborative research between programs.

Muijtjens et al. [38] investigated the effectiveness of single-point benchmarking and longitudinal benchmarking for inter-school educational evaluation; using data from progress tests assessing the graduation-level knowledge of all students from 3 Dutch co-operating medical schools. They argue that there are number of discrepancies that might undermine cross-institutional comparison and benchmarking in general, they include:

1   Different admission strategies favor recruitment of different student populations, leading to confusion of student effects and curriculum effects.

2   Differences in student and teacher experience with benchmarking instruments can create unfair disadvantages.

3   The test status, which can vary between schools from high-stakes summative tests to strictly formative tests.

4   Psychometric sources of error: single test scores are generally not sufficiently reliable and group and cohort effects can limit the generalizability of findings.

However, they believe that progress testing by Dutch medical schools presented an excellent authentic experimental set-up for benchmark testing as;

1   The student population of the schools is homogeneous, because admission to all Dutch medical schools are determined by a national lottery procedure.

2   All schools adhere to the same nationally agreed statutory objectives of undergraduate medical education. The cooperation on progress testing is based on these shared final objectives, joint item production, comparable test status and simultaneous assessment of all students at the schools.

They concluded that; the longitudinal nature of progress testing combined with multi-institutional cooperation, offers excellent opportunities for credible and defensible benchmarking. The noted however, that their study unequivocally shows that single-point benchmarking is dubious at best and its results should be interpreted with caution.

Benchmarking based on longitudinal data and cumulative deviations appears to be the method of preference wherever it is feasible, as it provides information that is superior in both richness and accuracy [38].

H   Curriculum mapping

The shift of emphasis from the educational process to the learning outcomes has had an impact on medical education throughout the world. Student progression towards the exit learning outcomes has proved to be a complex process. As many schools are moving towards outcome-based education models; the inclusion of outcomes in a curriculum map can help with curriculum evaluation and quality assurance. A curriculum map can be thought of as analogous to a roadmap of a curriculum, guiding its users – students, faculty members, teachers, and curriculum planners, evaluators and coordinators; through the various elements of the curriculum and their interconnections.

Curricular elements may include people (learners, teachers), activities (learning and assessment events), courses, outcomes and objectives, learning resources, topics and locations. Electronically speaking, a curriculum map is typically a relational database (or a number of databases that can communicate with one another) that contains information about the curriculum and people, and links between these various elements [45]. A curriculum map is needed to enable full benefit to be obtained from the outcome-based education and to allow both staff and students to understand the planned progression and the complex relationship between learning outcomes, learning opportunities, curriculum content and student assessment [24].

Some recent publications have outlined approaches taken by specific medical schools, whether they have created custom built systems or made use of existing solutions.(For references, I refer the reader to an article by Timothy G Willett [45]).

Staff and students can identify through the map the prerequisites for understanding each core clinical problem provided through the system-based courses.

The development of the system-based learning can be traced throughout all three phases of the curriculum. Students can identify their progression towards the learning outcomes through various educational opportunities and this progression can be fine-tuned by staff as necessary. The student assessment system and how the assessment relates to the outcomes of the curriculum, individual courses and the educational opportunities provided can be viewed as an aid to staff involved in the assessment system [24].

In summary, curriculum maps, like road maps, serve two key functions:

1   The curriculum map makes the curriculum more transparent to all the stakeholders: the teacher, the student, the curriculum developers, the manager, the profession and the public.
2   The curriculum map demonstrates the links between the different elements of the curriculum, e.g. between learning outcomes and learning opportunities and between the parts within one element, e.g. between different learning outcomes.

The windows through which the curriculum map can be explored may include:
(1) the expected learning outcomes; (2) curriculum content or areas of expertise covered; (3) student assessment; (4) learning opportunities; (5) learning location; (6) learning resources; (7) timetable; (8) staff; (9) curriculum management; (10) students. (For more reading on curriculum mapping, I refer the reader to Harden, 2001 (46))

CONCLUSION

Academic directors are continuously challenged by the need to monitor and evaluate the quality of their education programs with relatively little guidance from the literature on how to conduct this essential task. We have discussed key aspects of undergraduate medical curriculum evaluation and outlined a comprehensive framework for the evaluation and assessment that can be used throughout the spectrum of medical education; with a focus on outcomes, processes, and environments. This framework embraces the following pillars:

1   A curriculum has to be dynamic and responsive
2   Creating a culture of reflection and action involving all stakeholders is vital
3   Evaluation has to be comprehensive across the whole spectrum of medical education and to include; courses, clerkship, components of a residency based on accreditation requirements
4   It has to be a feasible and practical approach that is sufficiently rigorous to allow conclusions that can lead to action, and can be implemented across the spectrum of medical education for new and existing programs.

REFERENCES

[1]   Fitzpatrick, J. L., Randers, J. R., Worthen, B. R. (eds.), 2004. *Program evaluation: Alternative approaches and practical guidelines.* 3rd ed. Boston, MA: Pearson Education, Inc.

[2]   Dauphinee, W. D., Wood-Dauphinee, S., 2004. The need for evidence in medical education: The development of best evidence medical education as an opportunity to inform, guide, and sustain medical education research; *Academic Medicine*; 79:925-930.

[3]   Christiane Spiel, Barbara Schober and Ralph Reimann, 2006. Evaluation of curricula in higher education; challenges for evaluators; *Evaluation review*; 30(4):430-450.

[4]   Gerrity, Martha S. and John Mahaffy, 1998. Evaluating change in medical school curricula: How did we know where we were going? *Academic Medicine*; 73:55-59.

[5]   Australian Medical Council. *Assessment and Accreditation of Medical Schools: Standards and Procedures.* Available at: (http://www.amc.org.au/index.php/ar/bme). Accessed June 22, 2014.

[6]   The Liaison Committee for Medical Education for North American medical schools: *Functions and Structure of a Medical School.* Available at: (http://www.lcme.org/ publications.htm#standards-section). Accessed June 22, 2014.

[7]   Declan Kennedy, Áine Hyland and Norma Ryan, 2012. *Implementing Bologna in your institution: Writing and Using Learning Outcomes: a Practical Guide* (http://sss.dcu.ie/ afi/docs/bologna/writing_and_using_learning_outcomes.pdf). Accessed, June 27, 2014.

[8]   Shumway, M. and Harden, R. M., 2003. AMEE Guide No. 25: The assessment of learning outcomes for the competent and reflective physician; *Medical Teacher*; 25 (6): 569-584.

[9]   LCME (2003) Liaison Committee on Medical Education [website: http://www.lcme.org].

[10] AAMC, 1998. *Learning objectives for medical student education guidelines for medical schools: report I of the Medical School Objectives Project* (https://members.aamc.org/eweb/upload/Learning%20Objectives%20for%20Medical%20Student%20Educ%20Report%20I.pdf). Accessed June 22, 2014.

[11] *Accreditation Council for Graduate Medical Education (ACGME), Outcome Project, ACGME 2003* (http://www.ecfmg.org/echo/acgme-core-competencies.html). Note: This information was revised by ACGME in 2007 when it revised its Common Program Requirements. For more details and updates on the Common Program Requirements: General Competencies refer to the Outcome Project or "The Next Accreditation System (NAS)" on the ACGME-NAS (http://www.acgme.org/acgmeweb/tabid/435/ProgramandInstitutionalAccreditation/NextAccreditationSystem.aspx). Both Accessed June 28, 2014.

[12] IIME Core Committee, 2002. Global minimum essential requirements in medical education; *Medical Teacher*; 24(2): 130-135.

[13] The Medical Council of Canada, 2005. *Objectives for the Qualifying Examination* (http://mcc.ca/). Accessed June 28, 2014.

[14] The General Medical Council of UK, 2009. *Tomorrow's Doctors, Outcomes and standards for undergraduate medical education*, (http://www.gmc-uk.org/static/documents/content/Tomorrow_s_Doctors_0414.pdf). Accessed June 28, 2014.

[15] ACGME and ABMS, 2000. *Toolbox of Assessment Methods, A Product of the Joint Initiative, Accreditation Council for Graduate Medical Education (ACGME) Outcomes Project, American Board of Medical Specialties (ABMS)*, Version 1.1, September 2000 http://www.fammed.washington.edu/ebp/media/Toolbox[1].pdf. Accessed June 28, 2014.

[16] Scottish Deans Medical Curriculum Group, 2002. *The Scottish Doctor-Undergraduate Learning outcomes and their assessment: a foundation for competent and reflective practitioners* (http://www.scottishdoctor.org/). Accessed June 28, 2014.

[17] Cumming, A. 1., Ross, M., 2007. The Tuning Project for Medicine,learning outcomes for undergraduate medical education in Europe; *Med. Teach.* 29(7):636-41.

[18] Federation of Royal Colleges of Physicians, UK, 2006. *Generic Curriculum for the Medical Specialties*, (http://www.jrcptb.org.uk/trainingandcert/ST3-SpR/Documents/2007%20Generic%20Curriculum.pdf). Accessed online on June, 24, 2014.

[19] Mukhopadhyay, S. and Smith, S., 2010. Outcome-based education: Principles and practice; *Journal of Obstetrics and Gynaecology*; 30(8): 790-794.

[20] *USMLE Step 1; Content Description and General information* (http://www.usmle.org/pdfs/step-1/2014content_step1.pdf). Accessed online on June, 24, 2014.

[21] *NBME subject Exam's content outline:* (http://www.nbme.org/Schools/Subject-Exams/Subjects/Exams.html). Accessed, June 27, 2014.

[22] Ramsden, P., 2003. *Learning to Teach in Higher Education*, London: Routledge. 2nd edition.

[23] Biggs, J. 2003. *Teaching for Quality Learning at University*. Buckingham: Open University Press.

[24] Margery H. Davis and Ronald M. Harden, 2003. Planning and implementing an undergraduate medical curriculum: the lessons learned; *Medical Teacher*. 25(6): 596-608.

[25] David M. Fetterman, Jennifer Deitz and Neil Gesundheit, 2010. Empowerment Evaluation: A Collaborative Approach to Evaluating and Transforming a Medical School Curriculum; *Academic Medicine*; 85:813-820.

[26] Kathryn A. Gibson, Patrick Boyle, Deborah A. Black, Margaret Cunningham, Michael C. Grimm, and H. Patrick McNeil, 2088. Enhancing Evaluation in an Undergraduate Medical Education Program; *Academic Medicine*; 83: 787-793.

[27] Steven J. Durning, Paul Hemmer, Louis N. Pangaro, 2007. The structure of program evaluation: an approach for evaluating a course, clerkship, or components of a residency or fellowship training program; *Teaching and Learning in Medicine*; 19(3): 308-318.

[28] Marie E. Dagenais, Dana Hawley and James P. Lund, 2003. Assessing the Effectiveness of a New Curriculum: Part I; *Journal of Dental Education*; 67(1): 49-54.

[29] R. Pabst, H. Nave, H. J. Rothkötter, and T. Tschernig, 2001. Evaluation of the Medical Curriculum: Why, When, by Whom and for Whom Should Questionnaires Be Used; *European Journal of Morphology*; 39(4):237-239.

[30] Haydon, R., Donnely, M., Schwartz, R., Strodel, W., Jones, R., 1994. Use of standardized patients to identify deficits in student performance and curriculum effectiveness. *Am. J. Surg.*; 168:57-65.

[31] Klamen, D. L., Williams, R. G., 1997. The effect of medical education on students' patient- satisfaction ratings; *Academic Medicine*; 72(1):57-61.

[32] Cohen, D. S., Colliver, J. A., Marcy, M. S., Fried, E. T., Swartz, M. H., 1996. Psychometric properties of a standardized-patient checklist and rating-scale form used to assess interpersonal and communication skills; *Academic Medicine*; 71:S87-S89.

[33] Van Zanten, M., Norcini, J. J., Boulet, J. R., Simon, 2008. F. Overview of accreditation of undergraduate medical education programmes worldwide; *Medical Education*; 42: 930-937.

[34] Hans Karle, 2008. International recognition of basic medical education programmes; *Medical Education*; 42: 12-17.

[35] *The National Committee on Foreign Medical Education and Accreditation (NCFMEA)*. http://www.hepinc.com/node/488. Accessed, June 27, 2014.

[36] Hans Karle (2), 2008. World Federation for Medical Education Policy on International Recognition of Medical Schools' Programme; *Ann. Acad. Med. Singapore*; 37:1041-3.

[37] *AVICENNA Directories*. Available at (http://avicenna.ku.dk/). Accessed June 23, 2014.

[38] Arno M. M. Muijtjens, Lambert W. T. Schuwirth, Janke Cohen-Schotanus, Arnold J. N. M. Thoben and Cees P. M. van der Vleuten, 2008. Benchmarking by cross-institutional comparison of student achievement in a progress test; *Medical Education*; 42: 82-88.

[39] The National Commission for Assessment and Academic Accreditation (NCAAA). (http://ncaaa.org.sa/english/adefault.aspx). Accessed, June 27, 2014.

[40] Freeman, A., van der Vleuten, C., Nouns, Z., and Ricketts, C., 2010. Progress testing internationally; *Medical Teacher*; 32: 451-455.

[41] Freeman, A. and Ricketts, C., 2010. Choosing and designing knowledge assessments: Experience at a new medical school; *Medical Teacher*; 32: 578-581.

[42] Langer, M. and Swanson, D., 2010. Practical considerations in equating progress tests; *Medical Teacher*; 32: 509-512.

[43] Schuwirth, L., Bosman, G., Henning, R., Rinkel, R., and Wenink, A., 2010. Collaboration on progress testing in medical schools in the Netherlands; *Medical Teacher;* 32: 476-479.

[44] J. Yielder, W. Bagg and B. O'Connor, 2013. Progress testing: A potential for collaboration and benchmarking across Australian and New Zealand medical schools? *Focus on health professional education; a multi-disciplinary journal*; 15 (1): 81-87.

[45] Timothy G. Willett, 2008. Current status of curriculum mapping in Canada and the UK; *Medical Education*; 42: 786-793.

[46] R. M. Harden, 2001. AMEE Guide No. 21: Curriculum mapping: a tool for transparent and authentic teaching and learning; *Medical Teacher*; 23 (2).

In: Health and Disease
Editor: Paul Ganguly

ISBN: 978-1-63463-052-8
© 2015 Nova Science Publishers, Inc.

Chapter 12

MEDICAL CURRICULUM: STUDENTS' PERSPECTIVES

Ayman Mohamed Awad Mohamed, Mohammed Marwan Dabbagh, Al-Awwab Mohammad Dabaliz, Abdulazeez Abdulmajeed Barakat, Elhaitham Khaled Ahmed and Akef Obeidat*

Alfaisal University, Riyadh, Kingdom of Saudi Arabia

ABSTRACT

This chapter is different. This is simply because it is in fact not written by professionals or field experts like the authors of the other chapters of this book. On the contrary, it is written by students; on whom all what medical education actually revolves around. In essence, this chapter displays the perspective of a group of medical students who developed an interest in medical education throughout their medical school years as part of their extracurricular research activities and have thus developed some knowledge about what is going around in the world of medical education; that, in addition to their own experience as students of the century in a promising university like Alfaisal.

The chapter is structurally divided into five sections, each of which handles a major pillar of the medical curriculum. Furthermore, each section is further divided into five major topics, each of which discusses a critical challenge followed by proposed approach(s) and a number of interventions including student intervention, social intervention, and Electronic Resources Application - where applicable – which further enriches the chapter.

The authors' perspective has been influenced by comprehensive reading, students' experience in their own and other medical schools, and general knowledge about educational systems and protocols.

---

* E-mail address: aobeidat@alfaisal.edu.

SECTION I: CURRICULUM DESIGN AND CONTENT: LESSONS FROM THE FUTURE

A curriculum is definitely the cornerstone of any educational program. If not well designed and strategically planned; the system would have been academically insufficient. A well-structured curriculum must not only cover the academic domains, but rather extend to include community health needs where research, social accountability, and public awareness play a vital role. Apart from fulfilling the community needs, a modern curriculum should also empower its students with necessary knowledge and skills to become effective global citizens.

Nevertheless, no matter how well planned a curriculum is, still, there should be an effective and continuous bidirectional feedback exchange between the college's administration and its students; as the students are the direct receivers and their input is a direct reflection of the actual system effectiveness.

This section will discuss the following topics:
i.	Objectives, Outcomes and Continuity of Education
ii.	Basic Sciences vs Clinical Sciences
iii.	Student Selection and Progression
iv.	Integration of Research
v.	Roles of Physicians in the 21st Century

i. Objectives, Outcomes and Continuity of Education

Challenge: Lack of educational continuity and absence of specific objectives that are adequately detailed.

General consequences would include the possibility of disrupting the effective chronological sequence of information delivery and holistic knowledge structure along the continuum of education. It should be kept in mind that medical education is a continuous learning program where objectives are spread across the pre-medical, under-graduate, and post-graduate phases with different levels of depth and application. There must be an intra-phase continuum within each phase as well as an inter-phase continuum between the phases. Not having a properly detailed syllabii that does not take into account this intricate continuity of the courses and their balance and depth, several problems will manifest; such as:

1. Inadvertent, unnecessary repetition of information (inter- and intra-) phasically.
2. Over looked core concepts from the curriculum (inter- and intra-) phasically.
3. Lack of distinction between core (must know concepts) and redundant details.

In essence, proper continuity is impaired due to the deficiency of specific detailed objectives spanning all phases.

Looking at the way current curricula are designed and objectives are formulated, it is surprising that there is no structured approach to generate specific objectives but rather it is mainly dependent on the experience and subjective intervention of the curriculum committee or the group developing it.

The approach:
- Development of validated tools to objectively generate core and specific objectives:
  o Generation of core and specific objectives that are adequately detailed for all the three phases of education using these tools. The set of objectives must be decided upon before the start of any phase.
  o Distribution of the objectives among the different phases (pre-medical, under-graduate, and post-graduate) according to the appropriate respective phase level in a way that serves the continuum. The "spiral approach" is an example of the approach that can be used to serve this purpose.

- Personalized Track-Based Curricula (adaptive curriculum):
  o Where "ambition based tracks" are offered to the learner. In these tracks, the students get to choose a specific track from the very beginning according to their interest whether it is in a specific clinical field, such as neurology or cardiology, or a non-clinical medical field, such as research, medical education or medical management. In these tracks, the student is offered studying material related to the chosen tracks, in addition to other must know 'core' concepts that are taught in all tracks.

Student role: Involving students in the development and application of these tracks with the ensuing generation of objectives, followed by piloting it on volunteering students, and collecting their feedback on it before and throughout its application.

Electronic Resources Application: Using curriculum mapping tools.
Social Intervention: Including curricular objectives that serve the community.

ii. Basic Sciences vs. Clinical Sciences

Challenge: Lack of integration between basic and clinical sciences.

Course directors in the pre-clinical years frequently fail to point out the clinical relevance of their course objective. This leads to students' loss of interest in the course as they cannot appreciate its application in their future practice.

On the other hand, the mal-integration is also apparent during clinical years, as there is almost complete negligence of relevant basic sciences, which, negatively affects the student's understanding and performance.

Educators have attempted to overcome this mal-integration through the introduction of integrated curricula and the application of several modules such as Problem Based Learning in the pre-clinical years and Case Based Learning in the clerkship years; however, despite the fact that these attempts were important steps forward, they remain insufficient due to their limited application to either the pre-clinical phase or the clerkship phase without sufficient bridging between both phases.

The approach:

- Trans-disciplinary integration where there is complete horizontal integration between different disciplines, and complete vertical integration traversing basic and clinical sciences.

Electronic Resources Application: Production and usage of comprehensive customizable videos and 3D animations that clearly illustrate the different concepts in an integrated fashion.

iii. Student Selection and Progression

Challenge: Current selection criteria and progression predictors cover only some of the cognitive domain (i.e. academic) and neglect other important domains.

Planning the admission phase and the selection criteria are important bases for curriculum planning. This is to ensure that accepted students are able to undertake the requirements of the curriculum they will study and will make the most out of it. The admission requirements currently focus on assessing the applicants based on their academic merit and overlook other psychometric predictors that are related to additional cognitive outcomes in the curriculum. The fact that students come from different school educational systems impose a problematic challenge to the standardization of the criteria. Other non-cognitive based domains, such as affective and psychomotor domains are almost, completely, ignored from the selection criteria.

Absence of accurate performance predictors is not only limited to the admission stage, but rather continues throughout different stages of education. For example, many colleges depend on the student's GPA (Grade Point Average) as a single performance indicator to measure their progression. In other words, there are no sufficient progression predictors for the affective and psychomotor outcome domains that could be used to track the student's development throughout the years, resulting in less valuable feedback to the students.

Furthermore, current curricula undermine the individual differences between students in terms of talents and abilities; ignoring the important effect they might have on the development of the student's performance and even demotivating them to cultivate those talents; "One size does not fit all".

The approach:

- Individualized Curricula:
  o This is achieved by the development of validated tools to objectively assess students' abilities, talents and pace of progression, then utilizing this information in customizing the learning opportunities to build upon student's abilities, talents and learning styles to best fit their personal development.
  o This will allow for the introduction of "Individualized Pace-Based Tracks", which would give the opportunity to fast learners to shorten the duration of their training and slow learners more time to achieve necessary outcomes when needed. For example, fast learners might be able to complete their period of study in (3-4) years, while slow learners might take up to (5-6) years to complete with the same level of competence.

Student role: Providing information on common different learning styles, talents and abilities and tailoring them to best fit the cultural background along with providing feedback on their application.

Electronic Resources Application: Development and utilization of electronic tools to identify student learning styles, talents and abilities. Then cultivation of those optimal learning conditions for the students to do their best and monitor their progression using online and mobile applications.

Social Intervention: Considering personal talents and abilities in the admission criteria provides the opportunity for recruiting and accommodating a more diverse population of gifted students, which will in turn reflect positively on the medical practice in the community.

iv. Integration of Research

Challenge: Research outcomes are not integrated as core competencies in most medical curricula.

Despite the crucial role that research skills play on the development of desired skills and clinical outcomes, they are not yet considered as an essential part of medical curricula. Rather, many colleges still perceive research as a 'luxury' to have and not a necessity in the curricular structure.

Potential skills to be acquired by students' involved in research include: critical thinking, literature appraisal, practice of evidence based medicine, communication and teamwork skills. This is, in addition to its valuable contribution to academia, medical education, and health care through its scientific outcomes.

The approach:
- Integration of research education as a core accredited component of medical curricula throughout all educational phases including the pre-clinical and clinical sciences and in medical education.

Student role: Active participation of students in all types, forms and stages of research.

Electronic Resources Application: Providing advanced basic, clinical and educational research solutions in research training facilities in addition to accessibility to different databases and online research training programs.

Social Intervention: Directing both faculty and student research towards studying the health care needs of the community and its social impacts.

v. Roles of Physicians in the 21st Century

Challenge: Different roles of physicians are not adequately illustrated in current medical curricula.

Current curricula tend to over-emphasize the health care delivery role of the physician while disregarding most of the other vital roles of the physician and the different environments they will be working in.

A physician practicing in the 21st century is not only a health care provider; but rather a medical educator, a health policy maker, a public health advocate, a researcher, a leader, and a manager, just to list few.

Not to forget that he or she is a global citizen practicing medicine in trans-continental environments. Individuals from diverse cultural, political, religious, ethnic backgrounds and socioeconomic statuses need to be dealt with equally professionally by the physician. This necessitates broadening the intellectual horizons of the physician and his ability to effectively communicate his thoughts and messages. However, this can never be achieved without adequate exposure to humanities, which unfortunately, almost always, have no place in medical curricula.

The approach:
- Active integration of all competencies and roles of a physician of the 21st century in the curriculum.
- Providing opportunities for advanced exposure to those roles upon interest of the learner. This can be provided in the form of advanced electives or through dedicated interest based tracks.

Student role: Encouraging students to practice these different roles throughout their medical journey and collection of ensuing feedback.

Electronic Resources Application: Effective usage of distance learning and communication technologies to mimic trans-continental exposure to different working environments, endemics and cultures; for example, tropical diseases in Africa, alternative medicine in Arabian cultures, and acupuncture in Chinese culture.

Social Intervention: Utilizing training programs in the community services in such a way that it is helpful to the society and not merely a student training activity.

SECTION II: ASSESSMENT: HOW IT SHOULD BE DONE

Assessment is an important educational tool that curriculum planners use around the world. Simply put, it is used to evaluate the level of student attainment of the curriculum objectives. There should be a constructive alignment between the objectives in the syllabi, the material taught, and the assessment.

There are many assessment tools of different formats and styles with varying degrees of validity. It is the responsibility of the curriculum planners to choose the most suitable assessment tool that is fair and representative of the respective discipline or course it is assessing, in such a way that questions' quality and structure are consistent with the course design and objectives taking into account the natural distribution of the students' abilities.

In many instances, the assessment regime is structured in a way that it promotes unhealthy stress or tension in the students' lives to the extent of affecting their academic performance.

One of the most important rights of a student is to be able to have a transparent and detailed feedback on their exam's performance so that they are able to know their specific areas of weakness and work on improving them.

This section will discuss the following topics:
  i.   Constructive Alignment Between Assessment and Learning Outcomes
  ii. Methods of Assessment
  iii. Type and Quality of Questions
  iv. Grading Systems
  v.   Role of Feedback

i. Constructive Alignment between Assessment and Learning Outcomes

Challenge: Examinations are not aligned with intended and taught objectives.

Examinations are essential educational tools when they examine what has been taught and what the students have been instructed to study in order to measure their level of achievement of the curriculum's educational outcomes and point out areas of student weakness that requires further attention and development.

Mismatch between objectives and assessment, reduces the validity of such assessment tools and defeats their purpose.

One of the mismatch consequences is the lack of student orientation on what to expect from assessment, and this might adversely affect their performance.

The approach:
  • Establishing committees to oversee the constructive alignment between the declared and examined objectives, using blue prints for example. In addition, assuring that the students are well oriented on how learning objectives are to be taught and tested.
  • Deployment of periodic examination practice opportunities throughout the curriculum (formative assessment).
  • Development of tools to identify students who are at risk of facing difficulties and initiation of early preventative interventions that enable them to overcome such difficulties early on.

Student role: Involvement of students in the development of different assessment tools; in addition to collecting and implementing students' feedback on examination content and assessment tools.

Electronic Resources Application: Developing and using electronic analytic tools and applications to evaluate the student's achievement of the learning outcomes individually; in addition to the employment of tailored practice exercises and providing access to technologically advanced question banks.

ii. Methods of Assessments

Challenge: Using "one size fits all" assessment methods.

Using the same methods to evaluate disciplines that differ in nature and character is a major flaw in assessment and in curriculum planning; this is due to the fact that such methods will not accurately represent the actual outcome intended by curriculum planners from each discipline.

The adverse effect of utilizing the same methods to evaluate outcomes of various domains (like cognitive, affective, psychomotor, etc.) is that outcomes of such domains are not represented in most current assessment measurements, and thus are not evaluated. This in turn means that deciding what methods will be used to assess different subjects is an important area that curriculum planners need to pay more attention to at an early stage of curriculum planning.

The approach:
- Validating the use of different assessment methods against each domain of outcomes individually.
- Developing valid tools to appropriately assess other cognitive, affective and psychomotor domains, and providing customized toolkits for each subject to accord with its respective outcome domains.

Student role: Active utilization of students in medical education research targeting development and validation of assessment tools.

Electronic Resources Application: Development of online applications with outcome specific examination methodologies.

iii. Type and Quality of Questions

Challenge: Overuse of "recall type" questions.

According to Bloom's revised taxonomy, recall questions represent the lowest level of comprehension, which might not represent accurately the level of comprehension needed in most aspects of medical practice.

The approach:
- To introduce questions that represent different comprehension levels climbing up to higher levels on the revised Bloom's taxonomy.
- Assigning grade weightage to each exam question that corresponds well to its level of comprehension in the Bloom's taxonomy.

Students Intervention: The use of students volunteers to pilot different types of questions that assess different levels of comprehension, and accordingly assign a suitable percentage (weightage) of questions for each level of comprehension in each test.

Electronic Resources Application: Developing and using specific programs and applications to validate the effectiveness of questions by measuring different intended comprehension levels and outcomes.

iv. Grading Systems

Challenge: Exam-oriented teaching, leads to the development of grade-oriented students and unhealthy competition.

Grading systems serve as numerical representation of the student's knowledge and comprehension of the intended curriculum outcomes, playing an active role in the student's educational development. Planning how students achievements in a particular curriculum will be graded; is an essential element of curriculum planning.

Unfortunately, many grading systems add unnecessary psychological stress that eventually becomes demotivating to the student.

The approach:
- o Transformation of current numerical/Alphabetical grading system into Honor/Pass/Fail grading system. This change will promote teamwork, cooperation and collaboration spirits between students, reducing stress and maximizing benefits, which in turn results in transferring competition for grades into competition for achieving higher academic and non-academic curriculum outcomes.

Social Intervention: Shifting competition between students to community based projects that serve societal needs.

v. Role of Feedback

Challenge: Lack of comprehensive feedback systems.

The purpose of assessment is to provide comprehensive feedback as it sets the base upon which the student develops toward achieving the intended learning outcomes. Development of students depends on the quality and quantity of the provided feedback, and both of these variables are affected by methods of collection, analysis and reporting. This makes the development of an accurate and efficient feedback system absolutely essential and vital for the success of any proper curricular design. Consequently, planning the role of feedback and its collecting system is vital to any curriculum planning process.

Unfortunately, current feedback systems suffer noticeable deficiencies in terms of their collection, analysis and reporting back and forth between the college's administration and the students, and in most of the cases are limited to end-of-year or end-of-semester surveys.

The approach:
- o Development of a comprehensive 360-degree feedback system that provides continuous bidirectional feedback on all aspects of students' learning and

environment; Maastricht University's 360-degree feedback system as an example.

Student role: Involving students in continuous and periodic feedback programs and their collection.

Electronic Resources Application: Use of advanced electronic performance based feedback systems.

Section III: Student Support Systems: The Missing Piece of The Puzzle

As it is important to create a reliable curriculum, it is equally important to make sure that students are making the best of it. This entails the establishment of an efficient student support system that creates an environment that promotes students to excel with optimal performance capabilities. Such an environment should include a healthy balance between study, recreation, meditation, and various activities.

Furthermore, for students to acquire the best educational experience, they require some kind of professional coaching and guidance by a trained and experienced counselor (mentor).

Academically speaking, they also need to have clear consultations on how to study, from where to study, and what to study.

A well-planned student support system must also extend to provide career-counselling for students at large as well as individually.

This section will discuss the following topics:

i.   Academic Mentorship
ii.   Study Guides
iii. Psychological Support Systems
iv.   Social Factors
v.   Career Counseling

i. Academic Mentorship

Challenge: Lack of effective academic mentorship programs that extend throughout all the phases of the educational journey.

Mentorship is a cornerstone for student success. Its role in achieving the curriculum outcomes is vital and aught to be considered while planning the curriculum.

Unfortunately, current mentorship programs lack major components that assure its effectiveness. One of these is the continuity of mentorship throughout the span of the educational process; as some universities limit mentorship to the early phases of education only, or provide the same type of mentorship all throughout the educational program without the evolvement of the mentorship style to accord with the different demands for every phase.

Professional mentorship programs should give equal attention to all key stakeholders in the mentorship process, which include the mentor and the mentee. However, professional preparation of mentors is usually ignored as many universities assign the mentorship tasks to faculty who are not specially trained in mentorship skills, which in turn adversely affects the efficiency of such programs. One such adverse effect is that all students will be mentored in the same way without taking into account students' individual differences, as untrained mentors are unable to tailor their counseling to the individual needs of the students.

The approach:
- Development and implementation of structured and periodic academic mentorship programs that transcend throughout the different educational phases and are tailored to the specific needs of every phase of education and every individual student, along with the development of its associated feedback system.
- Development of mandatory professional mentorship training programs that enable mentors to individualize their mentorship practices efficiently.

Student role: Active involvement of senior students in the mentorship systems provided to their junior colleagues, in addition to the active and continuous implementation of the mentee's feedback.

Electronic Resources Application: Integrating the electronic mentorship tools into the students' electronic portfolios, in addition to using distance-learning technologies to extend the mentorship opportunities beyond the campus boundaries.

Social Intervention: involvement of members of the community in the mentorship programs.

ii. Study Guides

Challenge: Unavailability of study guides to support curriculum.

Despite the proven effectiveness of using study guides, it is unfortunate that many universities do not give it enough attention as they still view it as a luxury or a form of "spoon feeding".

Professional study guides play an important role in orienting the students towards knowing what is expected from them and directing them towards identifying "must know" core curricular components. Student guides play an important role in explaining how different components of the curriculum fit together.

The approach:
- Formulation of committees that specialize in the development and production of well-structured trans-phasic study guides that are comprehensive enough to cover all curricular components. Guides should include a clear specific learning objectives and outcomes in all domains of learning, how to achieve the desired level of competency in these outcomes, how each of these outcomes will be assessed, and the recommended academic resources.

Student role: Active involvement of the students in the development and improvement of the guides and their continuous update through class notes and other student activities.

Electronic Resources Application: The development and use of online and mobile electronic study guide utilities.

iii. Psychological Support Systems

Challenge: Unavailability of comprehensive students' psychiatric and psychological support systems.

The academic demand of medical studies and its competitive environment leads to higher levels of stress among medical students. If this problem is not appropriately addressed, it might be a major source of student demotivation, which might eventually escalate up to serious social and psychiatric problems. This also might affect students' achievement of the intended curriculum outcomes.

It is unfortunate that curriculum planners often ignore the dramatic effects that such systems might have on the students' progression.

The approach:
- Development and implementation of comprehensive individualized counseling systems covering psychological, psychiatric, medical, and socioeconomic aspects of the students' lives.

Student role: Involvement of the students in the promotion of peer to peer counseling services and in identifying student body needs and sources of stress that might go otherwise unnoticed.

iv. Social Factors

Challenge: The neglection of the social aspects of students' lives and their impact on students' progression.

It is unfortunate how curriculum planners often ignore social aspects of students' lives and possible external environmental factors that might contribute to that. This is obvious in the lack of attention to recreational activities, sports integration, hobby or talent cultivation, and financial needs.

The approach:
- Scheduling free time slots in the curriculum devoted to student recreation and student life.
- Implementation of adult educational games and competitions to selected components of the curriculum.
- Providing comprehensive scholarship opportunities and interest-free loans.
- Active integration of sports into student life, as it promotes teamwork, friendships, student well-being and health.

- Development of programs to identify student talents and develop them.
- Development of national and international structured volunteering programs in health related fields.

Student role: Active involvement and empowerment of student associations and student clubs in conducting students' social and sport activities as well as in identifying talent-developing opportunities.

Social Intervention: Employment of student social activities, volunteering programs and competitions to serve societal needs.

v. Career Counseling

Challenge: Unavailability of career counseling systems that comprehensively cover the different roles of a physician practicing in the 21st century.

Future employment is a major source of stress in student life, and many universities do not pay attention to career counseling and development programs that aim to prepare their potential graduates for their post graduate phase.

The approach:
- Development of efficient career counseling systems and offices that take into account the different possible clinical and non-clinical employment tracks and match that with the pre-determined curriculum goals and outcomes.
- Development of orientation sessions to help graduates go through licensing processes of different licencure bodies.
- Development of national and international partnerships and exchange programs for graduates' employment.

Electronic Resources Application: Using electronic career portal applications and comprehensive databases to help students identify appropriate employment requirements and the needed skills.

Social Intervention: Matching available employment opportunities with appropriate candidates to decrease unemployment rates.

SECTION IV: RESOURCES & TEACHING: THE WHO, WHAT AND HOW

The two main pillars of any organization, whether academic or not, are the availability of required resources and proper administration of those resources. For a college to have a good stance, it should have a well-established pool of resources that makes it independent and able to function well; given that proper administration is available.

The main resources required by a medical college include secure finances, competent faculty, and state of the art facilities; all of which are essential tools for a successful implementation of the college's curriculum.

This section will discuss the following topics:

   i. State of the Art Facilities
   ii. Financial Stability
   iii. Faculty and Human Capital Development
   iv. Different Teaching Styles
   v. Effective Teaching Resources

i. State of the Art Facilities

Challenge: As it is important to gain theoretical knowledge, applying it where possible is equally crucial. There is a clear deficiency in the availability of adequate facilities that support this in many medical schools.

There are various subject domains in the medical curriculum (both in basic and clinical sciences) and each requires a certain set of facilities and suitable tools to be taught or applied in practice. It is necessary to provide all required facilities to meet the objectives of the practical aspects of the curriculum. Unfortunately, this is not always taken into consideration in the curriculum design.

Other challenges are; the availability of teaching hospitals, proper organization, and dedicating more clinicians' time to students. These challenges are mostly due to not having a teaching hospital that is owned, run, and coordinated by the medical college itself; which creates a lot of incongruity between the curriculum and its actual outcomes.

The approach:
- Planning and providing the required facilities for each educational domain or course to ensure better implementation of the intended curriculum outcomes. For instance, for basic sciences, a medical college must have the following laboratories; anatomy, physiology, histology, microbiology, genetics, research facilities, functional to serve the curriculum's intended outcomes. Planning laboratories roles and place in the curriculum should be an important function carried out by the curriculum planning committees. These would certainly enrich the educational experience and benefit medical students by allowing them to appreciate the practical aspects of the theoretical information they are being continuously loaded with; and transforming it in their minds into more sensible knowledge that could be retained for a longer time. Also, clinical skill facilities such as simulators, 3D Labs, standardized patients, etc.; both in-house and at the teaching hospital are required for optimal performance and application.
- Development of integrated hospital units where health care delivery is taught in an integrated manner and not departmental based.

Student role: Students should be responsible enough to appreciate those facilities and treat them with appreciation. Peer to peer teaching should be encouraged at such facilities

Electronic Resources Application: Using advanced simulation, basic and clinical training laboratories equipped with advanced training softwares. These utilities must be always updated with the 21st century technology. The technicians and personnels responsible for running those utilities must be regularly trained to correctly use the devices and train the students.

ii. Financial Stability

Challenge: Financial stability is important for a college to pursue its ambitions, implement its curriculum, and to prosper. Lack of a stable funding source means financial insecurity, which would limit those capabilities and affect the delivery of the curriculum.

Therefore, sustained financial recourses unlock the abilities of curriculum planners to best choose or even develop teaching methods and tools to best meet the curriculum's intended outcomes.

The approach:
- Ownership of endowments would ensure sustained regular financial income, thus denoting financial security. Revenues should be invested to return profit.

Social intervention: Developing endowments that serve important social needs.

iii. Faculty and Human Capital Development

Challenge: Since students are the target of development in any educational system, it is equally important to develop the 'target-ers' of this system, the teachers.

Teaching in the 21st century has developed and evolved into a science on its own. It is no longer accepted that faculty depend solely on their experience and ignore the evidence-based practices concluded by educational research and institutes.

Furthermore, despite living in the digital era of human history, in many instances; faculty members are, unfortunately, lagging behind in terms of some very basic technology skills, which is appalling as technology in teaching has become an integral part of the day-to-day use.

More importantly, many faculty members use ineffective teaching tools or are poor at preparing innovative educational opportunities or resources.

The approach:
- While recruiting; preference should be given to faculty with medical education background.
- Conducting regular training programs that aim at enhancing teaching skills of faculty members and improve their communication skills with students.

Student role: Students ought to play a role in developing their faculty members' capabilities by providing them with continuous feedback on their teaching skills and other educational endevours.

Electronic Resources Application: Colleges need to invest more on professional development of their faculty pertaining to recent technological advances in the world of academia.

iv. Different Teaching Styles

Challenge: Every course in the college of medicine is unique on its own. However, majority of the core courses are taught with the same approach amongst most of the medical schools around the world.

The approach:
- Different medical schools need to adopt different teaching modalities that serve well their curricular structure and objectives. Needed resources that serve the purpose should be made available.

Student role: Student associations should also be ready to report to the college what they believe should be changed, amended, or removed from the teaching modalities in place.

Electronic Resources Application: Using social enterprise solutions can provide an effective mean for bidirectional feedback exchange between faculty and their students in regards to the best teaching tools and methods. Technical support to faculty should be available so that they can integrate several online and mobile applications into their teaching tools.

v. Effective Teaching Resources

Challenge: The medical field in particular is the least tolerant to mistakes as it deals directly with human lives. Having inadequate teaching/learning resources pertinent to certain fields of study certainly causes deterioration in the quality of education and hence debilitating the overall quality of the community healthcare on the long run. Planning how teaching resources and material to be developed and their role in delivering the curricular outcomes is of great value in the process of the curriculum design.

The approach:
- Medical colleges need to choose recommended teaching resources cautiously. Identification of the best resources is the key. Recommending resources to students' much better than leaving them explore on their own by trial and error.
- Developing integrated textbooks with smart learning tools and its customized online supplementary material.

Student role: Students should be encouraged to express their opinion about the different study resources recommended by the college and even to recommend other resources from what they have found interesting or valuable. Seniors are always the best advice-givers in such areas and should be always resorted to by their junior peers.

Electronic Resources Application: Providing online books and electronic teaching resources (especially the ones that are out of reach otherwise) via the college's e-library with free access for all students online.

Section V: Management and Leadership: The Struggle of the Mighty

Administration of the medical college is one of the most important factors that determine the success of the college in decision making, developing policies, improving the curriculum, and providing a healthy educational environment. The quality of management the college has, greatly affects the curriculum implementation and realization of its outcomes. Decision made by the college's administration should be based on feedback and consultations with all stakeholders. Therefore, there should be proper distribution of power along the hierarchy of decision making process among all stakeholders, including curriculum planners.

Moreover, all decisions should be channeled through the Quality Assurance office of the college for benchmarking.

This section will discuss the following topics:
i. Leadership Training
ii. Power Distribution
iii. Quality Assurance
iv. College's Relation with Other University's colleges and Departments
v. Effective Partnerships and international collaborations

i. Leadership Training

Challenge: Assigning administrative and managerial roles to faculty with little or no background in management.

Effective management of the college's tasks and projects requires competent administrators with professional management training and a healthcare-education background with sufficient experience in both, as this will assure the appropriateness of the decisions taken and their proper implementation.

Unfortunately, many colleges depend upon faculty's academic competence when assigning them administrative roles and ignore the importance of their managerial background and experience.

The approach:
• To develop mandatory management and leadership practical courses/workshops for faculty before assigning them any managerial/ administrative role.

Electronic Resources Application: Use of online training as part of periodic and continuous faculty development programs.

ii. Power Distribution

Challenge: Centralization of decision-making and restricting it to few individuals.

Limiting major decisions to few key individuals (e.g. committee or section heads) in any organization limits its capabilities to the experience and sometimes biasness of those individuals.

Medical colleges are not the exception, especially, when it comes to decisions relating to the curriculum and its implementation. Therefore, maintaining an appropriate balance of power distribution between administrators, curriculum planners and other college stakeholders is an important key for its success.

The approach:
- o Restructuring college's committees into task-based, well informed committees each is specialized in one of the college's major tasks. The membership of these committees should represent all college's stakeholders including college's administrators, quality assurance, faculty members, national and international experts, community representatives, and students. Decisions of all committees should be taken in consideration utterly by higher administration in the decision making process.

Student Intervention: Active representation of student body in all college's committees.

Social Intervention: Members from the community and other stakeholders should be added to the different college's committees.

iii. Quality Assurance

Challenge: The Quality Assurance Office is not utilized efficiently

The role of the Quality Assurance Office is to maintain and control the quality of actions being made and their outcomes throughout all the stages of the decision making process. This includes the quality of curriculum planning, execution and development.

Unfortunately, in many schools, the role of the Quality Assurance office is not well defined, especially its relation to the college's curriculum development and application.

As a result, this might lead to decisions taken by the administration that are not well researched or evidence based. Subsequently, the role of the Quality Assurance would be mainly to recommending crisis management measures.

The approach:
- Benchmarking process: The Quality Assurance Office should benchmark all college's aspects, including the curriculum to the best available national and international models and accreditation standards.
- Involve the Quality Assurance Office in the decision-making process.

Student Intervention:
- Active involvement of students in feedback generation and collection.
- Representation of student body in the committees of Quality Assurance Office.

Electronic Resources Application: Provide Quality Assurance body with the best available electronic resources to analyze and generate college's data, reports, and tools to monitor key performance indicators.

iv. College's Relation with Other University's Colleges and Departments

Challenge: Lack of workflow harmony in operational protocols between the medical college and other university's departments.

The academic nature of medicine and its curriculum requirements denotes special teaching systems that are very different from other fields of study. This mandates the use of special administrative structures, systems, academic and non-academic regulations that are different from those generally used in other university's colleges and departments, for example, unique admission processes and requirements, and different grading systems especially for clinical clerkships and internship.

However, many medical colleges are still structured to function under the same administrative and academic regulations as other colleges; which results frequently in conflicts that adversely affect the curriculum application and student experience at the college.

The approach:
- To give medical schools some sort of autonomy.

v. Effective Partnerships and international collaborations

Challenge: Lack of effective academic and non-academic partnerships.

Effective partnerships and international collaborations serve to provide students with training and career opportunities to meet curricular goals and outcomes.

Many medical schools either neglect the importance of this task or fail to build new partnerships, or frequently sign ineffective partnership agreements that add limited or no value to the college's vision and mission, intended outcomes, and future projections.

This is especially true when it comes to issues related to undergraduate and postgraduate curriculum development and student exchange opportunities. This in turn might confine the exposure of the students to the local training programs only and they lose the opportunity to experience international programs. This will reduce their chances to develop as global citizens and achieve the curriculum's globally-oriented outcomes.

The approach:
- Development of specialized medical partnership and international collaboration committees/offices to establish effective academic and non-academic, national and international partnerships.

Student Intervention: Active involvement of students in such committees/office

Social Intervention: Partnership with health related philanthropic associations and community bodies to serve the community through research, volunteering, advocacy and other related social needs.

QUESTIONS TO GUIDE FUTURE DISCUSSIONS

1. On what basis should curriculum planners decide upon the depth of intended objectives across the different phases of medical education?
2. How to assess students' interest in a specific field and track their evolvement as they progress? And how should "Personalized Track-Based Curricula" actively respond to this evolvement?
3. How do we generate and objectively assess learning outcomes related to affective and psychometric domains of learning?
4. What are the best indicators for student progression through the different phases of medical education?
5. What is the future of medical textbooks in the 21st century? How to develop them and what to add?
6. What are the roles of modern technologies and their effective uses in the individualization of teaching and learning?
7. What are the roles that adult learning theories play in the current trends in medical education?
8. What are the roles of medical students in medical education research? How to assess their positive effects on students' learning/teaching?
9. How early in the curriculum should components of undergraduate medical research be introduced? To what depth and how?
10. What are the effects of student associations/clubs on the development of the students' characters and achievements?

Table 1. Summary of the perspective of medical students on major aspects of medical curriculum

Section	Challenge	The Approach
Curriculum Design	Lack of educational continuity, absence of detailed objectives	objectively generate specific objectives and development of Personalized Track-Based Curricula
	detachment in the delivery between basic and clinical sciences	Complete horizontal and vertical integration in basic and clinical sciences
	Covers only parts of the cognitive domain and neglects the other important domains	Individualized Curricula
	The practice of Research is not integrated in medical curricula	Integration of research education and research practice in the curricula
	Not adequately illustrated in current medical curricula	Adequate basic and advanced exposure to medical oriented humanities and basic role of physicians
Assessment	Examinations do not match intended and taught objectives	A committee that reviews the alignment between the declared and examined objectives
	"One size fits all" assessment methods	Appropriately assess other specific domains and customize assessment for each discipline accordingly
	Overuse of recall type of questions	Introduce questions that represent different comprehension levels in a balanced manner

Section	Challenge	The Approach
	Development of grade-oriented students	Transformation of current ABC grading system into Honor/Pass/Fail grading system
	Lack of comprehensive feedback systems	Development of continuous bidirectional feedback on all aspects of students' learning
Student Support	Lack of effective academic mentorship programs	Development of Structured periodic academic mentorship and professional mentorship training
	Shortage of detailed study guides	Trans-phasic professionally structured and comprehensive study guides for all curricular components
	Unavailability of comprehensive psychological support systems	Development of comprehensive individualized counseling systems
	The negligence of the social lives and its effect on progression	Providing protected time periods devoted to student recreation and student life and scholarships
	Unavailability of career counseling systems	Counseling systems that take into account different possible clinical and non-clinical employment
Resources	Clear deficiency in the availability of adequate facilities	Providing the needed facilities for each educational domain or course
	Lack of a stable funding sources	Ownership of endowments would ensure sustained financial income thus denoting financial security
	Faculty members are outdated in terms of basic technology	Faculty with medical education background during recruitment process aided byperiodic training
	Majority of disciplines are taught in the same way	"one size does not fit all" when various courses' information delivery is concerned
	Scarcity of study resources in some areas	Recommended teaching resources must be chosen by the college cautiously
Management	Teaching faculty with little or no background in management	Management and leadership courses that are a prerequisite to administrative roles and assignment
	Centralization of decision-making and restricting it to limited individuals	Task based councilor committees represent all college stakeholders specialized in college major tasks.
	The role of Quality Assurance office is restricted to post-implementation actions	Benchmarking process, Channeling decisions and mandating their approvals and feedback collection
	Lack of harmony with other University's departments and effective partnerships	The autonomy of medical college, establishment of effective partnerships nationally and internationally

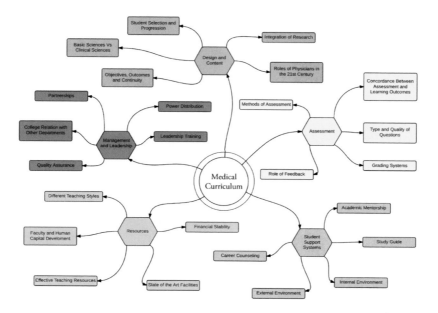

Figure 1. Map of the critical aspects of medical curriculum development based on the perspective of medical students.

Since this chapter is all about student perceptions, all concepts discussed, stemmed out from the authors discussions; accordingly; they are not referenced. However, the following are number of resources that we refer the readers to in order to compliment the concepts that were presented in this chapter.

REFERENCES

Butler, A., & Roediger, H. (2008). Feedback enhances the positive effects and reduces the negative effects of multiple-choice testing. *Memory & Cognition*, *36*(3), 604-616.

Catling, F., Williams, J., & Baker, R. (2014). A prescribing e-tutorial for medical students; *Clinical Teacher*, *11*, 33–37.

Garner, M., Gusberg, R., & Kim, A. (2014). The positive effect of immediate feedback on medical student education during the surgical clerkship; Journal *of Surgical Education*, *71*(3), 391-397.

Gormley, G., Collins, K., Boohan, M., Bickle, I., & Stevenson, M. Is there a place for e-learning in clinical skills? A survey of undergraduate medical students' experiences and attitudes. *Medical Teacher*, 31, *6-12.*

Harden, R. M. (2000). The integration ladder: A tool for curriculum planning and evaluation. *Medical Education.* 34:551-557.

Kaplowitz, J., & Wilkerson, L. (2002). Reaching and teaching new medical students. *Academic Medicine : Journal of the Association of American Medical Colleges*, *77*, 1173.

Kasule, O. H. (2013). Overview of medical student assessment: Why, what, who, and how. *Journal of Taibah University Medical Sciences;* 8(2) : 72–79.

Khan, M., & Aljarallah, B. (2011). Evaluation of modified essay questions (meq) and multiple choice questions (mcq) as a tool for assessing the cognitive skills of undergraduate medical students. *International Journal of Health Sciences*, *5*(1), 39-43.

Macnaughton, J. (2000). The humanities in medical education: context, outcomes and structures. *Medical Humanities*, *26*, 23–30.

Newbury, J. W., Shannon, S., Ryan, V., & Whitrow, M. (2005). Development of "rural week" for medical students: impact and quality report. *Rural and Remote Health*, *5*, 432.

Rees, C., Sheard, C., & McPherson, A. (2004). Medical students' views and experiences of methods of teaching and learning communication skills. *Patient Education and Counseling*, *54*, 119–121.

Reid, W. A., Duvall, E., & Evans, P. (2005). Can we influence medical students' approaches to learning? *Medical Teacher*, *27*, 401–407.

Rohe, D., Barrier, P., Clark, M., Cook, D., Vickers, K., & Decker, P. (2006). The benefits of pass-fail grading on stress, mood, and group cohesion in medical students. *Mayo Clinic Proceedings*, *81*(11), 1443-1448.

Sanson-Fisher, R. W., Rolfe, I. E., Jones, P., Ringland, C., & Agrez, M. (2002). Trialling a new way to learn clinical skills: Systematic clinical appraisal and learning. *Medical Education*, *36*, 1028–1034.

Stanger-Hall, K. F. (2012). Multiple-Choice Exams: An Obstacle for Higher-Level Thinking in Introductory Science Classes. *Cell Biology Education*; 11(3):294-306.

Strasser, R. P., Lanphear, J. H., McCready, W. G., Topps, M. H., Hunt, D. D., & Matte, M. C. (2009). Canada's new medical school: The Northern Ontario School of Medicine: social accountability through distributed community engaged learning. *Academic Medicine: Journal of the Association of American Medical Colleges, 84,* 1459–1464.

Supiano, M. A., Fantone, J. C., & Grum, C. (2002). A Web-based geriatrics portfolio to document medical students' learning outcomes. *Academic Medicine: Journal of the Association of American Medical Colleges, 77,* 937–938.

Varkey, P., Chutka, D. S., & Lesnick, T. G. (2006). The Aging Game: Improving Medical Students' Attitudes Toward Caring for the Elderly. *Journal of the American Medical Directors Association, 7,* 224–229.

Yates, M. S., Drewery, S., & Murdoch-Eaton, D. G. (2002). Alternative learning environments: what do they contribute to professional development of medical students? *Medical Teacher, 24,* 609–615.

Zink, T., Halaas, G. W., Finstad, D., & Brooks, K. D. (2008). The rural physician associate program: The value of immersion learning for third-year medical students. *Journal of Rural Health, 24,* 353–359.

INDEX

D

F

G

H

I

J

K

L